# Pocket Guide to Psychiatric Nursing

Gail W. Stuart, PhD, RN, CS, FAAN

Dean and Professor, College of Nursing
Professor, College of Medicine
Department of Psychiatry and Behavioral Sciences
Medical University of South Carolina
Charleston, South Carolina

Fifth Edition

 Mosby

*An Affiliate of Elsevier*

**M Mosby**

*An Affiliate of Elsevier*

*Vice President and Publishing Director, Nursing:* Sally Schrefer
*Senior Editor:* Terri Wood
*Project Manager:* Deborah Vogel
*Production Editor:* Kelley Barbarick
*Design Manager:* Amy Buxton

FIFTH EDITION
**Copyright © 2002 by Mosby, Inc.**

Previous editions copyrighted 1988, 1991, 1995, 1998

### NOTICE

Nursing is an ever-changing field. Standard safety precautions must be followed, but as new research and clinical experience broaden our knowledge, changes in treatment and drug therapy may become necessary or appropriate. Readers are advised to check the most current product information provided by the manufacturer of each drug to be administered to verify the recommended dose, the method and duration of administration, and contraindications. It is the responsibility of the licensed prescriber, relying on experience and knowledge of the patient, to determine dosages and the best treatment for each individual patient. Neither the publisher nor the editor assumes any liability for any injury and/or damage to persons or property arising from this publication.

Permissions may be sought directly from Elsevier's Health Sciences Rights Department in Philadelphia, USA: phone: (+1)215-238-7869, fax: (+1)215-238-2239, e-mail: healthpermissions@elsevier.com. You may also complete your request on-line via the Elsevier Science homepage (http://www.elsevier.com), by selecting 'Customer Support' and then 'Obtaining Permissions'.

Mosby, Inc.
*An Affiliate of Elsevier*
11830 Westline Industrial Drive
St. Louis, Missouri 63146

Printed in the United States of America

9997640276

03   04   05   GW/FF   9   8   7   6   5   4   3

# About the Author

**Dr. Gail Stuart** is dean and a tenured professor in the College of Nursing and a professor in the College of Medicine in the Department of Psychiatry and Behavioral Sciences at the Medical University of South Carolina. She received her Bachelor of Science degree in nursing from Georgetown University, her Master of Science degree in psychiatric nursing from the University of Maryland, and her doctorate in behavioral sciences from Johns Hopkins University, School of Hygiene and Public Health. She is an American Nurses Association Certified Specialist in psychiatric and mental health nursing, a fellow in the American Academy of Nursing, a member of Sigma Theta Tau, president-elect of the American College of Mental Health Administration, a Distinguished Practitioner in the National Academies of Practice, and a past president of the American Psychiatric Nurses Association. She has also been a van Ameringen fellow at the Beck Institute of Cognitive Therapy and Research and is a visiting professor at King's College, Institute of Psychiatry, at the Maudsley in London.

Dr. Stuart's current position at the Medical University of South Carolina is dean of the College of Nursing. Prior to that appointment she was the director of Doctoral Studies and coordinator of the Psychiatric–Mental Health Nursing Graduate Program. She was previously the associate director of the Center for Health Care Research where she worked as a member of an interdisciplinary research team focusing on issues of access, resource utilization, and healthcare delivery systems. She was also the administrator and chief executive officer of the Institute of Psychiatry at the Medical University where she was responsible for all clinical, fiscal, and human operations across the continuum of psychiatric care. Dr. Stuart has taught in undergraduate, graduate, and doctoral programs in nursing. She serves on numerous academic, pharmaceutical, and government boards and represents nursing on a variety of National Institute of Mental Health policy and research panels. She is a strong advocate for the specialty and is in great demand to speak and consult both nationally and internationally. She is a prolific writer and has published numerous articles, textbooks, and media productions. She has received many awards, including the American Nurses Association Distinguished Contribution to Psychiatric Nursing Award and the Psychiatric Nurse of the Year Award from the American Psychiatric Nurses Association. Dr. Stuart's clinical and research interests involve the study of depression, anxiety disorders, clinical outcomes, and mental health delivery systems.

# Preface

Running faster, working smarter. It seems like every psychiatric nurse I meet is experiencing the same demands of time, information, and technology. Add to that the increased emphasis placed on evidence-based practice, and one quickly realizes that the need to keep current with these changes is growing, but the time to do so is shrinking. This reality is the reason for this fifth edition of the *Pocket Guide to Psychiatric Nursing*. This new edition has a sharpened focus on presenting the most current, relevant, practical, and concise information about psychiatric nursing care. The compact format makes this content easily accessible to the nurse in the clinical setting. This pocket guide also serves as an abbreviated complement to the comprehensive text from which it is derived, *Principles and Practice of Psychiatric Nursing*, seventh edition. Thus the reader can learn more indepth information about any clinical aspect of psychiatric nursing care by accessing the larger textbook, and students can use this pocket guide as a review and synthesis of content presented in the larger text.

This fifth edition has updated content throughout, information about the latest psychotropic medications, and new tables that summarize the evidence on treatments for the various psychiatric disorders. It also includes information on alternative therapies and, at the end of each chapter, features World Wide Web sites that can be accessed on the Internet, which are related to the chapter's content. In this way readers can stay current with rapidly emerging developments in each clinical area. The text continues to focus on the essentials of psychiatric nursing and is organized around the nursing process, thus providing assistance with conceptualizing, planning, implementing, and documenting nursing care. Nursing treatment plan summaries are included to provide for the clinical application of the nursing process to specific nursing care problems. Both DSM-IV-TR medical and NANDA nursing diagnoses are included, enabling the nurse to maintain a nursing focus while understanding the medical approach as well. Each clinical chapter also includes a patient or family education plan. Whenever possible, tables and boxes are used to present material.

This pocket guide is divided into two parts. **Part I, Principles of Psychiatric Nursing Care**, consists of Chapters 1 through 8. This part is designed to focus on the basic concepts of psychiatric nursing regardless of the patient care need or the practice setting. Chapter 1 discusses roles and functions of psychiatric nurses. Chapter 2 presents aspects of the therapeutic nurse-patient relationship, while Chapter 3 presents the Stuart Stress Adaptation Model of Psychiatric Nursing Care. Chapter 4 describes the biopsychosocial context, Chapter 5 the environmental context, and Chapter 6 the legal-ethical context of psychiatric nursing care. Part I concludes with a discussion of the new ANA standards of psychiatric–mental health clinical nursing practice in Chapter 7 and the role of nursing throughout the continuum of psychiatric care in Chapter 8, including primary prevention, crisis resolution, and rehabilitation.

**Part II, Applying Principles in Nursing Practice**, comprises the major content of the book. Chapters 9 through 19 consider nursing approaches to patients with specific nursing care problems, including anxiety, psychophysiological illness, self-concept, disturbances of mood, self-destructive behavior, psychotic and personality disorders, impaired cognition, substance abuse, eating disorders, and variations in sexual responses. The concluding two chapters discuss two specific types of treatment: psychopharmacology and somatic and alternative therapies. These chapters are particularly useful to nurses working in settings that are shifting to a more biological focus on the treatment of mental illness, and they include many explanatory tables and charts.

Finally, I want to share with you a personal note of thanks for the wonderful interaction and dialogue you have provided me with over the years. Many of you remark how helpful my text has been to you in your clinical work. It is because of such exchanges that I remain committed to providing you the information that you need to give the best care possible to the patients and families with whom you work. Thus I dedicate this book to you and all our psychiatric nursing colleagues. Ours is a noble and caring mission. May we carry on with the knowledge, compassion, and commitment our patients so richly deserve.

**Gail Wiscarz Stuart**

# Contents

# PRINCIPLES OF PSYCHIATRIC NURSING CARE

# Roles and Functions of Psychiatric Nurses

## Psychiatric Nursing Defined and Described

Psychiatric nursing is an interpersonal process that strives to promote and maintain patient behavior that contributes to integrated functioning. The patient or client system may be an individual, family, group, organization, or community. The American Nurses' Association defines psychiatric and mental health nursing as

a specialized area of nursing practice employing theories of human behavior as its science and purposeful use of self as its art.[1]

The contemporary practice of psychiatric nursing occurs within a social and environmental context. The professional psychiatric nursing role has grown in complexity from its original historical elements. It now includes the dimensions of clinical competence, patient-family advocacy, fiscal responsibility, interdisciplinary collaboration, social accountability, and legal-ethical parameters.

The Center for Mental Health Services officially recognizes psychiatric and mental health nursing as one of the five core mental health disciplines. The psychiatric nurse uses knowledge from the psychosocial and biophysical sciences and theories of personality and human behavior to derive a theoretical framework on which to base nursing practice.

### Levels of Performance

The following four major factors help to determine the levels of function and types of activities engaged in by a psychiatric nurse:

1. The nurse practice act of one's state
2. The nurse's qualifications, including education, work experience, and certification status

3. The nurse's practice setting

4. The nurse's degree of personal competence and initiative

The following two levels of psychiatric–mental health clinical nursing practice have been identified[1]:

1. A *psychiatric–mental health registered nurse* (RN) is a licensed RN who has demonstrated clinical skills in psychiatric–mental health nursing that exceed those of a new nurse in the field. Certification is the formal process that validates the nurse's area of clinical expertise. The letter "C" placed after the RN (i.e., RN, C) designates basic-level certification status.

2. An *advanced practice registered nurse in psychiatric–mental health* (APRN-PMH) is a licensed RN who has, at a minimum, a master's degree, in-depth knowledge of psychiatric nursing theory, supervised clinical practice, and competence in advanced psychiatric nursing skills. Doctorally prepared psychiatric–mental health nurses in advanced practice have both a master's degree and a doctorate in nursing or a related field. The letters "CS" placed after the APRN (i.e., APRN, CS) designate that the nurse is a *certified specialist* in psychiatric–mental health nursing.

## Levels of Prevention

Psychiatric nursing interventions further include three areas of activity: primary, secondary, and tertiary prevention, as follows:

1. *Primary prevention* is a community concept that involves lowering the incidence of illness in a community by altering the causative factors before they have an opportunity to do harm. Primary prevention precedes illness and is applied to a generally healthy population. It includes health promotion and illness prevention.

2. *Secondary prevention* involves reducing the prevalence of actual illness by early detection and treatment of health problems.

3. *Tertiary prevention* involves reducing the impairment or disability that results from illness.

## Continuum of Care

Traditional settings for psychiatric nurses include psychiatric facilities, community mental health centers, psychiatric units in the general hospital, residential facilities, and private practice. With health care reform, however, alternative treatment settings throughout the continuum of mental health care have emerged for psychiatric nurses. Specifically, many hospitals have been transformed into integrated clinical systems that provide inpatient care, partial hospitalization or day treatment, residential care, home care, and outpatient or ambulatory care. Current community-based treatment settings have been expanded to include foster care or group homes, hospices, home health agencies, visiting nurse associations, emergency departments, shelters, nursing homes, primary care clinics, schools, prisons, industry, managed care facilities, and health maintenance organizations (HMOs).

## Competent Caring

The three domains of contemporary psychiatric nursing practice are: (1) direct care, (2) communication, and (3) management activities. The teaching, coordinating, delegating, and collaborating functions of the nurse's role are expressed within these overlapping domains of practice.

The various activities of psychiatric nurses within each one of these three domains can be further delineated. Box 1-1 lists the range of specific nursing activities that a psychiatric nurse could perform in each area. Although not all nurses participate in all these activities, they do reflect the current nature and scope of competent caring by psychiatric nurses. In addition, psychiatric nurses are able to do the following:

- Make biopsychosocial health assessments that are culturally sensitive.
- Design and implement treatment plans for patients and families with complex health problems and comorbid conditions.
- Engage in case management activities, such as organizing, accessing, negotiating, coordinating, and integrating services and benefits for individuals and families.
- Provide a health care map for individuals, families, and groups to guide them to community resources for mental health, including the most appropriate providers, agencies, technologies, and social systems.
- Promote and maintain mental health and manage the effects of mental illness through teaching and counseling.
- Provide care for physically ill patients with psychological problems and psychiatrically ill patients with physical problems.

## Box 1-1　Psychiatric Nursing Activities

Direct Care Activities

Activity therapy
Advocacy
Aftercare follow-up
Behavioral treatments
Case consultation
Case management
Cognitive treatments
Community assessment
Community-based care
Community education
Complementary interventions
Compliance counseling
Counseling
Crisis intervention
Discharge planning
Environmental change
Environmental safety
Family interventions
Group work
Health maintenance
Health promotion
Health teaching
High-risk assessment
Holistic interventions
Home health care
Individual counseling
Informed consent acquisition
Intake screening and evaluation
Interpretation of diagnostic and laboratory tests
Medication administration
Medication management
Mental health promotion
Mental illness prevention
Milieu therapy
Nutritional counseling
Ordering of diagnostic and laboratory tests
Parent education

*Continued*

## Box 1-1   Psychiatric Nursing Activities—cont'd

Direct Care Activities—cont'd

Patient triage
Physical assessment
Physiological treatments
Play therapy
Prescription of medications
Promotion of self-care activities
Provision of environmental safety
Psychiatric rehabilitation
Psychobiological interventions
Psychoeducation
Psychosocial assessment
Psychotherapy
Rehabilitation counseling
Relapse prevention
Research implementation
Social action
Social skills training
Somatic treatments
Stress management
Support of social systems
Telehealth

Communication Activities

Clinical case conferences
Development of treatment plans
Documentation of care
Forensic testimony
Interagency liaison
Peer review
Professional nurse networking
Report preparation
Staff meetings
Transcription of orders
Treatment team meetings
Verbal reports of care

*Continued*

## Box 1-1    Psychiatric Nursing Activities—cont'd

Management Activities
Budgeting and resource allocation
Clinical supervision
Collaboration
Committee participation
Community action
Consultation/liaison
Contract negotiation
Coordination of services
Delegation of assignments
Grant writing
Marketing and public relations
Mediation and conflict resolution
Mentorship
Needs assessment and forecasting
Organizational governance
Outcomes management
Performance evaluations
Policy and procedure development
Practice guidelines formulation
Professional presentations
Program evaluation
Program planning
Publications
Quality improvement activities
Recruitment and retention activities
Regulatory agency activities
Risk management
Software development
Staff scheduling
Staff and student education
Strategic planning
Unit governance
Utilization review

- Manage and coordinate systems of care integrating the needs of patients, families, staff, and regulators.

## Evidence-Based Practice

Accountability for patient care outcomes is a basic responsibility of professional nurses. Central to this accountability is the ability to examine nursing practice patterns, evaluate the nature of the data supporting them, and demonstrate sound clinical decision making in a way that can be empirically supported. This is the essence of evidence-based practice.

*Evidence-based practice* is the conscientious, explicit, and judicious use of the best evidence from systematic research to make decisions about the care of individual patients. It blends a nurse's clinical expertise with the best available research evidence. Evidence-based practice is also a method of self-directed, career-long learning as the nurse continuously seeks the best possible outcomes for patients through implementing effective interventions based on the most current research evidence. Evidence-based psychiatric nursing practice involves the following series of activities (Figure 1-1): (1) defining the clinical question; (2) finding the evidence; (3) analyzing the evidence; (4) using the evidence; and (5) evaluating the outcomes.

## Outcome Evaluation

Psychiatric nurses must be able to identify, describe, and measure the effect of the care they provide patients, families, and communities. *Outcomes* are those factors that affect the patient and family while they are involved in the health care system, including health status, functional status, quality of life, presence or absence of illness, type of coping response, and satisfaction with treatment. Outcome evaluation can focus on a clinical condition, an intervention, or the caregiving process.

One evolving framework for measuring nursing outcomes is the Iowa Nursing Intervention Project, which developed nursing intervention classification (NIC) codes[2] and nursing outcome classification (NOC) codes.[3] These lay out a taxonomy for nursing interventions and outcomes from a biopsychosocial perspective. They are a fertile area of potential nursing research that can document the nature and outcomes of psychiatric nursing practice.

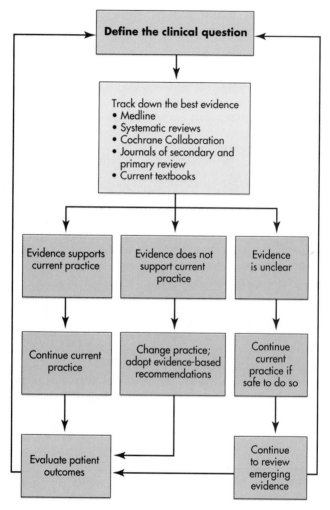

Figure 1-1
Developing evidence-based care.

Critically evaluating the outcomes of psychiatric nursing activities is a task for every psychiatric nurse regardless of role, qualifications, or practice setting. Psychiatric nurse clinicians, educators, administrators, and researchers all must assume responsibility for answering the question, What difference does psychiatric nursing care make?

*your* **INTERNET** connection

**American Nurses Association:**
www.ana.org

**American Nurses Credentialing Center:**
www.ana.org/ancc

**American Psychiatric Nurses' Association:**
www.apna.org

**Australian and New Zealand College of Mental Health Nurses:**
www.health.sci.utasedu.au/nursing/college

**Cochrane Collaboration:**
www.cochrane.org

**International Association of Forensic Nurses:**
www.forensicnurse.org

**International Nurses Society on Addictions:**
www.intnsa.org

**International Society of Psychiatric Nurses:**
www.ispn-psych.org

## References

1. American Nurses' Association: *Scope and standards of psychiatric–mental health clinical nursing practice,* Washington, DC, 2000, The Association.
2. McCloskey J, Bulechek G: *Nursing interventions classification (NIC),* St Louis, 2000, Mosby.

3. Johnson M et al: *Nursing outcomes classification (NOC),* St Louis, 2000, Mosby.

## Suggested readings

Baradell J, Hanrahan N: CPT coding and medicare reimbursement issues, *Clinical Nurse Specialist* 14(6):299-303, 2001.

Flaskerud J, Wuerker A: Mental health nursing in the 21st century, *Issues Ment Health Nurs* 20:5, 1999.

Lanza M: Power and leadership in psychiatric nursing: directions for the next century, parts I and II, *Perspect Psychiatr Care* 33:5, 1997.

McBride A, Austin J, editors: *Psychiatric–mental health nursing: integrating the behavioral and biological sciences,* Philadelphia, 1996, WB Saunders.

Merwin E, Mauck A: Psychiatric nursing outcome research: the state of the science, *Arch Psychiatr Nurs* 9:311, 1995.

Pearson L: Annual update of how each state stands on legislative issues affecting advanced nursing practice, *Nurse Pract* 26:18, 2001.

Shea C et al: *Advanced practice nursing in psychiatric and mental health care,* St Louis, 1999, Mosby.

Stuart G: Evidence-based psychiatric nursing practice: rhetoric or reality? *J Am Psychiatr Nurs Assoc* 7(4):2001.

Stuart G: Role utilization of nurses in public psychiatry, *Admin Policy Ment Health* 27(6):423-441, 2000.

Stuart G, Laraia M: *Principles and practice of psychiatric nursing,* ed 7, St Louis, 2001, Mosby.

# Therapeutic Nurse-Patient Relationship

The therapeutic nurse-patient relationship is a mutual learning experience and a corrective emotional experience for the patient. In this relationship the nurse uses the self and specified clinical techniques in working with the patient to bring about insight and behavioral change.

## Nature of the Relationship

The goals of a therapeutic relationship are directed toward the patient's growth and include the following:

1. Self-realization, self-acceptance, and increased self-respect
2. Clear sense of personal identity and improved personal integration
3. Ability to form intimate, interdependent, interpersonal relationships with a capacity to give and receive love
4. Improved functioning and increased ability to satisfy needs and achieve realistic personal goals

To achieve these goals, various aspects of the patient's life experiences are explored during the course of the relationship. The nurse allows for the patient's expression of perceptions, thoughts, and feelings and relates these to observed and reported actions. Areas of conflict and anxiety are clarified. It is also important for the nurse to identify and maximize the patient's ego strengths and to encourage socialization and family relatedness. Problems of communication are corrected and maladaptive behavior patterns modified as the patient tests out new patterns of behavior and more adaptive coping mechanisms. Figure 2-1 shows the elements that produce a therapeutic outcome.

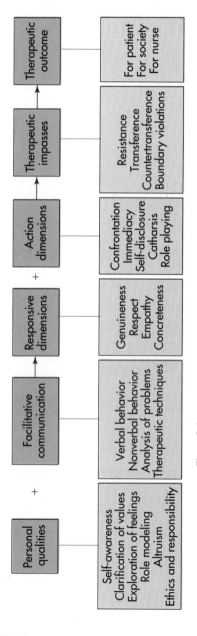

Figure 2-1
Elements affecting the nurse's ability to be therapeutic.

## Therapeutic Use of Self

The principal helping tool that the psychiatric nurse can use in practice is the self. Thus self-analysis is an essential aspect of therapeutic nursing care. Specific personal qualities needed by the nurse who wants to provide therapeutic care include the following:

1. Self-awareness
2. Clarification of values
3. Exploration of feelings
4. Ability to serve as role model
5. Altruistic motivations
6. Sense of ethics and responsibility

## Phases of the Relationship

The four sequential phases of the nurse-patient relationship are (1) preinteraction phase, (2) introductory or orientation phase, (3) working phase, and (4) termination phase. Table 2-1 summarizes the nurse's tasks in each phase of the relationship process.

# Facilitative Communication

Communication theory is relevant to psychiatric nursing practice for three major reasons. First, communication is the vehicle for establishing a therapeutic relationship because it involves conveying information and exchanging thoughts and feelings. Second, communication is the means by which people influence the behavior of others. Therefore communication is critical to the successful outcome of nursing intervention because the nursing process is directed toward promoting adaptive behavioral change. Finally, communication is the relationship itself; without it, a therapeutic nurse-patient relationship is not possible.

## Levels of Communication

*Verbal communication* occurs through the medium of words, spoken or written, and represents a small segment of total human communication. Validation of the meaning of verbal communication between the nurse and patient is essential.

*Nonverbal communication* involves all five senses and includes everything other than the written or spoken word. The five categories of nonverbal communication are as follows:

1. *Vocal cues* are paralinguistic or extraspeech noises and sounds.

Table 2-1   Nursing tasks in each phase of therapeutic relationship

| Phase | Task |
|---|---|
| Preinteraction | Explore own feelings, fantasies, and fears |
| | Analyze own professional strengths and limitations |
| | Gather data about patient when possible |
| | Plan for first meeting with patient |
| Introductory or orientation | Determine reason patient sought help |
| | Establish trust, acceptance, and open communication |
| | Explore patient's thoughts, feelings, and actions |
| | Identify patient's problems |
| | Define goals with patient |
| | Mutually formulate contract to include names, roles, responsibilities, expectations, purpose, meeting location, time of meetings, conditions for termination, and confidentiality |
| Working | Explore relevant stressors |
| | Promote patient's development of insight and use of constructive coping mechanisms. |
| | Discuss and overcome resistance behaviors |
| Termination | Establish reality of separation |
| | Review progress of therapy and attainment of goals |
| | Mutually explore feelings of rejection, loss, sadness, and anger and related behaviors |

2. *Action cues* are all body movements, including facial expression and posture.
3. *Object cues* are a person's intentional and nonintentional use of objects, such as dress and possessions.
4. *Space* is the physical distance between two people.
5. *Touch* is physical contact between two people and is the most personal nonverbal communication.

## The Communication Process

Human communication is a dynamic process that is influenced by the psychological and physiological conditions of the participants. The structural model of communication identifies the following five functional components:

1. *Sender*—originator of the message
2. *Message*—unit of information transmitted from the sender to the receiver
3. *Receiver*—perceiver of the message, whose behavior is influenced by the message
4. *Feedback*—response of the receiver to the sender
5. *Context*—setting in which the communication takes place

If a nurse evaluates the communication process with regard to these five structural elements, specific problems or potential errors can be identified.

## Therapeutic Communication Techniques

Two requirements of effective communication are (1) that it be aimed at preserving the self-respect of both the nurse and the patient and (2) that the communication of acceptance and understanding precedes any suggestions of information or more specific information. Various methods exist for recording nurse-patient communications, including videotape; sound recording; and verbatim, outline, and postinteraction notes. Table 2-2 identifies various therapeutic communication techniques with definitions, examples, therapeutic values, and nontherapeutic threats.

## Dimensions of the Relationship

The nurse must acquire certain skills or qualities to initiate and continue a therapeutic relationship. These skills incorporate verbal and nonverbal behavior and the attitudes and feelings behind the nurse's communication. They are broadly divided into responsive and action dimensions, as follows:

1. *Responsive dimensions* include genuineness, respect, empathic understanding, and concreteness. They are crucial in the orientation phase of the relationship to establish trust and open communication. They continue to be useful throughout the working and termination phases and allow the patient to achieve insight.

Table 2-2    Therapeutic communication techniques

| Technique | Definition | Example | Therapeutic Value | Nontherapeutic Threat |
|---|---|---|---|---|
| Listening | Active process of receiving information and examining one's reaction to messages received | Maintaining eye contact and receptive nonverbal communication | Nonverbally communicates nurse's interest and acceptance to patient | Failure to listen |
| Broad openings | Encouraging patient to select topic for discussion | "What are you thinking about?" | Indicates acceptance by nurse and value of patient's initiative | Domination of interaction by nurse; rejection of responses |
| Restating | Repeating to patient the main thought patient has expressed | "You say that your mother left you when you were 5 years old." | Indicates nurse is listening and validates, reinforces, or highlights something patient has said | Lack of validation of nurse's interpretation of message; being judgmental; reassuring; defending |
| Clarification | Attempting to put into words vague ideas or unclear thoughts of patient; asking patient to explain what is meant | "I'm not sure what you mean. Could you tell me that again?" | Helps to clarify patient's feelings, ideas, and perceptions; provides explicit correlation to patient's actions | Failure to probe; assumed understanding |

| Technique | Description | Example | Therapeutic value | Nontherapeutic threat |
|---|---|---|---|---|
| Reflection | Directing patient's ideas, feelings, questions, and content back to patient | "You're feeling tense and anxious, and it's related to a conversation you had with your mother last night?" | Validates nurse's understanding of what patient is saying and indicates empathy, interest, and respect for patient | Stereotyping patient's responses; inappropriate timing and depth of feeling; inappropriate response to patient's cultural experience and educational level |
| Focusing | Questions or statements that help patient expand on topic of importance | "I think we should talk more about your relationship with your father." | Allows patient to discuss central issues and keeps communication goal directed | Allowing abstractions and generalization; changing topics |
| Sharing perceptions | Asking patient to verify nurse's understanding of what patient is thinking or feeling | "You're smiling, but I sense that you're really very angry with me." | Conveys nurse's understanding and may clear up confusion | Challenging patient; accepting literal responses; reassuring; testing; defending |
| Identifying themes | Underlying issues or problems that emerge repeatedly | "I've noticed that in all the relationships you describe, you've been hurt by the man. Do you think this is an underlying issue?" | Allows nurse to best promote patient's exploration and understanding of important problems | Giving advice; reassuring; disapproving |

*Continued*

Table 2-2   Therapeutic communication techniques—cont'd

| Technique | Definition | Example | Therapeutic Value | Nontherapeutic Threat |
|---|---|---|---|---|
| Silence | Lack of verbal communication for therapeutic reason | Sitting with patient and nonverbally communicating interest and involvement | Allows patient time to think and gain insights, slows pace of interaction, and encourages patient to initiate conversation while nurse conveys support, understanding, and acceptance | Questioning patient; asking for "why" responses; failure to break nontherapeutic silence |
| Humor | Discharge of energy through comic enjoyment of the imperfect | "That gives a whole new meaning to the word *nervous*," said with shared kidding. | Can promote insight by making conscious repressed topics; can resolve paradoxes, temper aggression, and reveal new options; is a socially acceptable form of sublimation | Indiscriminate use; belittling of patient; screen to avoid nontherapeutic intimacy |

2. *Action-oriented dimensions* include confrontation, immediacy, nurse self-disclosure, emotional catharsis, and role playing. They must be implemented in the context of warmth, acceptance, and understanding established by the responsive dimensions. They help the therapeutic relationship progress by identifying obstacles to the patient's growth and by underscoring the need for not only internal understanding or insight but also external action and behavioral change.

Table 2-3 summarizes the responsive and action dimensions for therapeutic nurse-patient relationships.

# Therapeutic Impasses

Therapeutic impasses, or blocks in the progress of the nurse-patient relationship, are of three primary types: resistance, transference, and countertransference. They arise for a variety of reasons and may take many different forms, but they all stall the therapeutic relationship. Therefore the nurse should deal with them as soon as possible. These impasses provoke intense feelings in both the nurse and the patient that may range from anxiety and apprehension to frustration, love, or intense anger.

## Resistance

Resistance is the patient's attempt to remain unaware of anxiety-producing aspects within the self. It is a natural reluctance to or learned avoidance of verbalizing or even experiencing the troubled aspects of oneself. Ambivalent attitudes toward self-exploration, in which the patient both appreciates and avoids anxiety-producing experiences, are a normal part of the therapeutic process. A primary resistance is often the result of the patient's unwillingness to change when the need for change is recognized. Resistance behaviors are usually displayed by patients during the working phase of the relationship because it contains most of the problem-solving process. Box 2-1 lists forms of resistance displayed by patients.

## Transference

Transference is an unconscious response in which the patient experiences feelings and attitudes toward the nurse that were originally associated with significant figures in the patient's early life. The term refers to a group of reactions that attempt to reduce or allevi-

Table 2-3    Responsive and action-oriented dimensions for therapeutic nurse-patient relationships

| Dimension | Characteristics |
|---|---|
| **Responsive Dimensions** | |
| Genuineness | Implies that nurse is an open person who is self-congruent, authentic, and accessible |
| Respect | Suggests that patient is regarded as a person of worth who is valued and accepted without qualification |
| Empathic understanding | Viewing patient's world from patient's internal frame of reference, with sensitivity to patient's current feelings and with verbal ability to communicate this understanding in language appropriate to patient |
| Concreteness | Use of specific terminology rather than abstractions in discussion of patient's feelings, experiences, and behavior |
| **Action-Oriented Dimensions** | |
| Confrontation | Nurse's expression of perceived discrepancies in patient's behavior to expand patient's self-awareness |
| Immediacy | Current nurse-patient interaction in relationship is used to learn about patient's functioning in other interpersonal relationships |
| Nurse self-disclosure | Nurse reveals information about self and own ideas, values, feelings, and attitudes to facilitate patient's cooperation, learning, catharsis, or support |
| Emotional catharsis | Patient encouraged to talk about most bothersome aspects of life for therapeutic effect |
| Role playing | Acting out a particular situation to increase patient's insight into human relations and deepen patient's ability to see a situation from another point of view; also allows patient to experiment with new behavior in a safe environment |

---

**Box 2-1   Forms of Resistance**

- Suppression and repression of pertinent information
- Intensification of symptoms
- Self-devaluation and hopeless outlook on the future
- Forced flight into health, in which patient experiences sudden but short-lived recovery
- Intellectual inhibitions, which may be evident when patients say they have nothing on their mind or are unable to think about their problems; break appointments or arrive late for sessions; or are forgetful, silent, or sleepy
- Acting out or irrational behavior
- Superficial talk
- Intellectual insight, in which patient verbalizes self-understanding with correct use of terminology yet continues maladaptive behavior, or use of the defense of intellectualization when no insight exists
- Contempt for normality, which is evident when patient has developed insight but refuses to assume responsibility for change on the grounds that normality is not so appealing
- Transference reactions

---

ate anxiety. The outstanding traits defining transference are the inappropriateness of the patient's response in terms of intensity and the maladaptive use of the defense mechanism of displacement. Transference reactions are harmful to the therapeutic process only if they remain ignored and unexamined by the nurse. The two main types are hostile and dependent reactions.

## Countertransference

Countertransference is a therapeutic impasse created by the nurse, not the patient. It refers to a specific emotional response by the nurse to the patient that is inappropriate to the content and context of the therapeutic relationship or inappropriate in its emotional intensity. Countertransference is transference applied to the nurse. The nurse's responses are not justified by reality but rather reflect previous conflicts experienced with issues such as authority, gender assertiveness, and independence.

Countertransference reactions are usually one of three types: reactions of intense love or caring, reactions of intense hostility or hatred, and reactions of intense anxiety, often in response to a patient's resistance. Box 2-2 presents some forms of countertransference.

## Boundary Violations

Boundary violations occur when a nurse goes outside the boundaries of the therapeutic relationship and establishes a social, economic, or personal relationship with a patient. As a general rule, whenever the nurse is doing or thinking of doing something special, different, or unusual for a patient, a boundary violation usually is involved. Sexual contact of any kind is never therapeutic

---

**Box 2-2**    Forms of Countertransference Displayed by Nurses

- Difficulty empathizing with patient in certain problem areas
- Feeling depressed during or after session
- Carelessness about implementing contract, such as being late or running overtime
- Drowsiness during sessions
- Feeling angry or impatient because of patient's unwillingness to change
- Encouraging patient's dependency, praise, or affection
- Arguing with patient or tendency to "push" patient before ready
- Trying to help patient in matters not related to identified nursing goals
- Personal or social involvement with patient
- Dreaming about or preoccupation with patient
- Sexual or aggressive fantasies toward patient
- Recurrent anxiety, unease, or guilt related to patient
- Tendency to focus on only one aspect of information presented by patient or to view it only one way
- Need to defend nursing interventions with patient to others

and never acceptable within the nurse-patient relationship. Box 2-3 lists examples of possible boundary violations.

## Overcoming Therapeutic Impasses

To overcome therapeutic impasses, the nurse must be prepared to be exposed to powerful emotional feelings within the context of the nurse-patient relationship. Initially the nurse must have knowledge of the impasses and recognize behaviors that indicate their existence. Then the nurse can clarify and reflect on feeling and content to focus more objectively on what is happening.

The reasons behind the behavior are explored, and either the patient (for resistance and transference reactions) or the nurse (for countertransference reactions and boundary violations) accepts responsibility for the impasse and its negative impact on the therapeutic process. Finally, the goals of the relationship and the patient's needs and problems are reviewed. This should help the nurse reestablish a therapeutic alliance consistent with the process of the nurse-patient relationship.

---

### Box 2-3   Possible Boundary Violations Related to Psychiatric Nurses

- Patient takes nurse out to lunch or dinner
- Professional relationship turns into social relationship
- Nurse attends a party at patient's invitation
- Nurse regularly reveals personal information to patient
- Patient introduces nurse to family members, such as son or daughter, for the purpose of a social relationship
- Nurse accepts free gifts from patient's business
- Nurse agrees to meet patient for treatment outside the usual setting without therapeutic justification
- Nurse attends social functions of patient
- Patient gives nurse an expensive gift
- Nurse routinely hugs or has physical contact with patient
- Nurse does business with or purchases services from patient

*your* **INTERNET**
    c o n n e c t i o n

**Internet Mental Health:**
www.mentalhealth.com

**Knowledge Exchange Network:**
www.mentalhealth.org

**National Institute of Mental Health:**
www.nimh.nih.gov

**National Mental Health Association:**
www.nmha.org

## Suggested readings

Albert G: What are the characteristics of effective psychotherapists? The experts speak, *J Pract Psychiatry Behav Health* 3:35, 1997.

Bohart A, Greenberg L: *Empathy reconsidered*, Washington, DC, 1997, American Psychological Association.

Carkhoff R: *Helping and human relations,* vols 1 and 2, New York, 1969, Holt, Rinehart & Winston.

Eckroth-Bucher M: Philosophical basis and practice of self-awareness in psychiatric nursing, *J Psychosoc Nurs* 39(2):32, 2001.

Ens I: An analysis of the concept of countertransference, *Arch Psych Nurs* 12:273, 1998.

Krupnick J et al: The role of the therapeutic alliance in psychotherapy and pharmacotherapy outcome, *J Consult Clin Psychol* 64:532, 1996.

Nichols M: *The lost art of listening,* New York, 1995, Guilford.

Pilette P, Bereck C, Archber L: Therapeutic management of helping boundaries, *J Psychosoc Nurs* 33:40, 1995.

Reid W: Boundary issues and violations, *J Pract Psychiatry Behav Health* 4:173, 1999.

Reynolds W: *The measurement and development of empathy in nursing,* Aldershot, Hampshire, United Kingdom, 2000, Ashgate.

Stuart G, Laraia M: *Principles and practice of psychiatric nursing,* ed 7, St Louis, 2001, Mosby.

Suchman A: Control and relationship: two foundational values and their consequences, *Issues in Interdisciplinary Care* 3(2):145-150, 2001.

Sundeen S et al: *Nurse-client interaction: implementing the nursing process,* ed 6, St Louis, 1998, Mosby.

# The Stuart Stress Adaptation Model of Psychiatric Nursing Care

3

The *Report of the Surgeon General on Mental Health* is the first surgeon general's report ever issued on the topic of mental health and mental illness. It is based on an extensive review of the scientific literature and on consultations with mental health providers and consumers. This landmark document came with the following conclusions[1]:

- Mental health is fundamental to health.
- Mental disorders are real health conditions.
- The efficacy of mental health treatments is well documented.
- A range of treatments exists for most mental disorders.

## Defining Mental Health and Mental Illness

Health-illness and adaptation-maladaptation are distinct concepts. Each exists on a separate continuum. The health-illness continuum derives from a medical worldview. The adaptation-maladaptation continuum derives from a nursing worldview. Thus a person who has a medically diagnosed illness, whether physical or psychiatric, can adapt well to it. In contrast, a person who does not have a medically diagnosed illness may have many maladaptive coping responses. These two continuums reflect how nursing and medical models of practice complement each other.

### Mental Health

The following have been identified as criteria of mental health:

- Positive attitudes toward self
- Growth, development, and self-actualization

- Integration and emotional responsiveness
- Autonomy and self-determination
- Accurate reality perception
- Environmental mastery and social competence

## Mental Illness

One's definition of mental illness is derived from what one believes to be the causative factors. The following hypotheses have been proposed regarding influences on the occurrence of mental illness:

- The *biological hypothesis* proposes anatomical and physiological dysfunctions.
- The *learning hypothesis* proposes maladaptive learned behavioral patterns.
- The *cognitive hypothesis* proposes inaccuracies or deficits in knowledge or awareness.
- The *psychodynamic hypothesis* proposes intrapsychic conflicts and developmental deficits.
- The *environmental hypothesis* proposes stressors and aversive environmental responses.

Box 3-1 presents key facts about mental illness.

## Conceptual Models of Practice

Many mental health professionals practice within the framework of a conceptual model. A *model* is a means of organizing a complex body of knowledge, such as concepts related to human behavior. Using a model helps a clinician to develop a sound basis for assessment and intervention, as well as providing a way to evaluate the effectiveness of treatment. A number of conceptual models have been developed for psychiatric practice. Table 3-1 presents these models and associated theorists, their view of behavioral deviations, the therapeutic process, and the roles of the patient and therapist.

## The Stuart Stress Adaptation Model of Psychiatric Nursing Care

Psychiatric nurses can practice more effectively if their actions are based on a model that recognizes the presence of health or illness as an outcome of multiple characteristics of a person

*Text continued on p. 34*

## Box 3-1    Key Facts About Mental Illness

Extent and Severity of the Problem

- The full spectrum of mental disorders affects 22% of the adult population in a given year. This figure refers to all mental disorders and is comparable to rates for physical disorders when similarly broadly defined (e.g., respiratory disorders affect 50% of adults; cardiovascular diseases, 20%).
- Severe mental disorders (i.e., schizophrenia, manic-depressive illness, and severe forms of depression, panic disorder, and obsessive-compulsive disorder) affect 2.8% of the adult population (approximately 5 million people) and account for 25% of all federal disability payments.
- At least 7.5 million children in the United States under 18 years of age have a mental health problem severe enough to require treatment.
- Approximately 18 million persons in the United States 18 years of age and older experience problems as a result of alcohol use; 10.6 million of these have alcoholism.
- Most alcoholic persons improve through treatment, and evidence suggests that alcoholism treatment is effective in containing costs throughout the health care system and increasing worker productivity.
- An estimated 23 million people in the United States currently use illicit drugs.

Treatment Efficacy

- How *effective* are treatments for severe mental disorders compared with treatments for physical illness?

| Disorder | Treatment Success Rate (%) |
| --- | --- |
| Panic | 80 |
| Bipolar | 80 |
| Major depression | 65 |
| Schizophrenia | 60 |
| Obsessive-compulsive | 60 |
| Cardiovascular treatments | |
|     Atherectomy | 52 |
|     Angioplasty | 41 |

*From National Advisory Mental Health Council:* Am J Psychiatry *150:1447, 1993.*

Table 3-1    Models of psychiatric mental health practice

| Model (Major Theorists) | View of Behavioral Deviation | Therapeutic Process | Roles of Patient and Therapist |
|---|---|---|---|
| Psychoanalytical (S. Freud, Erikson, Klein, Horney, Fromm-Reichmann, Menninger) | Behavior is based on early development and inadequate resolution of developmental conflicts. Ego defenses unable to control anxiety. Symptoms result as effort to deal with anxiety and are related to unresolved conflicts. | Psychoanalysis uses techniques of free association and dream analysis. It interprets behavior, uses transference to revise earlier traumatic experiences, and identifies problem areas through interpretation of patient's resistances. | Patient verbalizes all thoughts and dreams and considers therapist's interpretations. Therapist remains remote to encourage development of transference and interprets patient's thoughts and dreams in terms of conflicts, transference, and resistance. |
| Interpersonal (Sullivan, Peplau) | Anxiety arises and is experienced interpersonally. The basic fear is fear of rejection. Person needs security and satisfaction that result from positive interpersonal relationships. | Relationship between therapist and patient builds feeling of security. Therapist helps patient experience trusting relationship and gain interpersonal satisfaction. Patient then assisted to develop close relationships outside therapy situation. | Patient shares anxieties and feelings with therapist. Therapist develops close relationship with patient; uses empathy to perceive patient's feelings and uses relationship as a corrective interpersonal experience. |

| Model | | | |
|---|---|---|---|
| Social (Szasz, Caplan) | Social and environmental factors create stress, which causes anxiety, resulting in symptom formation. Unacceptable (deviant) behavior is socially defined and meets needs of social system. | Patient helped to deal with social system. Crisis intervention may be used. Environmental manipulation and enlistment of special supports are also employed. Peer support is encouraged. | Patient actively presents problem to therapist and works with therapist toward resolution. Community resources are used. Therapist explores patient's social system and helps patient use resources available or create new resources. |
| Existential (Peris, Glasser, Ellis, Rogers, Frankl) | Life is meaningful when person can fully experience and accept the self. Behavioral deviation occurs when individual is thwarted in the effort to find and accept self. The self can be experienced through authentic relationships with other people. | Person aided to experience authenticity in relationships. Therapy is frequently conducted in groups. Patient is encouraged to explore and to accept self and helped to assume control of behavior. | Patient assumes responsibility for behavior and participates in meaningful experiences to learn about real self. Therapist helps patient to recognize value of self. Therapist clarifies realities of situation and introduces patient to genuine feelings and expanded awareness. |

Continued

Table 3-1  Models of psychiatric mental health practice—cont'd

| Model (Major Theorists) | View of Behavioral Deviation | Therapeutic Process | Roles of Patient and Therapist |
|---|---|---|---|
| Supportive (Werman, Rockland) | Problems are a result of biopsychosocial factors. Emphasis on current maladaptive coping responses. | Reality testing and self-esteem enhancing measures. Social supports are enlisted and adaptive coping responses reinforced. | Patient actively involved in treatment. Therapist is warm and empathic and allies with patient. |
| Communication (Berne, Watzlawick) | Behavioral disruptions occur when messages are not clearly communicated. Language can be used to distort meaning. Messages may be transmitted simultaneously at several levels. Verbal and nonverbal messages may lack congruence. | Communication patterns analyzed and feedback given to clarify problem areas. Transactional analysis focuses on games and learning to communicate directly without game playing. | Patient examines communication patterns, including games, and works to clarify own communication and validate messages from others. Therapist interprets communication pattern to patient and teaches principles of good communication. |

| Behavioral (Bandura, Pavlov, Wolpe, Skinner) | Behavior is learned. Deviation occurs because person has formed undesirable behavioral habits. Because behavior is learned, it can also be unlearned. Deviant behavior may be perpetuated because it reduces anxiety. If so, another anxiety-reducing behavior may be substituted. | Therapy is educational process. Behavioral deviations are not rewarded; more productive behaviors are reinforced. Relaxation therapy and assertiveness training are behavioral approaches. | Patient practices behavioral technique used; does homework and reinforcement exercises. Patient helps develop behavioral hierarchies. Therapist teaches patient about behavioral approach, helps develop behavioral hierarchy, and reinforces desired behaviors. |
| Medical (Meyer, Kraeplin, Spitzer, Frances) | Behavioral disruptions result from a biological disease. Symptoms result from a combination of physiological, genetic, environmental, and social factors. Deviant behavior relates to patient's tolerance for stress. | Diagnosis of illness is based on present condition and historical information plus diagnostic studies. Treatment may include somatic and pharmacological therapies in addition to various interpersonal techniques. | Patient practices prescribed therapy regimen and reports effects of therapy to therapist. Patient complies with long-term therapy if necessary. Therapist uses somatic and interpersonal therapies. Therapist diagnoses illness and prescribes therapeutic approach. |

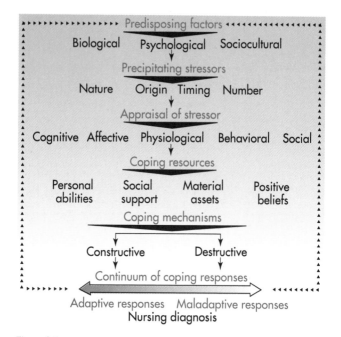

Figure 3-1
Biophysical components of the Stuart Stress Adaptation Model.

interacting with environmental factors. The Stuart Stress Adaptation Model of psychiatric nursing care integrates the biological, psychological, sociocultural, environmental, and legal-ethical aspects of nursing into a unified framework for practice (Figure 3-1). The model incorporates the theoretical basis, biopsychosocial components, continuum of coping responses, and nursing activities based on the patient's treatment stage: (1) health promotion, (2) maintenance, (3) acute, or (4) crisis (Figure 3-2). The full model is presented in Figure 3-3 and consists of the following components:

1. *Predisposing factors*—risk factors that influence both the type and the amount of resources the individual can use to cope with stress

| TREATMENT STAGE | CRISIS |
|---|---|
| Treatment Goal | Stabilization |
| Nursing Assessment | Risk Factors |
| Nursing Intervention | Manage Environment |
| Expected Outcome | No Harm to Self or Others |

| TREATMENT STAGE | ACUTE |
|---|---|
| Treatment Goal | Remission |
| Nursing Assessment | Symptoms and Coping Responses |
| Nursing Intervention | Mutual Treatment Planning, Modeling, and Teaching |
| Expected Outcome | Symptom Relief |

| TREATMENT STAGE | MAINTENANCE |
|---|---|
| Treatment Goal | Recovery |
| Nursing Assessment | Functional Status |
| Nursing Intervention | Reinforcement and Advocacy |
| Expected Outcome | Improved Functioning |

| TREATMENT STAGE | HEALTH PROMOTION |
|---|---|
| Treatment Goal | Optimal Level of Wellness |
| Nursing Assessment | Quality of Life and Well-Being |
| Nursing Intervention | Inspire and Validate |
| Expected Outcome | Attain Optimal Quality of Life |

Figure 3-2
Stages and activities of psychiatric nursing treatment.

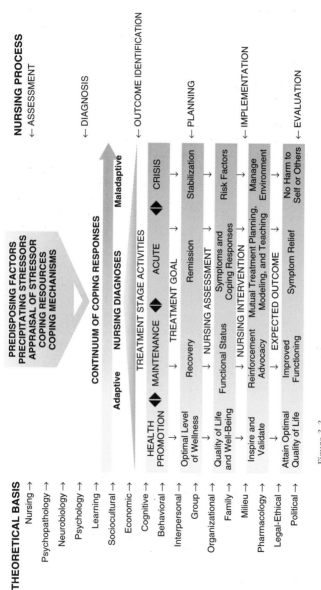

Figure 3-3
The Stuart Stress Adaptation Model of psychiatric nursing care.

2. *Precipitating stressors*—stimuli that the individual perceives as challenging, threatening, or demanding and that require excess energy for coping
3. *Appraisal of stressor*—evaluation of a stressor's significance for the individual's well-being in which the stressor assumes its meaning, intensity, and importance
4. *Coping resources*—evaluation of the individual's coping options and strategies
5. *Coping mechanisms*—any effort directed at stress management, including direct problem-solving efforts and ego defense mechanisms used to protect the self
6. *Continuum of coping responses*—range of adaptive to maladaptive human responses
7. *Treatment stage activities*—range of nursing functions related to treatment goal, nursing assessment, nursing intervention, and expected outcome

## Nursing and Medical Diagnoses

The continuum of coping responses is the subject of nursing diagnoses. The continuum may also include actual health problems that lead to a medical diagnosis. Nursing and medical diagnoses may complement each other, but one is not a component of the other. A patient with one specific medical diagnosis may have a number of complementary nursing diagnoses related to the range of health responses. Conversely, a patient may have a specific nursing diagnosis without any identified medical diagnoses.

### Nursing Diagnosis

A nursing diagnosis is a statement of the patient's nursing problem that includes both the adaptive or maladaptive health response and the contributing stressors.

The North American Nursing Diagnosis Association (NANDA) has identified, defined, and described a classification system of nursing diagnoses. Box 3-2 lists the NANDA nursing diagnoses.

### Medical Diagnosis

A medical diagnosis is the health problem or disease state of the patient. In the medical model of psychiatry, health problems are the mental disorders classified in the *Diagnostic and Statistical Manual of Mental Disorders,* ed 4, text revised (DSM-IV-TR).

## Box 3-2    NANDA Diagnoses

Activity intolerance
Activity intolerance, Risk for
Adjustment, Impaired
Airway clearance, Ineffective
Allergy response, Latex
Allergy response, Risk for latex
Anxiety
Anxiety, Death
Aspiration, Risk for
Attachment, Risk for impaired parent/infant/child
Autonomic dysreflexia
Autonomic dysreflexia, Risk for
Body image, Disturbed
Body temperature, Risk for imbalanced
Bowel incontinence
Breastfeeding, Effective
Breastfeeding, Ineffective
Breastfeeding, Interrupted
Breathing pattern, Ineffective
Cardiac output, Decreased
Caregiver role strain
Caregiver role strain, Risk for
Comfort, Impaired
Communication, Impaired verbal
Conflict, Decisional
Conflict, Parental role
Confusion, Acute
Confusion, Chronic
Constipation
Constipation, Perceived
Constipation, Risk for

Coping, Ineffective
Coping, Ineffective community
Coping, Readiness for enhanced community
Coping, Defensive
Coping, Compromised family
Coping, Disabled family
Coping, Readiness for enhanced family
Denial, Ineffective
Dentition, Impaired
Development, Risk for delayed
Diarrhea
Disuse syndrome, Risk for
Diversional activity, Deficient
Energy field, Disturbed
Environmental interpretation syndrome, Impaired
Failure to thrive, Adult
Falls, Risk for
Family processes: alcoholism, Dysfunctional
Family processes, Interrupted
Fatigue
Fear
Fluid volume, Deficient
Fluid volume, Excess
Fluid volume, Risk for deficient
Fluid volume, Risk for imbalanced
Gas exchange, Impaired
Grieving
Grieving, Anticipatory
Grieving, Dysfunctional

*From North American Nursing Diagnosis Association:* NANDA nursing diagnoses: definitions and classification 2000-2001, *Philadelphia, 2001, The Association.*

## Box 3-2  NANDA Diagnoses—cont'd

Growth and development, Delayed

Growth, Risk for disproportionate

Health maintenance, Ineffective

Health-seeking behaviors

Home maintenance, Impaired

Hopelessness

Hyperthermia

Hypothermia

Identity, Disturbed personal

Incontinence, Functional urinary

Incontinence, Reflex urinary

Incontinence, Stress urinary

Incontinence, Total urinary

Incontinence, Urge urinary

Incontinence, Risk for urge urinary

Infant behavior, Disorganized

Infant behavior, Risk for disorganized

Infant behavior, Readiness for enhanced organized

Infant feeding pattern, Ineffective

Infection, Risk for

Injury, Risk for

Injury, Risk for perioperative-positioning

Intracranial adaptive capacity, Decreased

Knowledge, Deficient

Loneliness, Risk for

Memory, Impaired

Mobility, Impaired bed

Mobility, Impaired physical

Mobility, Impaired wheelchair

Nausea

Neglect, Unilateral

Noncompliance

Nutrition: less than body requirements, Imbalanced

Nutrition: more than body requirements, Imbalanced

Nutrition: more than body requirements, Risk for imbalanced

Oral mucous membrane, Impaired

Pain, Acute

Pain, Chronic

Parenting, Impaired

Parenting, Risk for impaired

Peripheral neurovascular dysfunction, Risk for

Poisoning, Risk for

Post-trauma syndrome

Post-trauma syndrome, Risk for

Powerlessness

Powerlessness, Risk for

Protection, Ineffective

Rape-trauma syndrome

Rape-trauma syndrome, compound reaction

Rape-trauma syndrome, silent reaction

Relocation stress syndrome

Relocation stress syndrome, Risk for

Role performance, Ineffective

Self-care deficit, Bathing/hygiene

Self-care deficit, Dressing/grooming

Self-care deficit, Feeding

*Continued*

## Box 3-2    NANDA Diagnoses—cont'd

Self-care deficit, Toileting
Self-esteem, Chronic low
Self-esteem, Situational low
Self-esteem, Risk for situational low
Self-mutilation
Self-mutilation, Risk for
Sensory perception, Disturbed
Sexual dysfunction
Sexuality patterns, Ineffective
Skin integrity, Impaired
Skin integrity, Risk for impaired
Sleep deprivation
Sleep pattern, Disturbed
Social interaction, Impaired
Social isolation
Sorrow, Chronic
Spiritual distress
Spiritual distress, Risk for
Spiritual well-being, Readiness for enhanced
Suffocation, Risk for
Suicide, Risk for
Surgical recovery, Delayed
Swallowing, Impaired
Therapeutic regimen management, Effective

Therapeutic regimen management, Ineffective
Therapeutic regimen management, Ineffective community
Therapeutic regimen management, Ineffective family
Thermoregulation, Ineffective
Thought processes, Disturbed
Tissue integrity, Impaired
Tissue perfusion, Ineffective
Transfer ability, Impaired
Trauma, Risk for
Urinary elimination, Impaired
Urinary retention
Ventilation, Impaired spontaneous
Ventilatory weaning response, Dysfunctional
Violence, Risk for other-directed
Violence, Risk for self-directed
Walking, Impaired
Wandering

*From North American Nursing Diagnosis Association:* NANDA nursing diagnoses: definitions and classification 2000-2001, *Philadelphia, 2001, The Association.*

In the DSM-IV-TR the individual is evaluated on each of the following axes (Box 3-3):

Axis I Clinical disorders

Axis II Personality disorders

Axis III General medical conditions

Axis IV Psychosocial and environmental problems

Axis V Global assessment and functioning

*Text continued on p. 66*

## Box 3-3 DSM-IV-TR Classification

NOS = Not Otherwise Specified.

An x appearing in a diagnostic code indicates that a specific code number is required.

An ellipsis (. . .) is used in the names of certain disorders to indicate that the name of a specific mental disorder or general medical condition should be inserted when recording the name (e.g., 293.0 Delirium Due to Hypothyroidism).

If criteria are currently met, one of the following severity specifiers may be noted after the diagnosis:
    Mild
    Moderate
    Severe
If criteria are no longer met, one of the following specifiers may be noted:
    In Partial Remission
    In Full Remission
    Prior History

### Axis I Clinical Disorders

**Disorders usually first diagnosed in infancy, childhood, or adolescence**

*Mental retardation*

NOTE: These are coded on Axis II.
    317    Mild Mental Retardation
    318.0    Moderate Mental Retardation
    318.1    Severe Mental Retardation
    318.2    Profound Mental Retardation
    319    Mental Retardation, Severity Unspecified

*Learning disorders*
    315.00    Reading Disorders
    315.1    Mathematics Disorder
    315.2    Disorder of Written Expression
    315.9    Learning Disorder NOS

*From American Psychiatric Association:* Diagnostic and statistical manual of mental disorders, *ed 4, text revision (DSM-IV-TR), Washington, DC, 2000, The Association.* *Continued*

## Box 3-3    DSM-IV-TR Classification—cont'd

*Motor skills disorder*

    315.4    Developmental Coordination Disorder

*Communication disorders*

    315.31  Expressive Language Disorder

    315.31  Mixed Receptive-Expressive Language Disorder

    315.39  Phonological Disorder

    307.0    Stuttering

*Pervasive developmental disorders*

    307.9    Communication Disorder NOS

    299.00  Autistic Disorder

    299.80  Rett's Disorder

    299.10  Childhood Disintegrative Disorder

    299.80  Asperger's Disorder

    299.80  Pervasive Developmental Disorder NOS

*Attention-deficit and disruptive behavior disorders*

    314.xx  Attention-Deficit/Hyperactivity Disorder

       .01     Combined Type

       .00     Predominantly Inattentive Type

       .01     Predominantly Hyperactive-Impulsive Type

    314.9    Attention-Deficit/Hyperactivity Disorders NOS

    312.8    Conduct Disorder

             *Specify type:* Childhood-Onset Type/ Adolescent-Onset Type

    313.81  Oppositional Defiant Disorder

    312.9    Disruptive Behavior Disorder NOS

*Feeding and eating disorders of infancy or early childhood*

    307.52  Pica

    307.53  Rumination Disorder

    307.59  Feeding Disorder of Infancy or Early Childhood

*Tic disorders*

    307.23  Tourette's Disorder

    307.22  Chronic Motor or Vocal Tic Disorder

    307.21  Transient Tic Disorder

             *Specify if:* Single Episode/Recurrent

    307.20  Tic Disorder NOS

*From American Psychiatric Association:* Diagnostic and statistical manual of mental disorders, *ed 4, text revision (DSM-IV-TR), Washington, DC, 2000, The Association.*

## Box 3-3   DSM-IV-TR Classification—cont'd

*Elimination disorders*
| | |
|---|---|
| \_\_\_.\_ | Encopresis |
| 787.6 | With Constipation and Overflow Incontinence |
| 307.7 | Without Constipation and Overflow Incontinence |
| 307.6 | Enuresis (Not Due to a General Medical Condition) |
| | *Specify type:* Nocturnal Only/Diurnal Only/ Nocturnal and Diurnal |

*Other disorders of infancy, childhood, or adolescence*
| | |
|---|---|
| 309.21 | Separation Anxiety Disorder |
| | *Specify if:* Early Onset |
| 313.89 | Reactive Attachment Disorder of Infancy or Early Childhood |
| | *Specify type:* Inhibited Type/Disinhibited Type |
| 307.3 | Stereotypic Movement Disorder |
| | *Specify if:* With Self-Injurious Behavior |
| 313.9 | Disorder of Infancy, Childhood, or Adolescence NOS |

**Delirium, dementia, and amnestic and other cognitive disorders**

*Delirium*
| | |
|---|---|
| 293.0 | Delirium Due to . . . *[Indicate the General Medical Condition]* |
| \_\_\_.\_ | Substance Intoxication Delirium *(refer to Substance-Related Disorders for substance-specific codes)* |
| \_\_\_.\_ | Substance Withdrawal Delirium *(refer to Substance-Related Disorders for substance-specific codes)* |
| \_\_\_.\_ | Delirium Due to Multiple Etiologies *(code each of the specific etiologies)* |
| 780.09 | Delirium NOS |

*Dementia*
| | |
|---|---|
| 290.xx | Dementia of the Alzheimer's Type, with Early Onset *(also code 331.0 Alzheimer's disease on Axis III)* |
| .10 | Uncomplicated |
| .11 | With Delirium |

*Continued*

## Box 3-3    DSM-IV-TR Classification—cont'd

*Dementia—cont'd*

    .12    With Delusions

    .13    With Depressed Mood

         *Specify if:* With Behavioral Disturbance

290.xx  Dementia of the Alzheimer's Type. With Late Onset *(also code 331.0 Alzheimer's disease on Axis III)*

    .0    Uncomplicated

    .3    With Delirium

    .20    With Delusions

    .21    With Depressed Mood

         *Specify if:* With Behavioral Disturbance

290.xx  Vascular Dementia

    .40    Uncomplicated

    .41    With Delirium

    .42    With Delusions

    .43    With Depressed Mood

         *Specify if:* With Behavioral Disturbance

294.9   Dementia Due to HIV Disease *(also code 043.1 HIV infection affecting central nervous system on Axis III)*

294.1   Dementia Due to Head Trauma *(also code 854.00 head injury on Axis III)*

294.1   Dementia Due to Parkinson's Disease *(also code 332.0 Parkinson's disease on Axis III)*

294.1   Dementia Due to Huntington's Disease *(also code 333.4 Huntington's disease on Axis III)*

290.10  Dementia Due to Pick's Disease *(also code 331.1 Pick's disease on Axis III)*

290.10  Dementia Due to Creutzfeldt-Jakob Disease *(also code 046.1 Creutzfeldt-Jakob disease on Axis III)*

294.1   Dementia Due to . . . *[indicate the General Medical Condition not listed above] (also code the general medical condition on Axis III)*

*From American Psychiatric Association:* Diagnostic and statistical manual of mental disorders, *ed 4, text revision (DSM-IV-TR), Washington, DC, 2000, The Association.*

## Box 3-3   DSM-IV-TR Classification—cont'd

*Dementia—cont'd*

\_\_\_.\_   Substance-Induced Persisting Dementia (refer to Substance-Related Disorders for substance-specific codes)

\_\_\_.\_   Dementia Due to Multiple Etiologies *(code each of the specific etiologies)*

294.8   Dementia NOS

*Amnestic disorders*

294.0   Amnestic Disorder Due to . . . *[Indicate the General Medical Condition]*
*Specify if:* Transient/Chronic

\_\_\_.\_   Substance-Induced Persisting Amnestic Disorder *(refer to Substance-Related Disorders for substance-specific codes)*

294.8   Amnestic Disorder NOS

*Other cognitive disorders*

294.9   Cognitive Disorders NOS

**Mental disorders due to a general medical condition not elsewhere classified**

293.89   Catatonic Disorder Due to . . . *[Indicate the General Medical Condition]*

310.1   Personality Change Due to . . . *[Indicate the General Medical Condition]*
*Specify type:* Labile Type/Disinhibited Type/Aggressive Type/Apathetic Type/Paranoid Type/Other Type/Combined Type/Unspecified Type

293.9   Mental Disorder NOS Due to . . . *[Indicate the General Medical Condition]*

**Substance-related disorders**

[a]*The following specifiers may be applied to Substance Dependence:*

With Physiological Dependence/Without Physiological Dependence
Early Full Remission/Early Partial Remission
Sustained Full Remission/Sustained Partial Remission
On Agonist Therapy/In a Controlled Environment

*Continued*

## Box 3-3    DSM-IV-TR Classification—cont'd

**Substance-related disorders—cont'd**

*The following specifiers apply to Substance-Induced Disorders as noted:*

[I]With Onset During Intoxication/[W]With Onset During Withdrawal

*Alcohol-related disorders*

**Alcohol use disorders**

303.90    Alcohol Dependence[a]

305.00    Alcohol Abuse

**Alcohol-induced disorders**

303.00    Alcohol Intoxication

291.8     Alcohol Withdrawal
          *Specify if:* With Perceptual Disturbances

291.0     Alcohol Intoxication Delirium

291.0     Alcohol Withdrawal Delirium

291.2     Alcohol-Induced Persisting Dementia

291.1     Alcohol-Induced Persisting Amnestic Disorder

291.x     Alcohol-Induced Psychotic Disorder
    .5        With Delusions[I,W]
    .3        With Hallucinations[I,W]

291.8     Alcohol-Induced Mood Disorder[I,W]

291.8     Alcohol-Induced Anxiety Disorder[I,W]

291.8     Alcohol-Induced Sexual Dysfunction[I]

291.8     Alcohol-Induced Sleep Disorder[I,W]

291.9     Alcohol-Related Disorder NOS

*Amphetamine (or amphetamine-like)-related disorders*

**Amphetamine use disorders**

304.40    Amphetamine Dependence[a]

305.70    Amphetamine Abuse

**Amphetamine-induced disorders**

292.89    Amphetamine Intoxication
          *Specify if:* With Perceptual Disturbances

292.0     Amphetamine Withdrawal

292.81    Amphetamine Intoxication Delirium

292.xx    Amphetamine-Induced Psychotic Disorders
    .11       With Delusions[I]
    .12       With Hallucinations[I]

*From American Psychiatric Association:* Diagnostic and statistical manual of mental disorders, *ed 4, text revision (DSM-IV-TR), Washington, DC, 2000, The Association.*

## Box 3-3   DSM-IV-TR Classification—cont'd

**Amphetamine-induced disorders—cont'd**

292.84  Amphetamine-Induced Mood Disorder[I,W]

292.89  Amphetamine-Induced Anxiety Disorder[I]

292.89  Amphetamine-Induced Sexual Dysfunction[I]

292.89  Amphetamine-Induced Sleep Disorder[I,W]

292.9   Amphetamine-Induced Disorder NOS

*Caffeine-related disorders*

**Caffeine-induced disorders**

305.90  Caffeine Intoxication

292.89  Caffeine-Induced Anxiety Disorder[I]

292.89  Caffeine-Induced Sleep Disorder[I]

292.9   Caffeine-Related Disorder NOS

*Cannabis-related disorders*

**Cannabis use disorders**

304.30  Cannabis Dependence[a]

305.20  Cannabis Abuse

**Cannabis-induced disorders**

292.89  Cannabis Intoxication

  *Specify if:* Perceptual Disturbances

292.81  Cannabis Intoxication Delirium

292.xx  Cannabis-Induced Psychotic Disorder

  .11   With Delusions[I]

  .12   With Hallucinations[I]

292.89  Cannabis-Induced Anxiety Disorder[I]

292.9   Cannabis-Related Disorder NOS

*Cocaine-related disorders*

**Cocaine use disorders**

304.20  Cocaine Dependence[a]

305.60  Cocaine Abuse

**Cocaine-induced disorders**

292.89  Cocaine intoxication

  *Specify if:* With Perceptual Disturbances

292.0   Cocaine Withdrawal

292.81  Cocaine Intoxication Delirium

292.xx  Cocaine-Induced Psychotic Disorder

  .11   With Delusions[1]

  .12   With Hallucinations[1]

*Continued*

## Box 3-3    DSM-IV-TR Classification—cont'd

**Cocaine-induced disorders—cont'd**
292.84  Cocaine-Induced Mood Disorder[I,W]
292.89  Cocaine-Induced Anxiety Disorder[I,W]
292.89  Cocaine-Induced Sexual Dysfunction[I,W]
292.89  Cocaine-Induced Sleep Disorder[I,W]
292.9    Cocaine-Related Disorder NOS

*Hallucinogen-related disorders*
**Hallucinogen use disorders**
304.50  Hallucinogen Dependence[a]
305.30  Hallucinogen Abuse
**Hallucinogen-induced disorders**
292.89  Hallucinogen Intoxication
292.89  Hallucinogen Persisting Perception Disorder
         (Flashbacks)
292.81  Hallucinogen Intoxication Delirium
292.xx  Hallucinogen-Induced Psychotic Disorder
         Hallucinogen Intoxication Delirium
   .11      With Delusions[I]
   .12      With Hallucinations[I]
292.84  Hallucinogen-Induced Mood Disorders[I]
292.89  Hallucinogen-Induced Anxiety Disorder[I]
292.9    Hallucinogen-Related Disorder NOS

*Inhalant-related disorders*
**Inhalant use disorders**
304.60  Inhalant Dependence[a]
305.90  Inhalant Abuse
292.89  Inhalant Intoxication
292.81  Inhalant Intoxication Delirium
292.82  Inhalant-Induced Persisting Dementia
292.xx  Inhalant-Induced Psychotic Disorder
   .11      With Delusions[I]
   .12      With Hallucinations[I]
292.84  Inhalant-Induced Mood Disorder
292.89  Inhalant-Induced Anxiety Disorder
292.9    Inhalant-Related Disorder NOS

*From American Psychiatric Association:* Diagnostic and statistical manual of mental disorders, *ed 4, text revision (DSM-IV-TR), Washington, DC, 2000, The Association.*

## Box 3-3   DSM-IV-TR Classification—cont'd

*Nicotine-related disorders*
  **Nicotine use disorders**
  305.10  Nicotine Dependence[a]
  **Nicotine-induced disorders**
  292.0   Nicotine Withdrawal
  292.9   Nicotine-Related Disorder NOS
*Opioid-related disorders*
  **Opioid use disorders**
  304.00  Opioid Dependence[a]
  305.50  Opioid Abuse
  **Opioid-induced disorders**
  292.89  Opioid Intoxication
          *Specify if:* With Perceptual Disturbances
  292.0   Opioid Withdrawal
  292.81  Opioid-Intoxication Delirium
  292.xx  Opioid-Induced Psychotic Disorder
     .11     With Delusions[I]
     .12     With Hallucinations[I]
  292.84  Opioid-Induced Mood Disorder[I]
  292.89  Opioid-Induced Sexual Dysfunction[I,W]
  292.89  Opioid-Induced Sleep Disorder[I]
  292.9   Opioid-Related Disorder NOS
*Phencyclidine-related (or phencyclidine-like) disorders*
  **Phencyclidine use disorders**
  304.90  Phencyclidine Dependence[a]
  305.90  Phencyclidine Abuse
  **Phencyclidine-induced disorders**
  292.89  Phencyclidine Intoxication
          *Specify if:* With Perceptual Disturbances
  292.81  Phencyclidine Intoxication Delirium
  292.xx  Phencyclidine-Induced Psychotic Disorder
     .11     With Delusions[I]
     .12     With Hallucinations[I]
  292.84  Phencyclidine-Induced Mood Disorder[I]
  292.89  Phencyclidine-Induced Anxiety Disorder[I]
  292.9   Phencyclidine-Related Disorder NOS

*Continued*

## Box 3-3    DSM-IV-TR Classification—cont'd

*Sedative-, hypnotic-, or anxiolytic-related disorders*
  **Sedative, hypnotic, or anxiolytic use disorders**
  304.10  Sedative, Hypnotic, or Anxiolytic Dependence[a]
  305.40  Sedative, Hypnotic, or Anxiolytic Abuse
  **Sedative-, hypnotic-, or anxiolytic-induced disorders**
  292.89  Sedative, Hypnotic, or Anxiolytic Intoxication
  292.0   Sedative, Hypnotic, or Anxiolytic Withdrawal
          *Specify if:* With Perceptual Disturbances
  292.81  Sedative, Hypnotic, or Anxiolytic Intoxication
          Delirium
  292.81  Sedative, Hypnotic, or Anxiolytic Withdrawal
          Delirium
  292.82  Sedative-, Hypnotic-, or Anxiolytic-Induced
          Persisting Dementia
  292.83  Sedative-, Hypnotic-, or Anxiolytic-Induced
          Persisting Amnestic Disorder
  292.xx  Sedative-, Hypnotic-, or Anxiolytic-Induced
          Psychotic Disorder
      .11     With Delusions[I,W]
      .12     With Hallucinations[I,W]
  292.84  Sedative-, Hypnotic-, or Anxiolytic-Induced
          Mood Disorder[I,W]
  292.89  Sedative-, Hypnotic-, or Anxiolytic-Induced
          Anxiety Disorder[W]
  292.89  Sedative-, Hypnotic-, or Anxiolytic-Induced
          Sexual Dysfunction[I]
  292.89  Sedative-, Hypnotic-, or Anxiolytic-Induced
          Sleep Disorder[I,W]
  292.9   Sedative-, Hypnotic-, or Anxiolytic-Related
          Disorder NOS
*Polysubstance-related disorder*
  304.80  Polysubstance Dependence[a]
*Other (or unknown) substance-related disorders*
  **Other (or unknown) substance use disorders**
  304.90  Other (or Unknown) Substance Dependence[a]
  305.90  Other (or Unknown) Substance Abuse

*From American Psychiatric Association:* Diagnostic and statistical manual of mental disorders, *ed 4, text revision (DSM-IV-TR), Washington, DC, 2000, The Association.*

## Box 3-3   DSM-IV-TR Classification—cont'd

**Other (or unknown) substance-induced disorders**

292.89   Other (or Unknown) Substance Intoxication
*Specify if:* With Perceptual Disturbances

292.0    Other (or Unknown) Substance Withdrawal
*Specify if:* With Perceptual Disturbances

292.81   Other (or Unknown) Substance-Induced
Delirium

292.82   Other (or Unknown) Substance-Induced
Persisting Dementia

292.83   Other (or Unknown) Substance-Induced
Persisting Amnestic Disorder

292.xx   Other (or Unknown) Substance-Induced
Psychotic Disorder
   .11    With Delusions[I,W]
   .12    With Hallucinations[I,W]

292.84   Other (or Unknown) Substance-Induced Mood
Disorder[I,W]

292.89   Other (or Unknown) Substance-Induced
Anxiety Disorder[I,W]

292.89   Other (or Unknown) Substance-Induced
Anxiety Sexual Dysfunction[I]

292.89   Other (or Unknown) Substance-Induced Sleep
Disorder[I,W]

292.9    Other (or Unknown) Substance-Related
Disorder NOS

**Schizophrenia and other psychotic disorders**

295.xx   Schizophrenia

*The following Classification of Longitudinal Course
applies to all subtypes of Schizophrenia:*

Episodic With Interepisode Residual Symptoms (*specify
if:* With Prominent Negative Symptoms)/Episodic
With No Interepisode Residual Symptoms/
Continuous (*specify if:* With Prominent Negative
Symptoms)

Single Episode in Partial Remission (*specify if:* With
Prominent Negative Symptoms/Single Episode in
Full Remission)

*Continued*

## Box 3-3    DSM-IV-TR Classification—cont'd

**Schizophrenia and other psychotic disorders—cont'd**
   Other or Unspecified Pattern
       .30    Paranoid Type
       .10    Disorganized Type
       .20    Catatonic Type
       .90    Undifferentiated Type
       .60    Residual Type
   295.40 Schizophreniform Disorder
       *Specify if:* Without Good Prognostic Features/
       With Good Prognostic Features
   295.70 Schizoaffective Disorder
       *Specify type:* Bipolar Type/Depressive Type
   297.1  Delusional Disorder
       *Specify type:* Erotomanic Type/Grandiose Type/
       Jealous Type/Persecutory Type/Somatic Type/
       Mixed Type/Unspecified Type
   298.8  Brief Psychotic Disorder
       *Specify if:* With Marked Stressor(s)/Without
       Marked Stressor(s)/With Postpartum Onset
   297.3  Shared Psychotic Disorder
   293.xx Psychotic Disorder Due to . . . *[Indicate the*
       *General Medical Condition]*
       .81    With Delusions
       .82    With Hallucinations
   ___._   Substance-Induced Psychotic Disorder *(refer to*
       *Substance-Related Disorders for substance-*
       *specific codes)*
       *Specify if:* With Onset During Intoxication/With
       Onset During Withdrawal
   298.9  Psychotic Disorder NOS

**Mood disorders**
*Code current state of Major Depressive Disorder or*
*Bipolar I Disorder in fifth digit:*
   1 = Mild
   2 = Moderate
   3 = Severe, Without Psychotic Features

*From American Psychiatric Association:* Diagnostic and statistical manual of mental disorders, *ed 4, text revision (DSM-IV-TR), Washington, DC, 2000, The Association.*

## Box 3-3   DSM-IV-TR Classification—cont'd

**Mood disorders—cont'd**

    4 = Severe, With Psychotic Features
        *Specify:* Mood-Congruent Psychotic Features/Mood-
        Incongruent Psychotic Features
    5 = In Partial Remission
    6 = In Full Remission
    0 = Unspecified
*The following specifiers apply (for current or most recent episode) to Mood Disorders as noted:*
    [a]Severity/Psychotic/Remission Specifiers/[b]Chronic/
    [c]With Catatonic Features/[d]With Melancholic Features/
    [e]With Atypical Features/[f]With Postpartum Onset
*The following specifiers apply to Mood Disorders as noted:*
    [g]With or Without Full Interepisode Recovery/
    [h]With Seasonal Pattern/[i]With Rapid Cycling

*Depressive disorders*

    296.xx   Major Depressive Disorder
      .2x    Single Episode[a,b,c,d,e,f]
      .3x    Recurrent[a,b,c,d,e,f,g,h]
    300.4    Dysthymic Disorder
            *Specify if:* Early Onset/Late Onset
            *Specify:* With Atypical Features
    311       Depressive Disorder NOS

*Bipolar disorders*

    296.xx   Bipolar I Disorder.
      .0x    Single Manic Episode[a,c,f]
            *Specify if:* Mixed
      .40    Most Recent Episode Hypomanic[g,h,i]
      .4x    Most Recent Episode Manic[a,c,f,g,h,i]
      .6x    Most Recent Episode Mixed[a,c,f,g,h,i]
      .5x    Most Recent Episode
            Depressed[a,b,c,d,e,f,g,h,i]
      .7     Most Recent Episode Unspecified[g,h,i]
    296.89   Bipolar II Disorder[a,b,c,d,e,f,g,h,i]
            *Specify* (current or most recent episode):
            Hypomanic/Depressed

*Continued*

## Box 3-3    DSM-IV-TR Classification—cont'd

*Bipolar disorders—cont'd*
- 301.13  Cyclothymic Disorder
- 296.80  Bipolar Disorder NOS
- 293.83  Mood Disorder Due to . . . *[Indicate the General Medical Condition]*
  *Specify type:* With Depressive Features/With Major Depressive–Like Episode/With Manic Features/With Mixed Features
- \_\_\_.\_    Substance-Induced Mood Disorder *[refer to Substance-Related Disorders for substance-specific codes]*
  *Specify type:* With Depressive Features/With Manic Features/With Mixed Features
  *Specify if:* With Onset During Intoxication/With Onset During Withdrawal
- 296.90  Mood Disorder NOS

**Anxiety disorders**
- 300.01  Panic Disorder Without Agoraphobia
- 300.21  Panic Disorder With Agoraphobia
- 300.22  Agoraphobia Without History of Panic Disorder
- 300.29  Specific Phobia
  *Specify type:* Animal Type/Natural Environment Type/Blood-Injection-Injury Type/Situational Type/Other Type
- 300.23  Social Phobia
  *Specify if:* Generalized
- 300.3  Obsessive-Compulsive Disorder
  *Specify if:* With Poor Insight
- 309.81  Posttraumatic Stress Disorder
  *Specify if:* Acute/Chronic
  *Specify if:* With Delayed Onset
- 308.3  Acute Stress Disorder
- 300.02  Generalized Anxiety Disorder

*From American Psychiatric Association:* Diagnostic and statistical manual of mental disorders, *ed 4, text revision (DSM-IV-TR), Washington, DC, 2000, The Association.*

## Box 3-3   DSM-IV-TR Classification—cont'd

**Anxiety disorders—cont'd**

293.89  Anxiety Disorder Due to . . . *[Indicate the General Medical Condition]*
*Specify if:* With Generalized Anxiety/With Panic Attacks/With Obsessive-Compulsive Symptoms

___.__  Substance-Induced Anxiety Disorder *(refer to Substance-Related Disorders for substance-specific codes)*
*Specify if:* With Generalized Anxiety/With Panic Attacks/With Obsessive-Compulsive Symptoms/With Phobic Symptoms
*Specify if:* With Onset During Intoxication/With Onset During Withdrawal

300.00  Anxiety Disorder NOS

**Somatoform disorders**

300.81  Somatization Disorder

300.81  Undifferentiated Somatoform Disorder

300.11  Conversion Disorder
*Specify if:* With Motor Symptom or Deficit/With Sensory Symptom or Deficit/With Seizures or Convulsions/With Mixed Presentation

307.xx  Pain Disorder
 .80  Associated With Psychological Factors
 .89  Associated With Both Psychological Factors and a General Medical Condition
*Specify if:* Acute/Chronic

300.7  Hypochondriasis
*Specify if:* With Poor Insight

300.7  Body Dysmorphic Disorder

300.89  Somatoform Disorder NOS

**Factitious disorders**

300.xx  Factitious Disorder
 .16  With Predominantly Psychological Signs and Symptoms
 .19  With Predominantly Physical Signs and Symptoms

*Continued*

## Box 3-3   DSM-IV-TR Classification—cont'd

**Factitious disorders—cont'd**
    .19    With Combined Psychological and Physical
           Signs and Symptoms
  300.19  Factitious Disorder NOS

**Dissociative disorders**
  300.12  Dissociative Amnesia
  300.13  Dissociative Fugue
  300.14  Dissociative Identity Disorder
  300.6   Depersonalization Disorder
  300.15  Dissociative Disorder NOS

**Sexual and gender identity disorders**
*Sexual dysfunctions*
*The following specifiers apply to all primary Sexual*
*Dysfunctions:*
  Lifelong Type/Acquired Type/Generalized Type/
  Situational Type Due to Psychological Factors/Due to
  Combined Factors

**Sexual desire disorders**
  302.71  Hypoactive Sexual Desire Disorder
  302.79  Sexual Aversion Disorder

**Sexual arousal disorders**
  302.72  Female Sexual Arousal Disorder
  302.72  Male Erectile Disorder

**Orgasm disorders**
  302.73  Female Orgasmic Disorder
  302.74  Male Orgasmic Disorder
  302.75  Premature Ejaculation

**Sexual pain disorders**
  302.76  Dyspareunia (Not Due to a General Medical
          Condition)
  306.51  Vaginismus (Not Due to a General Medical
          Condition)

**Sexual dysfunctions due to a general medical condition**
  625.8   Female Hypoactive Sexual Desire Disorder
         Due to . . . *[Indicate the General Medical*
         *Condition]*

*From American Psychiatric Association:* Diagnostic and statistical manual of mental disorders, *ed 4, text revision (DSM-IV-TR), Washington, DC, 2000, The Association.*

## Box 3-3   DSM-IV-TR Classification—cont'd

*Sexual dysfunctions—cont'd*

609.89  Male Hypoactive Sexual Desire Disorder Due
to . . . *[Indicate the General Medical Condition]*

607.84  Male Erectile Disorder Due to . . . *[Indicate the
General Medical Condition]*

625.0   Female Dyspareunia Due to . . . *[Indicate the
General Medical Condition]*

608.89  Male Dyspareunia Due to . . . *[Indicate the
General Medical Condition]*

625.8   Other Female Sexual Dysfunction Due to
. . . *[Indicate the General Medical Condition]*

608.89  Other Male Sexual Dysfunction Due to . . . *[In-
dicate the General Medical Condition]*

___.__   Substance-Induced Sexual Dysfunction *(refer to
Substance-Related Disorders for substance-
specific codes)*
*Specify if:* With Impaired Desired/With Im-
paired Arousal/With Impaired Orgasm/With
Sexual Pain
*Specify if:* With Onset During Intoxication

302.70  Sexual Disfunction NOS

*Paraphilias*

302.4   Exhibitionism

302.81  Fetishism

302.89  Frotteurism

302.2   Pedophilia
*Specify if:* Sexually Attracted to Males/Sexually
Attracted to Females/Sexually Attracted to Both
*Specify type:* Exclusive Type/Nonexclusive Type

302.83  Sexual Masochism

302.84  Sexual Sadism

302.3   Transvestic Fetishism
*Specify if:* With Gender Dysphoria

302.82  Voyeurism

302.9   Paraphilia NOS

*Continued*

## Box 3-3    DSM-IV-TR Classification—cont'd

*Gender identity disorders*

3022.xx Gender Identity Disorder
- .6      In Children
- .85     In Adolescents or Adults
  *Specify if:* Sexually Attracted to Males/Sexually Attracted to Females/Sexually Attracted to Both/Sexually Attracted to Neither
- 302.6   Gender Identity Disorder NOS
- 302.9   Sexual Disorder NOS

**Eating disorders**

- 307.1   Anorexia nervosa
  *Specify type:* Restricting Type: Binge-Eating/Purging Type
- 307.51  Bulimia Nervosa
  *Specify type:* Purging Type/Nonpurging Type
- 307.50  Eating Disorder NOS

**Sleep Disorders**

*Primary sleep disorders*

**Dyssomnias**
- 307.42  Primary Insomnia
- 307.44  Primary Hypersomnia
  *Specify if:* Recurrent
- 347     Narcolepsy
- 780.59  Breathing-Related Sleep Disorder
- 307.45  Circadian Rhythm Sleep Disorder
  *Specify type:* Delayed Sleep Phase Type/Jet Lag Type/Shift Work Type/Unspecified Type
- 307.47  Dyssomnias NOS

**Parasomnias**
- 307.47  Nightmare Disorder
- 307.46  Sleep Terror Disorder
- 307.46  Sleepwalking Disorder
- 307.47  Parasomnia NOS

*Sleep disorders related to another mental disorder*

- 307.42  Insomnia Related to . . . *[Indicate the Axis I or Axis II Disorder]*

*From American Psychiatric Association:* Diagnostic and statistical manual of mental disorders, *ed 4, text revision (DSM-IV-TR), Washington, DC, 2000, The Association.*

## Box 3-3   DSM-IV-TR Classification—cont'd

*Sleep disorders related to another mental disorder—cont'd*

   307.44   Hypersomnia Related to . . . *[Indicate the Axis I or Axis II Disorder]*

*Other sleep disorders*

   780.xx   Sleep Disorder Due to . . . *[Indicate the General Medical Condition]*
      .52   Insomnia Type
      .54   Hypersomnia Type
      .59   Parasomnia Type
      .59   Mixed Type
    \_\_\_.\_   Substance-Induced Sleep Disorder *(refer to Substance-Related Disorders for substance-specific codes)*
        *Specify type:* Insomnia Type/Hypersomnia Type/Parasomnia Type/Mixed Type
        *Specify if:* With Onset During Intoxication/With Onset During Withdrawal

**Impulse control disorders not elsewhere classified**

   312.34   Intermittent Explosive Disorder
   312.32   Kleptomania
   312.33   Pyromania
   312.31   Pathological Gambling
   312.39   Trichotillomania
   312.30   Impulse Control Disorder NOS

**Adjustment disorders**

   309.xx   Adjustment Disorder
      .0   With Depressed Mood
      .24   With Anxiety
      .28   With Mixed Anxiety and Depressed Mood
      .3   With Disturbance of Conduct
      .4   With Mixed Disturbance of Emotions and Conduct
      .9   Unspecified
        *Specify if:* Acute/Chronic

*Continued*

## Box 3-3    DSM-IV-TR Classification—cont'd

**Personality disorders**
*NOTE: These are coded on Axis II.*

|  |  |
|---|---|
| 301.0 | Paranoid Personality Disorder |
| 301.20 | Schizoid Personality Disorder |
| 301.22 | Schizotypal Personality Disorder |
| 301.7 | Antisocial Personality Disorder |
| 301.83 | Borderline Personality Disorder |
| 301.50 | Histrionic Personality Disorder |
| 301.81 | Narcissistic Personality Disorder |
| 301.82 | Avoidant Personality Disorder |
| 301.6 | Dependent Personality Disorder |
| 301.4 | Obsessive-Compulsive Personality Disorder |
| 301.9 | Personality Disorder NOS |

**Other conditions that may be a focus of clinical attention**
*Psychological factors affecting medical condition*

. . . *[Specified Psychological Factor]* . . . affecting *[Indicate the General Medical Condition] Choose name based on nature of factors:*
Mental Disorder Affecting Medical Condition
Psychological Symptoms Affecting Medical Condition
Personality Traits or Coping Style Affecting Medical Condition
Maladaptive Health Behaviors Affecting Medical Condition
Stress-Related Physiological Response Affecting Medical Condition
Other or Unspecified Psychological Factors Affecting Medical Condition

*Medication-induced movement disorders*

|  |  |
|---|---|
| 332.1 | Neuroleptic-Induced Parkinsonism |
| 333.92 | Neuroleptic Malignant Syndrome |
| 333.7 | Neuroleptic-Induced Acute Dystonia |
| 333.99 | Neuroleptic-Induced Acute Akathisia |
| 333.82 | Neuroleptic-Induced Tardive Dyskinesia |
| 333.1 | Medication-Induced Postural Tremor |
| 333.90 | Medication-Induced Movement Disorder NOS |

*From American Psychiatric Association:* Diagnostic and statistical manual of mental disorders, *ed 4, text revision (DSM-IV-TR), Washington, DC, 2000, The Association.*

## Box 3-3   DSM-IV-TR Classification—cont'd

*Other medication-induced disorders*

    995.2    Adverse Effects of Medication NOS

*Relational problems*

    V61.9    Relational Problem Related to a Mental Disorder or General Medical Condition

    V61.20  Parent-Child Relational Problem

    V61.1    Partner Relational Problem

    V61.8    Sibling Relational Problem

    V62.81  Relational Problem NOS

*Problems related to abuse or neglect*

    V61.21  Physical Abuse of Child *(code 995.5 if focus of attention is on victim)*

    V61.21  Sexual Abuse of Child *(code 995.5 if focus of attention is on victim)*

    V61.21  Neglect of Child *(code 995.5 if focus of attention is on victim)*

    V61.1    Physical Abuse of Adult *(code 995.81 if focus of attention is on victim)*

    V61.1    Sexual Abuse of Adult *(code 995.81 if focus of attention is on victim)*

*Additional conditions that may be a focus of clinical attention*

    V15.81  Noncompliance With Treatment

    V65.2    Malingering

    V71.01  Adult Antisocial Behavior

    V71.02  Childhood or Adolescent Antisocial Behavior

    V62.89  Borderline Intellectual Functioning
            Note: *This is coded on Axis II.*

    780.9    Age-Related Cognitive Decline

    V62.82  Bereavement

    V62.3    Academic Problem

    V62.2    Occupational Problem

    313.82  Identity Problem

    V62.89  Religious or Spiritual Problem

    V62.4    Acculturation Problem

    V62.89  Phase of Life Problem

*Continued*

### Box 3-3   DSM-IV-TR Classification—cont'd

**Additional codes**

| | |
|---|---|
| 300.9 | Unspecified Mental Disorder (nonpsychotic) |
| V71.09 | No Diagnosis or Condition on Axis I |
| 799.9 | Diagnosis or Condition Deferred on Axis I |
| V71.09 | No Diagnosis on Axis II |
| 799.9 | Diagnosis Deferred on Axis II |

Axis II Personality Disorders

| | |
|---|---|
| 301.0 | Paranoid Personality Disorder |
| 301.20 | Schizoid Personality Disorder |
| 301.22 | Schizotypal Personality Disorder |
| 301.7 | Antisocial Personality Disorder |
| 301.83 | Borderline Personality Disorder |
| 301.5 | Histrionic Personality Disorder |
| 301.81 | Narcissistic Personality Disorder |
| 301.82 | Avoidant Personality Disorder |
| 301.65 | Dependent Personality Disorder |
| 301.45 | Obsessive-Compulsive Personality Disorder |
| 301.9 | Personality Disorder NOS |

Axis III General Medical Conditions (with ICD-9-CM codes)

Infectious and Parasitic Diseases (001-139)

Neoplasms (140-239)

Endocrine, Nutritional, and Metabolic Diseases and Immunity Disorders (240-279)

Diseases of the Blood and Blood-Forming Organs (280-289)

Diseases of the Nervous System and Sense Organs (320-389)

Diseases of the Circulatory System (390-459)

Diseases of the Respiratory System (460-519)

Diseases of the Digestive System (520-579)

Diseases of the Genitourinary System (580-629)

Complications of Pregnancy, Childbirth, and the Puerperium (630-676)

Diseases of the Skin and Subcutaneous Tissue (680-709)

*From American Psychiatric Association:* Diagnostic and statistical manual of mental disorders, *ed 4, text revision (DSM-IV-TR), Washington, DC, 2000, The Association.*

## Box 3-3    DSM-IV-TR Classification—cont'd

Axis III General Medical Conditions (with ICD-9-CM codes) —cont'd

Diseases of the Musculoskeletal System and Connective Tissue (710-739)

Congenital Anomalies (740-759)

Certain Conditions Originating in the Perinatal Period (760-779)

Symptoms, Signs, and Ill-Defined Conditions (780-799)

Injury and Poisoning (800-999)

Axis IV Psychosocial and Environmental Problems

- **Problems with primary support group**—e.g., death of a family member; health problems in family; disruption of family by separation, divorce, or estrangement; removal from the home; remarriage of parent; sexual or physical abuse; parental overprotection; neglect of child; inadequate discipline; discord with siblings; birth of a sibling
- **Problems related to the social environment**—e.g., death or loss of friend; inadequate social support; living alone; difficulty with acculturation; discrimination; adjustment to life cycle transition (e.g., retirement)
- **Educational problems**—e.g., illiteracy; academic problems; discord with teachers or classmates; inadequate school environment
- **Occupational problems**—e.g., unemployment; threat of job loss; stressful work schedule; difficult work conditions; job dissatisfaction; job change; discord with boss or co-workers
- **Housing problems**—e.g., homelessness; inadequate housing; unsafe neighborhood; discord with neighbors or landlord
- **Economic problems**—e.g., extreme poverty; inadequate finances; insufficient welfare support
- **Problems with access to health care services**—e.g., inadequate health care services; transportation to health care facilities unavailable; inadequate health insurance

*Continued*

## Box 3-3    DSM-IV-TR Classification—cont'd

Axis IV Psychosocial and Environmental Problems—cont'd

- **Problems related to interaction with the legal system crime**—e.g., arrest; incarceration; litigation; victim of crime

Axis V Global Assessment of Functioning (GAF) Scale*

Consider psychological, social, and occupational functioning on a hypothetical continuum of mental health-illness. Do not include impairment in functioning due to physical (or environmental) limitations.

Code (NOTE: Use intermediate codes when appropriate, e.g., 45, 68, 72.)

| | |
|---|---|
| 100 | Superior functioning in a wide range of activities, life's problems never seem to get out of hand, is sought out by others because of many positive |
| 91 | qualities. No symptoms. |
| 90 | Absent or minimal symptoms (e.g., mild anxiety before an exam), good functioning in all areas, interested and involved in a wide range of activities, socially effective, generally satisfied with life, no more than everyday problems or concerns (e.g., |
| 81 | an occasional argument with family members). |

*From American Psychiatric Association:* Diagnostic and statistical manual of mental disorders, *ed 4, text revision (DSM-IV-TR), Washington, DC, 2000, The Association.*

*The rating of overall psychological functioning on a scale of 0-100 was operationalized by Luborsky in the Health-Sickness Rating Scale (Luborsky L: Clinicians' judgments of mental health, *Arch Gen Psychiatry* 7:407-417, 1962). Spitzer and colleagues developed a revision of the Health-Sickness Rating Scale called the Global Assessment Scale (GAS) (Endicott J, Spitzer RL, Fleiss JL, Cohen J: The global assessment scale, a procedure for measuring overall severity of psychiatric disturbance, *Arch Gen Psychiatry* 33:766-771, 1976). A modified version of the GAS was included in DSM-III-R as the Global Assessment of Functioning (GAF) Scale.

**Box 3-3**    DSM-IV-TR Classification—cont'd

Code

| | |
|---|---|
| 80 | If symptoms are present, they are transient and expectable reactions to psychosocial stressors (e.g., difficulty concentrating after family argument); no more than slight impairment in social, occupational, or school functioning (e.g., temporarily |
| 71 | falling behind in schoolwork). |
| 70 | Some mild symptoms (e.g., depressed mood and mild insomnia) OR some difficulty in social, occupational, or school functioning (e.g., occasional truancy, theft within the household), but generally functioning pretty well, has some meaningful inter- |
| 61 | personal relationships. |
| 60 | Moderate symptoms (e.g., flat affect and circumstantial speech, occasional panic attacks) OR moderate difficulty in social, occupational, or school functioning (e.g., few friends, conflicts with peers |
| 51 | or co-workers). |
| 50 | Serious symptoms (e.g., suicidal ideation, severe obsessional rituals, frequent shoplifting) OR any serious impairment in social, occupational, or school functioning (e.g., no friends, unable to keep |
| 41 | a job). |
| 40 | Some impairment in reality testing or communication (e.g., speech is at times illogical, obscure, or irrelevant) OR major impairment in several areas, such as work or school, family relations, judgment, thinking, or mood (e.g., depressed man avoids friends, neglects family, and is unable to work; child frequently beats up younger children, is |
| 31 | defiant at home, and is failing at school). |
| 30 | Behavior is considerably influenced by delusions or hallucinations OR serious impairment in communication or judgment (e.g., sometimes incoherent, acts grossly inappropriately, suicidal preoccupation) OR inability to function in almost all areas |
| 21 | (e.g., stays in bed all day; no job, home, or friends) |

---

### Box 3-3    DSM-IV-TR Classification—cont'd

Code

| | |
|---|---|
| 20 | Some danger of hurting self or others (e.g., suicide attempts without clear expectation of death, frequently violent, manic excitement) OR occasionally fails to maintain minimal personal hygiene (e.g., smears feces) OR gross impairment in communication (e.g., largely incoherent or mute). |
| 11 | |
| 10 | Persistent danger of severely hurting self or others (e.g., recurrent violence) OR persistent inability to maintain minimal personal hygiene OR serious suicidal act with clear expectation of death. |
| 1 | |
| 0 | Inadequate information. |

---

*From American Psychiatric Association:* Diagnostic and statistical manual of mental disorders, *ed 4, text revision (DSM-IV-TR), Washington, DC, 2000, The Association.*

*your* **INTERNET**
c o n n e c t i o n

**Center for Mental Health Services:**
www.mentalhealth.org/cmhs

**Internet Mental Health:**
mentalhealth.com

**Mental Health Infosource:**
mhsource.com

**Mental Health Net:**
www.mentalhelp.net

**Psych Central:**
psychcentral.com

**US Department of Health and Human Services:**
www.hhs.gov

**Virtual Office of the Surgeon General:**
www.surgeongeneral.gov/sgoffice.htm

# Reference

1. US Department of Health and Human Services: *Mental health: a report of the surgeon general,* Rockville, Md, 1999, National Institute of Mental Health.

## Suggested readings

Chodoff P: The changing role of dynamic psychotherapy in psychiatric practice, *Psychiatric Services* 51:1404-1407, 2000.

Dyer J, McGuinness T: Resilience: analysis of concept, *Arch Psychiatr Nurs* 10:276, 1996.

Harris E, Barraclough B: Excess mortality of mental disorder, *Br J Psychiatry,* 173:11, 1998.

Jorm A: Public knowledge and beliefs about mental disorders, *British J of Psychiatry* 177:396-401, 2000.

Kendler K: Social support: a genetic-epidemiologic analysis, *Am J Psychiatry* 154:1398, 1997.

Kessler R et al: Lifetime and 12-month prevalence of DSM-R psychiatric disorders in the United States, *Arch Gen Psychiatry* 51:8, 1994.

Monat A, Lazarus R: *Stress and coping,* New York, 1991, Columbia University Press.

Murray C, Lopez A: *The global burden of disease: a comprehensive assessment of mortality and disability from disease, injuries, and risk factors in 1990 and projected to 2020,* Cambridge, Mass, 1996, Harvard University Press.

Neugebauer R: Mind matters: the importance of mental disorders in public health's 21st century mission, *Am J Public Health* 89:1309, 1999.

Stuart G, Laraia M: *Principles and practice of psychiatric nursing,* ed 7, St Louis, 2001, Mosby.

Tucker G: Putting DSM-IV in perspective, *Am J Psychiatry* 155:159, 1998.

Ustun T: The global burden of mental disorders, *Am J Public Health* 89:1315, 1999.

# Biopsychosocial Context of Psychiatric Nursing Care

4

The practice of contemporary psychiatric nursing requires that the nurse use a model of care that integrates the biological, psychological, and sociocultural aspects of the individual in assessing, planning, and implementing nursing interventions.

## Biological Context of Care

New tools and techniques help to explain how the brain works and how the brain, mind, and body interact. The psychiatric nurse must have a working knowledge of the normal structure and function of the brain, particularly mental functions, just as the cardiac care nurse must know how the heart works. Psychiatric nurses can then interpret expanding biological information and its potential for effective treatments to consumers of mental health services and to other health care providers, thus further reinforcing nurses' role as patient advocates.

## Neuroimaging Techniques

Brain imaging techniques allow for direct viewing of the structure and function of the intact, living brain. These techniques not only help in diagnosing some brain disorders but also map the regions of the brain and correlate them with function. They provide pictures of the working brain. Table 4-1 describes some of these important imaging techniques.

Table 4-1  Brain imaging techniques

| Technique | How it Works | What it Images |
|---|---|---|
| Computed tomography (CT) | Series of radiographs that are computer-constructed into "slices" of the brain that can be stacked by the computer, giving a three-dimensional view. | Brain structure |
| Magnetic resonance imaging (MRI) | Magnetic field surrounding the head induces brain tissues to emit radio waves that are computerized for clear, detailed construction of sectional images of the brain. | Brain structure; newer functional MRI (FMRI) techniques show brain activity |
| Brain electrical activity mapping (BEAM) | CT techniques are used to display data derived from electroencephalographic (EEG) recordings of brain electrical activity that can be sensory-evoked by specific stimuli (e.g., flash of light, sudden sound) or cognitive-evoked by specific mental tasks. | Brain activity/function |
| Positron emission tomography (PET) | Injected radioactive substance travels to the brain and shows up as a bright spot on the scan; different substances are taken up by the brain in different amounts, depending on type of tissue and level of activity. | Brain activity/function |
| Single-photon emission computed tomography (SPECT) | Similar to PET, but SPECT uses more stable substances and different detectors to visualize blood flow patterns. | Brain activity/function |

## Genetics of Mental Illness

The ongoing search for the gene or genes that cause mental illness has been difficult and inconclusive to date. The complexity of human emotions and behavior is most likely governed by a variety of genes and their interplay with each other, environmental factors, personality, and life experiences.

There are several proposed uses of genetics in psychiatry. These include the following:

- *New drugs* will target molecular regulators of gene expression that control neuroproteins and neuroenzymes in brain regions shown to be abnormal in a particular psychiatric illness.

- *Gene therapy,* the introduction of genes into existing cells to prevent or cure disease, may one day be commonplace for the treatment of psychiatric illness. Studies using "candidate genes" (cloned human genes that are functionally related to the disease of interest) are used in research procedures in the laboratory and are becoming more available for psychiatric research.

## Circadian Rhythms

Recent biological research has suggested that body rhythms are governed by internal circadian pacemakers located in specific areas of the brain and that they are subject to change by specific external cues. Circadian rhythm is like a network of internal clocks that time and coordinate events within the body according to an approximate 24-hour cycle. These rhythms affect every aspect of health and well-being, including lifestyle, sleep, moods, eating, drinking, fertility, and illness. Recent research suggests that one of the most important internal timekeepers is located in the hypothalamus of the brain.

## Psychoneuroimmunology

Psychoneuroimmunology is a field that explores the interactions among the central nervous system, the endocrine system, and the immune system; the impact of behavior/stress on these interactions; and how psychological and pharmacological interventions may modulate these interactions. Although the evidence is compelling that psychosocial stressors can temporarily impair the immune response and thus contribute to the development of a variety of illnesses, the role for autoimmunity in the major psychiatric illnesses is unclear. Efforts to relate specific stressors to specific diseases have not generally been successful, but stress is recognized as a potential key to understanding the development and course of many illnesses.

## Biological Assessment of the Psychiatric Patient

Psychiatric nurses should include a thorough biological assessment in their evaluation of psychiatric patients. Undiagnosed physical illness can be costly and dangerous if undetected or treated incorrectly. The psychiatric nurse is well suited to screen for the major signs of physical or organic disorders that may complicate a patient's psychiatric status, to identify physical illnesses that may have been overlooked, or to refer a patient for a thorough medical diagnostic workup if indicated.

A complete health care history of the patient, lifestyle review, physical examination, analysis of laboratory values, and discussion of presenting symptoms and coping responses are essential elements of a baseline assessment (Box 4-1). The nurse should be able to perform a basic physical examination to assess for gross abnormalities and be able to interpret the results of existing, more complex examinations. Appearance, gait, coordination, bilateral strength, tremors and tics, speech, and symptoms such as headaches, blurred vision, dizziness, vomiting, motor weakness, disorientation, confusion, and memory problems should be assessed in detail.

Only after a patient has been carefully screened can the nurse determine which of the patient's presenting problems are amenable to psychiatric intervention and which may require a consultant in another specialty.

## Psychological Context of Care

All nurses, regardless of clinical setting, should be proficient in assessing a patient's psychological status and should incorporate the findings into the patient's plan of care. The mental status examination is a cornerstone in the evaluation of any patient with a medical, neurological, or psychiatric disorder that affects thoughts, emotions, or behavior. It is used to detect changes or abnormalities in a person's intellectual functioning, thought content, judgment, mood, and affect and can be used to suggest possible brain lesions. In this way the mental status examination

## Box 4-1    Biological Assessment of the Psychiatric Patient

Health Care History

**General health care**

Regular and specialty health care providers

Frequency of health care visits

Date of last examination

Any unusual circumstances of birth, including mother's preterm habits and condition

Allergies

Immunizations

Papanicolaou smear and mammogram

Chest x-ray exam and electrocardiogram (ECG)

Tuberculosis (TB) test

**Hospitalizations, surgeries and medical procedures**

When; why indicated; treatments; outcome

**Brain impairment**

Diagnosed brain problem

Head trauma

Details of accidents or periods of unconsciousness for any reason: blows to head, electrical shocks, high fevers, seizures, fainting, dizziness, headaches, falls

**Cancer**

Full history, particularly metastases (lung, breast, melanoma, gastrointestinal tract, and kidney are most likely to metastasize)

Results of treatment (chemotherapy, surgeries)

**Lung problems**

Details of any condition or event that restricts airflow to lungs for more than 2 minutes or adversely affects oxygen absorption (brain uses 20% of body's oxygen), such as with chronic obstructive pulmonary disease, near drowning, near strangulation, high-altitude oxygen deprivation, resuscitation events

**Cardiac problems**

Childhood illnesses such as scarlet or rheumatic fever

History of heart attacks, strokes, or hypertension

Arteriosclerotic conditions

**Box 4-1    Biological Assessment of the Psychiatric Patient—cont'd**

Health Care History—cont'd

**Diabetes**
  Stability of glucose levels
**Endocrine disturbances**
  Thyroid and adrenal function
**Menstrual history**
  Age of first menstrual period
  Regularity of menstrual periods, impact on lifestyle
  Date of last menstrual period, duration
**Menopausal history**
  Assess for premenstrual syndromes
**Sexual history**
  Sexual function and activity
  Screen for sexual dysfunction
  Safe-sex practices and sexually transmitted diseases
**Reproductive history**
  Number of pregnancies, births, children and their ages
  Birth control methods

Lifestyle

**Eating**
  Details of unusual or unsupervised diets, appetite,
    weight changes, cravings, and caffeine intake
**Medications**
  Full history of current and past psychiatric medications
    given to patient and first-degree relatives
  Full history of current use of nonpsychiatric prescrip-
    tion medicines, over-the-counter medicines, and
    herbal and other alternative remedies
**Substance use**
  Alcohol, drug, caffeine, and tobacco use
**Toxins**
  Overcome by automobile exhaust or natural gas
  Exposure to lead, mercury, insecticides, herbicides,
    solvents, cleaning agents, lawn chemicals
  Fetal alcohol syndrome

*Continued*

## Box 4-1    Biological Assessment of the Psychiatric Patient—cont'd

Lifestyle—cont'd

**Occupation (current and past)**
Chemicals in workplace (e.g., farming, painting)
Work-related accidents (e.g., construction, mining)
Military experiences
Stressful job circumstances

**Injury**
Contact sports and sports-related injuries
Exposure to violence or abuse
Rape or molestation

**Impact of culture, race, ethnicity, and gender**

Physical Examination

**Review of physiological systems**
Integumentary: skin, nails, hair, scalp
Head: eyes, ears, nose, mouth, throat, neck
Breasts
Respiratory
Cardiovascular
Hematolymphatic
Gastrointestinal tract
Urinary tract
Genital
Neurological, soft signs, and cranial nerves
Musculoskeletal
Nutritive
Restorative: sleep and rest
Endocrine
Allergic and immunological
Gait, coordination, and balance

Laboratory Values

Hematology: complete blood count (CBC) and sedimentation rate, screen for anemia
Chemistry, blood urea nitrogen (BUN), glucose, thyroid, adrenal, liver and kidney function

## Box 4-1  Biological Assessment of the Psychiatric Patient—cont'd

Laboratory Values—cont'd

Serology, especially syphilis screen, human immunodeficiency virus (HIV), hepatitis
Urinalysis, screen for drugs
Stool tests for occult blood

Presenting Symptoms and Coping Responses

Description: nature, frequency, intensity
Threats to safety of self or others
Functional status
Quality of life
Support system

is to psychiatric nursing what the physical examination is to general medical nursing.

## Interviewing Skills

The goal-directed patient interview can be facilitated in the following ways:

1. Address the patient by name and introduce yourself and state the purpose of the interview.
2. Demonstrate awareness of and respect for the patient and a sensitivity to the patient's feelings by assuming a warm, empathic approach.
3. Select an environment that provides privacy, physical comfort, and minimal distractions.
4. Listen to what the patient is saying and note underlying themes and omissions.
5. Observe verbal content and nonverbal communication.
6. Allow sufficient time for the interview, and avoid a tense, hurried approach.
7. Monitor your feelings and anxieties in the patient interview.
8. Use secondary sources of information (e.g., medical history, psychological evaluation, social history) as a supplement to, not a substitute for, your clinical impressions and evaluation.

## Mental Status Examination

The mental status exam represents a cross section of the patient's psychological life and the sum of the nurse's observations and impressions at that moment. It is not an evaluation of how that patient was in the past or will be in the future. The examination is an evaluation of the patient's current state. The elements of the examination depend on the patient's clinical presentation and the patient's educational and cultural background. It includes observing the patient's behavior and describing it in an objective, nonjudgmental manner. The mental status examination includes information pertaining to the categories listed in Box 4-2.

---

### Box 4-2    Categories of the Mental Status Examination

General Description

Appearance
Speech
Motor activity
Interaction during interview

Emotional State

Mood
Affect

Experiences

Perceptions

Thinking

Thought content
Thought process

Sensorium and Cognition

Level of consciousness
Memory
Level of concentration and calculation
Information and intelligence
Judgment
Insight

---

## Appearance

In the mental status examination the nurse notes the patient's general appearance.

### *Observations*

The following physical characteristics of the patient should be included:

- Apparent age
- Manner of dress
- Cleanliness
- Posture
- Unusual gait
- Facial expressions
- Eye contact
- Pupil dilation or constriction
- General state of health and nutrition

**NURSE ALERT.**   Dilated pupils are sometimes associated with drug intoxication, whereas pupil constriction may indicate narcotic addiction. Stooped posture is often seen in depressed individuals. Manic patients may dress in colorful or unusual attire.

## Speech

Speech is usually described in terms of rate, volume, and characteristics. *Rate* refers to the speed of the patient's speech, and *volume* refers to how loudly a patient talks.

### *Observations*

Speech can be described as follows:

- Rate—rapid or slow
- Volume—loud or soft
- Amount—minimal (paucity), mute, or pressured
- Characteristics—stuttering, slurring of words, or unusual accents

**NURSE ALERT.** Speech disturbances are often caused by specific brain disturbances. For example, mumbling may occur in patients with Huntington's chorea, and slurring of speech is common in intoxicated patients. Manic patients often show pressured speech, and depressed patients often have paucity of speech.

## Motor activity

*Motor activity* refers to the patient's physical movement.

### Observations

The nurse should record the following:

- Level of activity—lethargic, tense, restless, or agitated
- Type of activity—tics, grimaces, or tremors
- Unusual gestures or mannerisms—compulsions

**NURSE ALERT.** Excessive body movement may be associated with anxiety, mania, or stimulant abuse. Minimal body activity may suggest depression, organicity, catatonic schizophrenia, or drug-induced stupor. Tics and grimaces may suggest adverse effects to medications. Repeated motor movements or compulsions may indicate obsessive-compulsive disorder. Repeated picking of lint or dirt off clothing is sometimes associated with delirium or toxic conditions.

## Interaction during the interview

*Interaction* describes how the patient relates to the nurse during the interview.

### Observations

Has the patient been hostile, uncooperative, irritable, guarded, apathetic, defensive, suspicious, or seductive? The nurse may explore this area by asking, "You seem irritated about something; is that an accurate observation?"

> **NURSE ALERT.**    Suspiciousness may be evident in the paranoid or substance-abusing patient. Irritability may suggest an anxiety disorder. Apathy may be associated with depression and seductive behavior with bipolar illness.

## Mood

*Mood* is the patient's self-report of the prevailing emotional state and reflects the patient's life situation.

### Observations

Mood can be evaluated by asking a simple, nonleading question such as, "How are you feeling today?" Does the patient report feeling sad, fearful, hopeless, euphoric, or anxious? Asking the patient to rate mood on a scale of 0 to 10 can help provide the nurse with an immediate reading of the patient's mood.

If the potential for suicide is suspected, it is essential that the nurse inquire directly regarding the patient's thoughts about self-destruction. Suicidal and homicidal thoughts must be addressed directly. To judge a patient's suicidal or homicidal risk, the nurse should assess the patient's plans, ability to carry out those plans (e.g., availability of guns), attitude about death, and available support systems.

> **NURSE ALERT.**    Most people with depression describe feeling hopeless, and 25% of those with depression have suicidal ideation. Suicidal ideation is also common in patients with anxiety disorders and schizophrenia. Elation is most common in those with mania.

## Affect

*Affect* is the patient's prevailing emotional tone as observed by the nurse during the interview.

*Observations*

Affect can be described in terms of the following:

- Range
- Duration
- Intensity
- Appropriateness

Does the patient report significant life events without any emotional response, indicating flat affect? Does the patient's response appear restricted or blunted in some way? Does the patient demonstrate great lability in expression by quickly shifting from one affect to another? Is the patient's response incongruent with speech content? For example, does the patient report being persecuted by the police and then laugh?

> **NURSE ALERT.** Labile affect is often seen in manic patients, and a flat, incongruent affect is often evident in schizophrenic patients.

## Perceptions

The two major types of perceptual problems are hallucinations and illusions. *Hallucinations* are defined as false sensory impressions or experiences. *Illusions* are false perceptions or false responses to a sensory stimulus.

*Observations*

Hallucinations may occur in any of the five major sensory modalities, as follows:

- Auditory (sound)
- Visual (sight)
- Tactile (touch)
- Gustatory (taste)
- Olfactory (smell)

Command hallucinations are those that tell the person to do something, such as kill him or herself, harm another, or join someone in the afterlife. The nurse might inquire about the patient's perceptions by asking, "Do you ever see or hear things?" or "Do you have strange experiences as you fall asleep or on awakening?"

**NURSE ALERT.**   Auditory hallucinations are the most common and suggest schizophrenia. Visual hallucinations suggest organicity. Tactile hallucinations suggest organic mental disorder, cocaine abuse, or delirium tremens.

## Thought content

*Thought content* refers to the specific meaning expressed in the patient's communication—the "what" of the patient's thinking.

### Observations

Although the patient may talk about a variety of subjects during the interview, the nurse should note several content areas in the mental status examination (Box 4-3). They may be complicated and are often concealed by the patient.

**NURSE ALERT.**   Obsessions and phobias are symptoms associated with anxiety disorders. Delusions, depersonalization, and ideas of reference suggest schizophrenia and other psychotic disorders.

## Thought process

*Thought process* refers to the "how" of the patient's self-expression. A patient's thought process is observed through speech. The patterns or forms of verbalization, rather than the content, are assessed.

### Observations

A number of problems can be assessed that involve a patient's thinking (Box 4-4). The nurse can ask various questions to evaluate the patient's thought process. Does the patient's thinking proceed in a systematic, organized, and logical manner? Is the patient's self-expression clear? Is it relatively easy for the patient to move from one topic to another?

## Box 4-3    Thought Content Descriptors

**Delusion**—false belief that is firmly maintained even though it is not shared by others and is contradicted by social reality

    **Religious delusion**—belief that one is favored by a higher being or is an instrument of that being

    **Somatic delusion**—belief that one's body or parts of one's body are diseased or distorted

    **Grandiose delusion**—belief that one possesses greatness or special powers

    **Paranoid delusion**—excessive or irrational suspiciousness and distrustfulness of others, characterized by systematized delusions that others are "out to get them" or are spying on them

    **Thought broadcasting**—delusion about thoughts being aired to the outside world

    **Thought insertion**—delusion that thoughts are placed into the mind by outside people or influences

**Depersonalization**—feeling of having lost self-identity and that things around the person are different, strange, or unreal

**Hypochondriasis**—somatic overconcern with and morbid attention to details of body functioning

**Ideas of reference**—incorrect interpretation of casual incidents and external events as having direct personal references

**Magical thinking**—belief that thinking equates with doing; characterized by lack of realistic relationship between cause and effect

**Nihilistic ideas**—thoughts of nonexistence and hopelessness

**Obsession**—idea, emotion, or impulse that repetitively and insistently forces itself into consciousness, although it is unwelcome

**Phobia**—morbid fear associated with extreme anxiety

## Box 4-4  Thought Process Descriptors

**Circumstantial**—thought and speech associated with excessive and unnecessary detail that is usually relevant to a question; an answer is ultimately given

**Flight of ideas**—overproductive speech characterized by rapid shifting from one topic to another and fragmented ideas

**Loose associations**—lack of a logical relationship between thoughts and ideas that renders speech and thought inexact, vague, diffuse, and unfocused

**Neologisms**—new word or words created by patient, often a blend of other words

**Perseveration**—involuntary, excessive continuation or repetition of a single response, idea, or activity; may apply to speech or movement, but most often verbal

**Tangential**—similar to circumstantial, but patient never returns to central point and never answers original question

**Thought blocking**—sudden stopping in the train of thought or in midst of a sentence

**Word salad**—series of words that seem completely unrelated

---

**NURSE ALERT.**   Circumstantial thinking may be a sign of defensiveness or paranoid thinking. Loose associations and neologisms suggest schizophrenia or other psychotic disorders. Flight of ideas indicates mania. Perseveration is often associated with brain damage and psychotic disorders. Word salad represents the highest level of thought disorganization (see Box 4-4.)

### Level of consciousness

Mental status examinations routinely assess a patient's orientation to the current situation.

*Observations*

A variety of terms can be used to describe a patient's level of consciousness, such as confused, sedated, or stuporous. In addition, the patient should be questioned regarding orientation to time, place, and person. The nurse usually can determine this by the patient's answers to the following three simple questions:

1. Person—What is your name?
2. Place—Where are you today (e.g., what city, what particular building)?
3. Time—What is today's date?

If the patient answers correctly, the nurse can note "oriented times three." Level of orientation can also be pursued in greater depth, but this area may be confounded by sociocultural factors.

---

**NURSE ALERT.**    Patients with organic mental disorder may give grossly inaccurate answers, with orientation to person remaining intact longer than orientation to time or place. Patients with schizophrenic disorders may say they are someone else or somewhere else or reveal a personalized orientation to the world.

---

## Memory

A mental status examination can provide a quick screen of potential memory problems but not a definitive answer to whether a specific impairment exists. Neuropsychological assessment is required to specify the nature and extent of memory impairment. Memory is broadly defined as the ability to recall past experiences.

*Observations*

The following areas must be tested:

- *Remote memory*—recall of events, information, and people from the distant past
- *Recent memory*—recall of events, information, and people from the past week or so
- *Immediate memory*—recall of information or data to which a person was just exposed

Recall of remote events involves reviewing information from the patient's history. This part of the evaluation can be woven into the history-taking portion of the nursing assessment. This involves asking the patient questions about time and place of birth, names of schools attended, date of marriage, ages of family members, and so forth. The problem with an evaluation of the patient's remote memory is that the nurse is often unable to tell if the patient is reporting events accurately. Thus the nurse may need to check past records or have family or friends confirm this historical information.

Recent memory can be tested by asking the patient to recall the events of the past 24 hours. A reliable informant may be needed to verify this information. Another test of recent memory is to ask the patient to remember three words (e.g., object, color, address) and then repeat them 15 minutes later in the interview.

Immediate recall can be tested by asking the patient to repeat a series of numbers either forward or backward within 10 seconds. The nurse should begin with a short series of numbers and proceed to longer lists.

**NURSE ALERT.** Loss of memory occurs with organicity, dissociative disorder, and conversion disorder. Patients with Alzheimer's dementia retain remote memory longer than recent memory. Anxiety and depression can impair immediate retention and recent memory.

### Level of concentration and calculation

*Concentration* is the patient's ability to pay attention during the course of the interview. *Calculation* is the person's ability to do simple math.

#### Observations

The nurse should note the patient's level of distractibility. Calculation can be assessed by asking the patient to do the following:
1. Count from 1 to 20 rapidly
2. Do simple calculations, such as $2 \times 3$ or $21 + 7$
3. Serially subtract 7 from 100

If patients have difficulty subtracting 7 from 100, they can be asked to subtract 3 from 20 in the same way. Finally, more functional calculation skills can be assessed by asking practical questions such as, "How many nickels are there in $1.35?"

**NURSE ALERT.**    Many psychiatric illnesses impair the ability to concentrate and complete simple calculations. It is particularly important to differentiate among organic mental disorder, anxiety, and depression.

### Information and intelligence

Information and intelligence are controversial areas of assessment, and the nurse should be cautious about judging intelligence after the brief and limited contact typical of the mental status examination. The nurse should also remember that information in this category is highly influenced by sociocultural factors of the nurse, the patient, and the treatment setting.

#### Observations

The nurse should assess the last grade of school completed, the patient's general fund of knowledge, and the patient's use of vocabulary. It is also critical that the nurse assess the patient's level of literacy. The ability to conceptualize and abstract can be tested by having the patient explain a series of proverbs. The patient can be given an example of a proverb with its interpretation and then asked to explain what several proverbs mean. Frequently used proverbs include the following:

- When it rains, it pours.
- A stitch in time saves nine.
- A rolling stone gathers no moss.
- The proof of the pudding is in the eating.
- People who live in glass houses shouldn't throw stones.
- A bird in the hand is worth two in the bush.

If the patient's educational level is below the eighth grade, asking the patient to list similarities between a series of paired objects may better help the nurse assess the ability to abstract. The following paired objects are frequently used:

- Bicycle and bus
- Apple and pear
- Television and newspaper

A higher-level reply addresses function, whereas a description of structure indicates more concrete thinking. To determine a patient's fund of general knowledge, the nurse can ask the patient to name the last five presidents, the mayor, five large cities, or the occupation of a well-known person.

> **NURSE ALERT.** The patient's educational level and any learning disabilities should be carefully evaluated. Mental retardation should be ruled out whenever possible.

## Judgment

*Judgment* involves making decisions that are constructive and adaptive. It involves the ability to understand facts and draw conclusions from relationships.

### Observations

Judgment can be evaluated by exploring the patient's involvement in activities, relationships, and vocational choices. For example, is the patient regularly involved in illegal or dangerous activities or frequently engaged in destructive relationships with others? It is also useful to determine if the judgments are deliberate or impulsive. Finally, several hypothetical situations can be presented for the patient to evaluate, such as the following:

1. What would you do if you found a stamped, addressed envelope lying on the ground?
2. How would you find your way out of a forest in the daytime?
3. What would you do if you entered your house and smelled gas?
4. If you won $10,000, what would you do with it?

> **NURSE ALERT.** Judgment is impaired in intoxicated patients and those with organic mental disorders, schizophrenia, psychotic disorders, and borderline or below average IQ. It may also be a problem for manic patients and those with personality disorders.

### Insight

*Insight* refers to the patient's understanding of the nature of the illness.

#### Observations

The nurse must determine if the patient accepts or denies the presence of illness. In addition, the nurse should inquire if the patient blames the problem on someone else or some external factors. Several questions may help to determine the patient's degree of insight. What does the patient think about what the nurse has been told? What does the patient want others, including the nurse, to do about it?

> **NURSE ALERT.** Impaired insight is associated with many psychiatric illnesses, including organic mental disorder, psychosis, substance abuse, eating disorders, personality disorders, and borderline or lower IQ. Whether or not a patient sees the need for treatment also critically affects the therapeutic alliance, setting of mutual goals, implementation of the treatment plan, and future adherence to it.

## Behavioral Rating Scales

A variety of behavioral rating scales and measurement tools are available as additional methods of assessment. Rating scales help clinicians perform the following:

1. Measure the extent of a patient's problems
2. Make an accurate diagnosis

3. Track patient progress over time
4. Document the efficacy of treatment

Frequently used scales include the following:

1. Beck Depression Inventory—self-reporting, 13-item scale designed to measure depth of depression and to screen depressed patients rapidly
2. Brief Psychiatric Rating Scale (BPRS)—clinician-administered, 18-item scale that provides rapid and efficient evaluation of treatment response by focusing on adult psychopathology
3. Clinical Global Impressions (CGI)—clinician-administered, three-item scale measuring severity of illness, global improvement, and efficacy of drug regimen
4. Hamilton Anxiety Scale (HAM-A)—clinician-administered, 14-item scale for patients with a diagnosis of anxiety
5. Hamilton Psychiatric Rating Scale for Depression (HAM-D)—clinician-administered, 21-item scale for assessing severity of an adult patient's depression and for showing changes in condition
6. Manic-State Rating Scale—clinician-administered, 26-item scale that measures manic symptoms, including frequency and intensity of behavior
7. Nurses' Observation Scale for Inpatient Evaluation (NOSIE)—30-item scale measuring patient behavior in adult and geriatric wards, with nursing personnel providing measures of patients' strengths and pathological states
8. Self-Report Symptom Check List-90 (SCL-90)—self-reporting, 90-item scale that presents a list of problems and complaints and asks the patient how bothersome these problems, if present, have been during the past week

## Sociocultural Context of Care

In each patient interaction the psychiatric nurse should be aware of the broader world in which the patient lives. The nurse should realize that the patient's perception of health and illness, help-seeking behavior, and treatment adherence depends on the individual's unique beliefs, social norms, and cultural values. The culturally sensitive nurse understands the importance of social and cultural forces for the individual, recognizes the uniqueness of these aspects, respects nurse-patient differences, and incorporates sociocultural information into psychiatric nursing care.

## Sociocultural Risk Factors

Sociocultural risk factors for psychiatric illness include the following:
1. Age
2. Ethnicity
3. Gender
4. Education
5. Income
6. Belief system

These predisposing factors can significantly increase the potential for developing a psychiatric disorder, decrease the potential for recovery, or both. No one or two of these factors alone can adequately describe the sociocultural context of psychiatric nursing care. Together, however, they provide a sociocultural profile of the patient that is essential to quality psychiatric nursing practice.

## Sociocultural Stressors

Lack of awareness of these risk factors and their effect on the individual, along with lack of respect for sociocultural differences, can result in inadequate nursing care. Table 4-2 lists some sociocultural stressors that also can hinder the quality of psychiatric care.

## Sociocultural Assessment

Assessment of the patient's sociocultural risk factors and stressors greatly enhances the nurse's ability to establish a therapeutic alliance, identify the patient's problems, and develop a psychiatric nursing treatment plan that is accurate, appropriate, and culturally relevant. Box 4-5 presents questions that the nurse might ask regarding each of the risk factors identified.

The psychotherapeutic treatment process also is influenced by the cultural and ethnic context of both the patient and the health care provider. Together the nurse and patient need to agree on the nature of the patient's coping responses, the means for solving problems, and the expected outcomes of treatment.

## Box 4-5   Questions Related to Sociocultural Risk Factors

### Age

What is the patient's current stage of development?
What are the developmental tasks of the patient?
Are those tasks age-appropriate for the patient?
What are the patient's attitudes and beliefs regarding the specific age group?
With what age-related stressors is the patient currently coping?
What impact does the patient's age have on mental and physical health?

### Ethnicity

What is the patient's ethnic background?
What is the patient's ethnic identity?
Is the patient traditional, bicultural, multicultural, or culturally alienated?
What are the patient's attitudes, beliefs, and values regarding the specific ethnic group?
With what ethnic-related stressors is the patient currently coping?
What impact does the person's ethnicity have on mental and physical health?

### Gender

What is the patient's gender?
What is the patient's gender identity?
How does the patient define gender-specific roles?
What are the patient's attitudes and beliefs regarding males and females and masculinity and femininity?
With what gender-related stressors is the patient currently coping?
What impact does the person's gender have on mental and physical health?

*Continued*

### Box 4-5   Questions Related to Sociocultural Risk Factors—cont'd

Education

What is the patient's educational level?

What were the patient's educational experiences like?

What are the patient's attitudes and beliefs regarding education in general and the patient's own education in particular?

With what education-related stressors is the patient currently coping?

What impact does the patient's education have on mental and physical health?

Income

What is the patient's income?

What is the source of the patient's income?

How does the patient describe the specific income group?

What are the patient's attitudes and beliefs regarding personal socioeconomic status?

With what economic-related stressors is the patient currently coping?

What impact does the patient's income have on mental and physical health?

Belief System

What are the patient's beliefs about health and illness?

What was the patient's religious or spiritual upbringing?

What are the patient's current religious or spiritual beliefs?

Who is the patient's regular health care provider?

With what belief system–related stressors is the patient currently coping?

What impact does the patient's belief system have on mental and physical health?

Table 4-2   Sociocultural stressors

| Stressor | Definition |
| --- | --- |
| Disadvantagement | Lack of socioeconomic resources that are basic to biopsychosocial adaptation |
| Stereotype | Depersonalized conception of individuals within a group |
| Intolerance | Unwillingness to accept different opinions or beliefs from people of different backgrounds |
| Stigma | Attribute or trait deemed by the individual's social environment to be different and diminishing |
| Prejudice | Preconceived, unfavorable belief about individuals or groups that disregards knowledge, thought, or reason |
| Discrimination | Differential treatment of individuals or groups not based on actual merit |
| Racism | Belief that inherent differences among the races determine individual achievement and that one race is superior |

*your* INTERNET
c o n n e c t i o n

American Psychological Association PsychNET:
www.apa.org

Dana Brain Web:
www.dana.org/brainweb

EthnoMed Ethnic Medicine Guide:
www.healthlinks.washington.edu/clinical/ethnomed

National Center for Cultural Competence:
www.dml.georgetown.edu/nccc/index.html

## Suggested readings

American Psychiatric Association: Practice guideline for psychiatric evaluation of adults, *Am J Psychiatry* 152(Suppl 11):67, 1995.

Baker F, Bell C: Issues in the psychiatric treatment of African Americans, *Psychiatr Serv* 50(3):362, 1999.

Center for Mental Health Services: *Cultural competence standards*, Rockville, Md, 1998, Substance Abuse and Mental Health Services Administration

Coleman F, Kay J: The biology of the brain. In Kay J, Tasman A: *Psychiatry: behavioral science and clinical essentials*, Philadelphia, 2000, WB Saunders.

Collins F: Medical and societal consequences of the Human Genome Project, *N Engl J Med* 341:28, 1999.

Goldstein M, Griswold K: Cultural sensitivity and aging, *Psychiatr Serv* 49(6):769, 1998.

Goleman D: *Working with emotional intelligence*, New York, 1998, Bantam.

Flaskerud J: Ethnicity, culture and neuropsychiatry, *Issues Ment Health Nurs*, 21:5, 2000.

Herrera J et al: *Cross Cultural Psychiatry*, New York, 1999, John Wiley & Sons.

Hudak C, Gallo B: Quick review of neurodiagnostic testing, *Am J Nurs* 97:16cc, 1997.

Janca A, Andrews G: Computers in psychiatric care, *Curr Opin Psychiatry* 12:701, 1999.

Koenig H, McCullogh M, Larson D: *Handbook of religion and health*, Oxford, 2001, Oxford University Press.

Lin K, Cheung F: Mental health issues for Asian Americans, *Psychiatr Serv* 50(6):774, 1999.

Nolte J: *The human brain: an introduction to its functional anatomy*, ed 4, St Louis, 1999, Mosby.

Ruiz P: New clinical perspectives in cultural psychiatry, *J Pract Psychiatry Behav Health* 4(3):150, 1998.

SAMHSA: *Developing culturally competent systems of care for state mental health services*, Washington, DC, 1998, Western Interstate Commission for Higher Education.

Slick L: Staying one step ahead of the body clock. *Advances for Nurses* 3(2):27, 2001.

Stuart G, Laraia M: *Principles and practice of psychiatric nursing*, ed 7, St Louis, 2001, Mosby.

Strub R: *The mental status examination in neurology*, Philadelphia, 2000, FA Davis.

Tseng W, Streltzer J: *Culture and psychopathology: a guide to clinical assessment*, New York, 1997, Brunner/Mazel.

Tuck I et al: Spiritual interventions provided by mental health nurses, *West J Nurs Res* 19(3):351, 1997.

# Environmental Context of Psychiatric Nursing Care

5

## Managed Care

Managed care is a reality of the current health care environment. In a well-functioning system of managed care, a defined group of people receive treatment services that are clinically necessary and medically appropriate, have defined benefit parameters, are provided over a predetermined time, are in compliance with quality standards, and have anticipated and measurable outcomes. Currently the term *managed care,* as applied to mental and substance abuse disorders, has been replaced by *managed behavioral health care,* which refers to these disorders together as one set of health problems.

## Defining Characteristics

Managed care differs significantly from the traditional fee-for-service health care delivery system (Table 5-1). Managed care involves a major shift away from the person as customer to the *population* as customer. It deemphasizes high-cost, episodic, inpatient admissions and procedures in favor of creating a full continuum of care and then selecting the correct level of care and treatment setting. Whereas the traditional system fostered duplication of services and technology among hospitals, managed care stimulates the consolidation of services, formation of networks, and use of primary care networks to provide both referral and gatekeeping activities.

Table 5-1   Comparison of traditional and managed care health delivery systems

| Characteristic | Traditional System | Managed Care System |
|---|---|---|
| Provider focus | Specialized care of individual patient | Total care of member population |
| Pricing | Separate physician and hospital fee schedules | Discounts, case rates, capitation |
| Market share | Number of admissions<br>Number of procedures<br>Number of visits | Number of covered lives |
| Management focus | High inpatient occupancy rate | Low inpatient occupancy rate<br>Correct level of care |
| Service line | Acute care programs as driving forces<br>Inconsistent integration<br>Physician dependent<br>Individual services | Continuum of care:<br>Inpatient<br>Partial hospitalization Outpatient<br>Residential<br>Home |

| | | |
|---|---|---|
| Cost management | Payers assume admission rate risk<br>Provider assumes length-of-stay risk | Provider networks assume all utilization risks<br>Admission rate<br>Length of stay |
| Costs | Cost per procedure<br>Cost per hospitalization | Cost per life<br>Inpatient days per 1000<br>Visits per 1000 |
| Competition | Multiple hospitals for communities<br>Duplication of services and technology | Increased consolidation and network formation as occupancy declines<br>Closures<br>Alternative uses of hospitals |
| Characteristic outcomes | Qualitative measures:<br>Reputation<br>Facilities | Quantitative measures:<br>Quality<br>Cost |
| Referral base | Focus on high-tech capabilities<br>Separate physician and hospital marketing efforts | Ability to form primary care networks<br>Mutual goals and strategies of providers and hospitals |

Managed care is not a single entity; rather, it can assume various types or forms (Box 5-1). *Managed competition* is a purchasing strategy in which managed care organizations contract with several hospitals that provide cost-effective, comprehensive services. Consumers are then informed about the hospitals from which they may receive services, even though the facility may not be the patient's preferred choice.

## Financial Aspects

A managed care system uses the following three major payment mechanisms:

1. *Discounted fee-for-service payment plan,* in which clinicians are paid for all services that have been authorized and provided to a consumer. The payment rate is discounted or is less than the clinician's standard fee schedule and often includes a provision for a copayment that must be collected from the consumer at each visit.

---

### Box 5-1    Types of Managed Care Plans

- Health maintenance organizations (HMOs) are organized delivery systems that provide care to a defined population, usually for a predetermined fixed amount (capitation rate). Consumers enrolled in HMOs are restricted to using HMO providers.
- Preferred provider organizations (PPOs) are plans that contract with a limited number of clinicians, most often physicians, and hospitals who provide care at discounted rates. Members of these plans are given financial incentives to use the "preferred providers" but are not prevented from using any provider of choice. Insurers or employers select the providers to be included in their preferred plan.
- Point-of-service plans (POSs) allow consumers to choose between delivery systems at the time they seek care. In a triple-option plan, for example, people can choose among an HMO, PPO, or fee-for-service plan. Financial incentives are usually provided to encourage people to use the least expensive option.

---

2. *Case rate system,* in which the clinician is paid a flat fee for a predefined episode of care. The most well-known case rate system is Medicare's diagnosis-related groups (DRGs), in which Medicare pays a flat fee for a particular hospitalization episode regardless of how many days the person was hospitalized. This system shifts the financial risk to the provider because the provider receives a flat fee regardless of the actual cost of care.

3. *Capitation system,* in which the consumer pays a fixed fee—a per member, per month (PMPM) premium. In return the managed care company that receives the PMPM fee agrees to provide all the medically necessary health care required by all the covered customers in the group. In this case, most of the financial risk lies with the managed care company, who must deliver all necessary health care within the premiums received by their population pool. HMOs are the best-known examples of capitated payment systems.

Managed care exerts cost control measures in the following ways:

- *Preadmission certification* takes into account the patient's medical and psychiatric status and level of functioning; socioenvironmental factors; and procedural issues associated with treatment. The managed care reviewer's role is to determine the most appropriate form of treatment and the proper treatment setting. In this way the reviewer acts as a gatekeeper on issues of cost and quality.

- *Utilization review* evaluates the appropriateness and necessity of services and procedures. It is a way of monitoring the care and services administered and has the most immediate impact on patient care. The patient's treatment plan, diagnostic and therapeutic interventions, and discharge planning are continuously monitored by a third party. This third party determines reimbursement for treatment based on current standards of care. The review and approval can be done before providing the services *(precertification review),* at the time the service is rendered *(concurrent review),* or after the service has been provided *(retrospective review),* which may be used retroactively to deny payment.

- *Case management* typically is targeted to those patients who have treatment complications, have high-expense episodes of care, or need alternative, less expensive treatments or settings. This group often includes patients with serious and persistent mental illness. Case management focuses on achieving desirable patient outcomes, appropriate lengths of stay, efficient use of resources, and patient involvement and satisfaction.

## Access to Services

*Access* can be defined as the degree to which services and information about care are conveniently and easily obtained. It is an important part of any effective mental health care delivery system. Today more than half the people who seek health care for mental disorders are treated by primary care practitioners. However, many who appear to need care do not receive it, either from a primary care or specialty provider. When access to mental health care is made difficult, the overall costs of general medical care increase because those with behavioral health care problems are high-level users of medical services. An ideal comprehensive health care system would (1) provide multiple points of entry for treatment, including direct access through self-referral; (2) adequately fund behavioral health care benefits and services; (3) reimburse all types of providers for their services; and (4) find ways of measuring and reinforcing standards for the accessibility, appropriateness, quality, and effectiveness of treatment.

## Employee Assistance Programs

Employee assistance programs (EAPs) are work site–based programs designed to help identify and resolve behavioral, health, and productivity problems that may affect employees' well-being or job performance. Their focus is wide-ranging, covering alcohol and other drug abuse, physical and emotional health, and marital, family, financial, legal, and other personal concerns. As such, they are important points of access to behavioral health care.

## Treatment Parity

Many people who need treatment for mental illnesses and chemical dependency disorders do not receive it because their insurance policies deny or restrict coverage for such treatment. A law passed by the U.S. Congress in 1996 ended the cash benefits and Medicare and Medicaid coverage for persons whose disability is based on drug addiction or alcoholism.

Currently more than half the states have some degree of mental health parity, with fairness bills pending in many other state legislatures. State laws differ in conditions served, specificity of parity, minimum benefits, approved providers, managed care usage, exemptions, and populations covered.

Ideally parity would include insurance coverage for mental and addictive disorders that is equal to that provided for any physical disease or illness in terms of service, dollar limits, deductibles, and copayments. Yet many current parity provisions are much narrower. For example, the federal parity law allows for the use of a wide range of cost control mechanisms for mental health services, such as higher deductibles or copayments and limits on services or hospital days, that differ from those used for physical health services. In addition, current exemptions to many state insurance regulations severely limit the number of people covered by parity laws, as well as the services they may receive. Finally, parity that covers only "medical treatment" of a particular mental illness may minimize or exclude preventive services and psychosocial treatments that are necessary to maintain a person's functional capacities. Thus although progress is being made in mandating behavioral health benefits, much additional work remains.

## Telepsychiatry

An exciting development in the field that may have important implications for access to care is the emergence of telepsychiatry. Telepsychiatry connects people by audiovisual communication and is seen as one means of providing expert health care services to patients distant from a source of care. It is suggested for the diagnosis and treatment of patients in remote locations or where psychiatric expertise is scarce. The high cost of providing the needed technology, particularly by public mental health systems with limited resources, has hampered its widespread use. In addition, issues of reliability of diagnosis, effectiveness of treatment, and patient satisfaction need further study.

## Clinical Appropriateness

*Clinical appropriateness* refers to the degree to which the type, amount, and level of clinical services are delivered to promote the most positive clinical outcomes for the consumer. To meet managed care's criteria of clinical appropriateness, behavioral health care organizations are developing diversified but fully integrated continuums of care by expanding their own services, contracting with other health care organizations, or affiliating with area providers. These continuums of care must be capable of providing services and alternative levels of care to children, adolescents, adults, and elderly people requiring either psychiatric or substance abuse services. The goal is to provide "one-stop shopping" for managed behavioral care consumers and to secure market dominance in a particular geographical area. The levels of care for each stage of treatment expected in an integrated continuum of care are listed in Table 5-2.

## Practice Guidelines

Practice guidelines in psychiatric care are strategies for mental health care delivery developed to facilitate clinical decision making and to provide patients with critical information concerning their treatment options. The goals of practice guidelines are as follows:

- Document preferred or "best" practices
- Increase consistency of care
- Facilitate outcome research
- Enhance quality of care provided
- Improve staff productivity
- Reduce costs

Practice guidelines can be developed in a variety of ways. The best mental health practice guidelines are based on a scientific review of the available clinical research literature in order to establish which treatments have been documented to be safe and effective for particular conditions. Guidelines have been developed by professional associations, managed care companies, and academic centers using techniques such as expert consensus and data analysis. Regardless of how they are developed, it is essential that they be updated regularly to keep up with the latest findings in the field.

## Clinical Pathways

A clinical pathway identifies the key clinical processes and corresponding timelines to which the patient must adhere to achieve standard outcomes within a specified time. It is a written plan that serves as a map and timetable for the efficient, effective delivery of health care. Valid clinical pathways are developed over time by a multidisciplinary team. They can be constructed around diagnoses from the *Diagnostic and Statistical Manual of Mental Disorders* (DSM-IV-TR), North American Nursing Diagnosis Association (NANDA) diagnoses, clinical conditions, treatment stages, clinical interventions, or targeted behaviors. They are most often used in inpatient settings, serve as a shortened version of the multidisciplinary plan of care for a patient, and require close team cooperation and monitoring of ongoing quality improvement. Some clinical settings have computerized their pathways to enhance the consistency and efficiency of care provided.

The key elements of the clinical pathway are (1) identifying a target population; (2) describing the expected outcome of treatment in a measurable, realistic, and patient-centered way; (3) specifying treatment strategies and interventions; and (4) documenting patient care activities, variances, and goal achievement. At this time, great variability exists in the format and use of clinical pathways in psychiatric care.

## Clinical Algorithms

Clinical, treatment, or medication algorithms take practice guidelines to a greater level of specificity by providing step-by-step information on issues such as treatment options, treatment sequencing, preferred dosage, and progress assessment. They thus provide clinicians with a framework that can enhance treatment planning and decision making for individual patients.

Algorithms are rule-based deductive systems that can help the clinician select from large databases of information relevant to decision making. Algorithms are cognitive tools for the clinician. They are intended to assist, not limit, clinical decision making. A clinical algorithm can be represented by a flowchart that identifies what clinical process might follow from a patient's clinical status and response to prior treatments, thereby providing a more specific statement of priority, or what to do next if the treatment is not effective, than the many options recommended by guidelines.

## Outcomes Measurement

Outcomes are the extent to which services are cost effective and have a favorable effect on the consumer's symptoms, functioning, and well-being. Outcomes include all those factors affecting the

Table 5-2   Levels of care for each stage of treatment in an integrated behavioral continuum of care

| Stages of Treatment | Crisis | Acute | Maintenance | Health Promotion |
|---|---|---|---|---|
| **Goal** | Stabilization | Remission | Recovery | Optimal level of wellness |
| **Expected Outcome** | No harm to self or others | Symptom relief | Improved functioning | Optimal quality of life |
| **Level of Care** | Inpatient hospitalization<br>24-hour mobile emergency intervention<br>Crisis stabilization unit and beds<br>23-hour observation beds<br>Outpatient detoxification<br>Telephone access and triage | Partial hospitalization<br>Intensive remission-oriented outpatient care<br>Assertive community treatment<br>Intensive in-home intervention<br>23-hour respite beds<br>Telepsychiatry | Rehabilitative day treatment<br>Multimodal recovery-oriented outpatient<br>Relapse prevention<br>Rehabilitation-oriented residential<br>Supported independent living | Education<br>Respite care<br>Drop-in centers<br>Peer support<br>Social activities<br>School<br>Employment<br>Housing |

patient and family while they are involved in the health care system, such as health status, functional status, quality of life, presence or absence of illness, type of coping response, and satisfaction with treatment. Outcome evaluation can focus on a clinical condition, an intervention, or a caregiving process. The variety of outcomes that can be examined include clinical, functional, satisfaction, and financial indicators related to the provision of psychiatric care (Box 5-2). The specific purposes of outcomes measurement are as follows:

- Evaluate the outcomes of care
- Suggest changes in treatment
- Evaluate program effectiveness
- Profile the practice pattern of providers
- Determine the most appropriate level of care
- Predict the path of a patient's illness and recovery
- Contribute to quality improvement programs

## Accountability Issues

Driven by the demand to demonstrate quality and reduce costs, the behavioral health-care environment is confronted by new issues of accountability.

### Consumer Empowerment

Consumer empowerment has been an emerging movement over the past decade. The term *consumer* is one in a long list of labels that users of psychiatric services have applied to themselves. Other terms include *client, customer, patient, ex-patient,* and *survivor.* The term *consumer* is most often used when it applies to empowerment.

With managed care it is clear that individuals will have limits placed on their choice of providers, service settings, and sometimes even treatment options. If limited options are available, patients may be unable to take advantage of newer treatments that may help them. Partly in response to these concerns, the Center for Mental Health Services has developed a set of principles that emphasizes the need for comprehensive services, continuity of care, and responsiveness to the needs of service recipients. Also, a number of mental health organizations, including the American Psychiatric Nurses' Association, have endorsed a bill of rights for managed care. All these initiatives reflect a focused effort to protect patients and balance the issues of cost and quality in the current psychiatric care environment.

## Provider Concerns

Providers are increasingly aware of their responsibility to provide cost-effective care within an environment of shrinking psychiatric resources. New dilemmas arise for clinicians who must balance a responsibility to both an individual patient and a population of patients. Also, managed care has increased the tension between patient advocacy and resource allocation, because providers may feel the need to serve the organization's "bottom line" and thus may jeopardize the individual patient's interests.

When mental health clinicians become part of networks or organized systems of care, they become subject to the review of others. Their activities are often routinely measured, and they are held accountable for the type and amount of care they deliver. Many mental health professionals view this negatively, but others see it as a positive trend leading to an overall improvement in behavioral health care services.

Providers also struggle with (1) the ambiguity of many of the rules, regulations, and expectations of this new health care environment; (2) the overreliance of managed care on treatment protocols that diminish professional judgment and minimize individual patient or clinical factors; and (3) the reduced clinician productivity resulting from administrative burdens and excessive documentation. Finally, providers' roles and functions are often subject to confusion, and the realities of the new environment often escalate conflict among the mental health disciplines rather than enhance interdisciplinary collaboration.

## Service Settings

Mental health facilities have been criticized for denying inpatient care or transferring patients to another facility for economic reasons when it is not in the patient's best interests. Another effect of managed care has been the layoffs and downsizing of inpatient facilities because of decreased inpatient census and increased managed competition. The resulting shortage of staff and the increased work the remaining members are asked to assume may adversely affect the care provided. In addition, although staffing is decreas-

## Box 5-2  Categories of Outcome Indicators

Clinical Outcome Indicators
- High-risk behaviors
- Symptomatology
- Coping responses
- Relapse
- Recurrence
- Readmission
- Number of treatment episodes
- Medical complications
- Incidence reports
- Mortality

Functional Outcome Indicators
- Functional status
- Social interaction
- Activities of daily living
- Occupational abilities
- Quality of life
- Family relationships
- Housing arrangement

Satisfaction Outcome Indicators

**Patient/family satisfaction with:**
- Outcomes
- Providers
- Delivery system
- Caregiving process
- Organization

Financial Outcome Indicators
- Cost per treatment episode
- Revenue per treatment episode
- Length of inpatient stay
- Use of health care resources
- Costs related to disability

ing, the acuity of inpatient disorders is increasing, which more urgently demands an adequate number of well-trained staff to deliver quality patient care.

Another challenge to service setting accountability arises with information management. Computerized patient records are providing standardized formats for easier data collection and analyses. Clinical, financial, and administrative information systems are being integrated to measure outcomes related to quality and costs of care. Important accountability issues are related to confidentiality, appropriate uses of data, and protection of data, particularly in an area as sensitive as psychiatric and substance abuse disorders.

## Accrediting Organizations

Accrediting organizations for managed care include the Utilization Review Accreditation Committee (URAC), the Joint Commission on Accreditation of Healthcare Organizations (JCAHO), and the National Committee on Quality Assurance (NCQA). NCQA is an independent, nonprofit HMO-accrediting organization composed of independent health care quality experts, employers, labor union officials, and consumers. In 1991 NCQA adopted standards that assess performance in the following six areas:

1. Quality improvement and information
2. Utilization management
3. Credentialing of providers
4. Members' rights and responsibilities
5. Preventive health services
6. Medical records

NCQA accreditation is designed for most managed care companies. NCQA has the longest performance record in managed care accreditation, and its accreditation is mandated by law in many states.

## Nursing Roles in Managed Care

Nurses bring great assets to the managed care arena through their rich blend of skills and expertise. Although nursing activity varies greatly based on education, experience, certification, service setting, and geographical location, psychiatric nurses have assumed many roles in managed care, including the following:

- Psychiatric–mental health clinician
- Case manager

- Evaluation and triage nurse
- Utilization review nurse
- Patient educator
- Risk manager
- Quality improvement officer
- Marketing and development specialist
- Corporate manager and executive

Throughout all the changes in the mental health care environment, individuals, families, and communities continue to experience significant emotional problems. Thus the need for psychiatric nurses, as competent and caring professionals, will also continue. Nurses must be proactive, however, in realigning their positions within the changing environment.

## *your* INTERNET connection

American Association of Managed Care Nurses:
www.aamcn.org

American Managed Behavioral Healthcare Association:
www.ambha.org

Employee Assistance Professionals Association:
www.eap-association.com

Institute for Behavioral Health Care:
www.ibh.com

National Association of Psychiatric Health Systems:
www.naphs.org

National Committee for Quality Assurance (NCQA):
www.ncqa.org

National Guideline Clearinghouse:
www.guideline.gov

Telemedicine Information Exchange:
tie.telemed.org

## Suggested readings

American College of Mental Health Administration (ACMHA): *Moving forward practice guidelines in mental health and addiction services,* Pittsburgh, 2000, ACMHA.

Chan S, Wong K: The use of critical pathways in caring for schizophrenic patients in a mental hospital, *Arch Psychiatr Nurs* 13(3):145, 1999.

Center for Mental Health Services: *Mental health, United States, 1998,* Washington, DC, 1998, US Government Printing Office.

Coughlin KM: *Behavioral outcomes & guidelines sourcebook: 2000 edition,* New York, 1999, Faulkner & Gray.

Cummings N: Spectacular accomplishments and disappointing mistakes: the first decade of managed behavioral care, *Behav Healthc Tomorrow* August 1998, p 61.

Druss B, Rosenheck R: Mental disorders and access to medical care in the United States, *Am J Psychiatry* 155(12):1775, 1998.

Dykes PC: *Psychiatric clinical pathways: an interdisciplinary approach,* Gaithersburg, Md, 1998, Aspen.

Fletcher J: Mental health nurses: guardians of ethics in managed care, *J Psychsoc Nurs* 36(7):34, 1998.

Frueh C et al: Procedural and methodological issues in telepsychiatry research and program development, *Psychiatr Serv* 51(12):1522, 2000.

Geller J et al: A national survey of "consumer empowerment" at the state level, *Psychiatr Serv* 49(4):498, 1998.

Gilbert D et al: Texas medication algorithm project: definitions, rationale, and methods to develop medication algorithms, *J Clin Psychiatry* 59(7):345, 1998.

Goldman H: The obligation of mental health services to the least well off, *Psychiatr Serv* 50(5):659, 1999.

Hall L, Beinecke R: Consumer and family views of managed care, *New Dir Ment Health Serv* 78:77, 1998.

Hoge M et al: Ten dimensions of public-sector managed care, *Psychiatr Serv* 50(1):51, 1999.

Institute of Medicine: *Crossing the quality chasm,* Washington, DC, 2001, National Academy Press.

Institute of Medicine: *Managing managed care: quality improvement in behavioral health,* Washington, DC, 1997, National Academy Press.

Jenkins R, White P: Telehealth advancing nursing practice, *Nursing Outlook* 49:100-105, 2001.

Levinson C, Druss B: The evolution of mental health parity in American politics, *Admin Pol Ment Health* 28(2):139, 2000.

Mechanic D: Emerging trends in mental health policy and practice, *Health Aff* 17(6):82, 1998.

Mechanic D: *Mental health and social policy: the emergence of managed care,* Needham Heights, Mass, 1999, Allyn and Bacon.

Schreter R: Trends in managed care, 2000 edition, *Psychiatr Serv* 51(12):1493, 2000.

Sederer L, Dickey B: *Outcomes assessment in clinical practice,* Baltimore, 1996, Williams & Wilkins.

Sing M et al: *The costs and effects of parity for mental health and substance abuse insurance benefits,* Rockville, Md, 1998, US Department Health and Human Services.

Speer D: *Mental health outcome evaluation,* San Diego, 1998, Academic Press.

Stuart G, Laraia M: *Principles and practice of psychiatric nursing,* ed 7, St Louis, 2001, Mosby.

# Legal-Ethical Context of Psychiatric Nursing Care

6

The practice of psychiatric nursing is influenced by the law, particularly regarding the rights of patients and the quality of their care. Many of the laws vary from state to state, and nurses are required to become familiar with the legal provisions of their own state. Knowledge of the law enhances the freedom of both the nurse and the patient.

## Hospitalization and Community Treatment

The process of hospitalization can be traumatic or supportive, depending on the institution, attitude of family and friends, response of the staff, and type of admission. Table 6-1 presents characteristics that distinguish between the two types of admission to psychiatric hospitals: voluntary and involuntary.

### Involuntary Admission (Commitment)

The legal basis for involuntary confinement is either the police power of the state for the protection of society or *parens patriae,* the state's duty to protect citizens who cannot protect themselves. Figure 6-1 lists common procedural elements of the commitment process. Action is begun with a petition by a relative, friend, public official, physician, or any interested citizen stating that the person is mentally ill and in need of treatment. An examination of the patient's mental status is then completed by one or two physicians.

The decision as to whether the patient requires hospitalization is then made, and who decides this determines the nature of the

Table 6-1   Characteristics of the two types of admission to psychiatric hospitals

|  | Voluntary Admission | Involuntary Admission |
| --- | --- | --- |
| Admission | Written application by patient | Application did not originate with patient |
| Discharge | Initiated by patient | Initiated by hospital or court but not by patient |
| Status of civil rights | Retained in full by patient | Patient may retain none, some, or all, depending on state law |
| Justification | Voluntarily seeks help | Mentally ill and one or more of the following: 1. Dangerous to self or others 2. Needs treatment 3. Unable to meet own basic needs |

commitment. Medical certification means that physicians make the decision. Court or judicial commitment is decided by a judge or jury in a formal hearing. The patient may retain legal counsel to prepare for the hearing. Administrative commitment is determined by a special tribunal of hearing officers.

If the individual is determined to be (1) dangerous to self or others, (2) mentally ill and in need of treatment, or (3) unable to meet basic needs such as food and shelter, that person is hospitalized.

## Discharge

Voluntary patients of lawful age may initiate their own discharge. Most states require that patients give written notice of their desire for discharge. For patients who are leaving against medical advice, most hospitals request they sign a form stating this. If voluntary patients elope from the hospital, they can be brought back only if they again voluntarily agree. If they refuse to return to the hospital, they must be discharged or involuntary commitment procedures must be initiated. Involuntary patients have lost the right to leave the hospital when they wish. If a committed patient elopes from the hospital, the staff has the legal obligation to notify the police and committing courts.

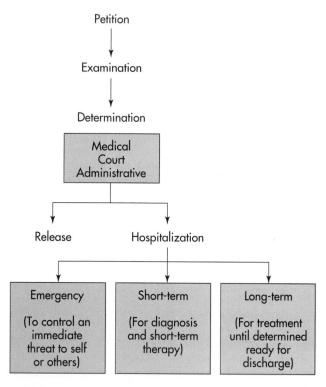

Figure 6-1
Diagram of the involuntary commitment process.

## Involuntary Community Treatment

Involuntary community treatment can be provided for those in need through (1) outpatient commitment, (2) preventive commitment, and (3) conditional release from the hospital. These initiatives arose from the mandate to offer psychiatric patients treatment in the least restrictive setting.

*Outpatient commitment* is the process by which the courts can order patients "committed" to a course of outpatient treatment specified by their clinicians. This type of commitment provides an alternative to inpatient treatment for those who meet the involuntary commitment criterion of dangerousness to self or others.

*Preventive commitment* permits commitment for outpatients who do not yet meet the usual commitment criteria but will do so soon without intervention. The criteria used for preventive commitment are sometimes referred to as a *predicted deterioration standard.* In this case a person is believed to need treatment to prevent a relapse, which would likely result in the individual becoming imminently dangerous.

*Conditional release* involves continued supervision of a person who has been released from the hospital. The hospital or court informs the person of the conditions for release, such as reporting to a medication clinic. Violation of these conditions usually results in rehospitalization. This approach is used primarily to determine if the individual is able to function in the community under supervision.

These initiatives are alternatives to address the pressing problem of the homeless but nondangerous mentally ill individual who is in need of psychiatric treatment and stabilization in the community. They may be most beneficial for revolving-door patients—those who stop taking their medication shortly after discharge, rapidly deteriorate, and soon require rehospitalization.

## Ethical Considerations

All nurses must analyze their beliefs regarding voluntary and involuntary hospitalization and community treatment of psychiatric patients. Psychiatric nurses, patients, families, and citizens need to address such issues as the value of commitment, goals of hospitalization, treatment received while hospitalized, community alternatives, and quality of life. Nurses are responsible for reviewing commitment procedures in their state and working for the necessary clinical, ethical, and legal reforms.

# Patients' Rights

Box 6-1 lists patients' rights that have been adopted by many states. Some of these rights that are especially important to psychiatric nurses are discussed next.

*Right to communicate with people outside the hospital.* The patient is free to visit and hold telephone conversations in privacy and send unopened letters to anyone.

*Right to personal effects.* The patient has the right to bring a limited amount of personal items. This does not hold the hospital

---

### Box 6-1 Rights of Psychiatric Patients

- Right to communicate with people outside the hospital through correspondence, telephone, and personal visits
- Right to keep clothing and personal effects with them in the hospital, except for potentially dangerous objects
- Right to religious freedom
- Right to be employed, if possible
- Right to manage and dispose of property
- Right to execute wills
- Right to enter into contractual relationships
- Right to make purchases
- Right to education
- Right to habeas corpus
- Right to independent psychiatric examination
- Right to civil service status
- Right to retain licenses, privileges, or permits established by law, such as a driver's or professional license
- Right to sue or be sued
- Right to marry and divorce
- Right not to be subject to unnecessary mechanical restraints
- Right to periodic review of status
- Right to legal representation
- Right to privacy
- Right to informed consent
- Right to treatment
- Right to refuse treatment
- Right to treatment in the least restrictive setting

---

responsible for their safety, however, and does not relieve the hospital staff of ensuring the patient's safety.

*Right to execute wills.* A person's competency to make a will is known as "testamentary capacity." Persons can make a valid will if they (1) know that they are making a will, (2) know the nature and extent of their property, and (3) know who their friends and relatives are and what the relationship means. Each of these criteria must be met and documented for the will to be considered valid.

*Right to habeas corpus.* All patients retain this right, which allows for a court of law to require the speedy release of individuals who can show they are being deprived of their liberty and detained illegally.

*Right to independent psychiatric examination.* The patient may demand a psychiatric examination by a physician of choice. If this physician determines that the patient is not mentally ill, the person must be released.

*Right to privacy.* The individual may keep some personal information completely secret from others.

*Confidentiality.* The principle of confidentiality allows the disclosure of certain information to another person, but this is limited to strictly authorized individuals. *Privileged communication* is a legal phrase that applies only in court-related proceedings. It means that the listener cannot disclose information from an individual unless the speaker gives permission. Privileged communication does not apply to hospital charts, and most states do not provide for privileged communication between nurses and patients. In addition, therapists have the responsibility to breach the confidentiality of the relationship to warn a potential victim of impending violence by a patient.

*Right to informed consent.* A physician must explain the treatment to the patient, including its possible complications, side effects, and risks. The physician must obtain the patient's consent, which must be competent, understanding, and voluntary. Box 6-2 lists the reasonable information to be disclosed in obtaining informed consent.

*Right to treatment.* Criteria for adequate treatment are defined in three areas: (1) a humane psychological and physical environment, (2) a qualified staff with a sufficient number of members to administer treatment, and (3) individualized treatment plans.

*Right to refuse treatment.* Patients may refuse treatment unless they have been legally determined to be incompetent. A determination of *incompetency* requires that the person has a mental disorder resulting in a defect in judgment and that this defect makes this person incapable of handling personal affairs. Incompetency can only be reversed through another court hearing.

## Ethical Considerations

Ensuring patients' rights is often complicated by ethical considerations that the nurse must carefully examine. Many ethical dilem-

## Box 6-2   Obtaining Informed Consent

Information to Disclose

- **Diagnosis:** description of patient's problem
- **Treatment:** nature and purpose of proposed treatment
- **Consequences:** risks and benefits of proposed treatment, including physical and psychological effects, costs, and potential problems
- **Alternatives:** viable alternatives to proposed treatment and their risks and benefits
- **Prognosis:** expected outcome with treatment, with alternative treatment, and without treatment

Principles of Informing

- Assess the patient's ability to give informed consent.
- Simplify language so that laypersons can understand.
- Offer opportunities for the patient and family to ask questions.
- Test the patient's understanding after the explanation.
- Reeducate as often as needed.
- Document all relevant factors, including what was disclosed; patient's understanding, competency, and voluntary agreement to treatment; and the actual consent.

mas arise from health care professionals' "paternalistic" attitude toward their patients, which reduces adult patients to the status of children and interferes with their freedom of action. Ethical questions can also arise for the psychiatric nurse when implementing patients' rights, such as the right to treatment, right to refuse treatment, and right to treatment in the least restrictive setting. All nurses participate in some therapeutic psychiatric regimens with ambiguous scientific and ethical bases. Thus each nurse must analyze such ethical dilemmas as freedom of choice versus coercion, helping versus imposing values, and focusing on cure versus prevention. Nurses assume an active role in defining adequate treatment and allocating important resources for mentally ill patients.

# Legislative Initiatives

Other legislation has also changed the nature of psychiatric care and service delivery in the United States.

## Protection and Advocacy Act

Under the Protection and Advocacy for Mentally Ill Individuals Act of 1986, all states must designate an agency that is responsible for protecting the rights of mentally ill patients. The following three areas of advocacy would help to maximize the fulfillment of patients' rights:

1. Educating mental health staff and implementing policies and procedures that recognize and protect patients' rights
2. Establishing an additional procedure to permit the speedy resolution of problems, questions, or disagreements that occur based on legal rights
3. Providing access to legal services when patients' rights have been denied

## Americans with Disabilities Act

The Americans with Disabilities Act (ADA), passed in 1990, protects more than 43 million people in the United States with one or more physical or mental disabilities from discrimination in jobs, public services, and accommodations. It prohibits discrimination against these persons in hiring, firing, training, compensation, and advancement in employment. Employers are prohibited from asking job applicants whether they have a disability, and medical examinations and questions about disability may be required only if the concerns are job related and necessary.

## Advanced Directives

Advanced directives came about as a result of the Patient Self-Determination Act (PSDA) of 1990. Written while a person is competent, these documents specify how decisions about treatment should be made if the person were to become incompetent. Use of advanced directives seems particularly appropriate for persons with mental illness who may alternate between periods of competence and incompetence. They could, for example, formalize a patient's wishes about forced medication or treatment setting.

## Psychiatry and Criminal Responsibility

Three sets of criteria are used in the United States to determine the criminal responsibility of an offender with a mental illness (Table 6-2). Of these, the American Law Institute's test (ALI) is the most frequently used. The two types of insanity defense are as follows:

1. Not guilty by reason of insanity (NGBI)
2. Guilty but mentally ill (GBMI)

Both outcomes typically result in the hospitalization of patients in state mental hospitals or treatment facilities provided in a penal institution.

## Legal Role of the Nurse

The psychiatric nurse has rights and responsibilities attendant to each of three legal roles: nurse as provider, nurse as employee, and nurse as citizen. Nurses may experience a conflict of interest among these rights and responsibilities. Professional nursing judgment requires a careful examination of the context of nursing care, the possible consequences of nursing actions, and the feasible alternatives the nurse might employ.

Table 6-2    Three sets of criteria typically used to determine criminal responsibilities of a mentally ill offender

| Name of Test | Criteria |
|---|---|
| M'Naghten rule | 1. The individual did not know the nature and quality of the act.<br>2. The individual did not know that the act was wrong. |
| Irresistible impulse test | An individual is impulsively driven to commit the criminal act with lack of premeditation and a strong urge to do so. This test is seldom used without other criteria. |
| American Law Institute's test | An individual lacks the capacity to "appreciate" the wrongfulness of the act or to "conform" conduct to the requirements of the law. It excludes the psychopath and is a popular criterion for determining criminal responsibility. |

Malpractice

Malpractice involves the failure of a professional person to provide the type of care given by members of the person's profession in the community, resulting in harm to the patient. Most malpractice claims are filed under the law of negligent tort. A tort is a civil wrong for which the injured party is entitled to compensation. Under the law of negligent tort the plaintiff must prove the following:

1. A legal duty of care existed.
2. The nurse performed the duty negligently.
3. Damages were incurred by the patient as a result.
4. The damages were substantial.

*your*INTERNET
connection

**American Society for Bioethics and Humanities:**
www.asbh.org

**Bazelon Center for Mental Health Law:**
www.bazelon.org

**Medical-Legal Consulting Institute, Inc.:**
www.legalnurse.com

**Thomas, Legislative Information on the Internet:**
thomas.loc.gov

**US Department of Justice, Americans with Disabilities Act:**
www.usdoj.gov/crt/ada/adahom1.htm

## Suggested readings

Applebaum P: A "health information infrastructure" and the threat to confidentiality of health records, *Psychiatr Serv* 49(1): 27, 1998.

Appelbaum P: Discrimination in psychiatric disability coverage and the Americans with Disabilities Act, *Psychiatr Serv* 49(7):875, 1998.

Allen M, Smith V: Opening Pandora's box: the practical and legal dangers of involuntary outpatient commitment, *Psychiatric Services* 52(3):342, 2001.

Bazelon Center for Mental Health Law: *Psychiatric advance directive,* Washington, DC, 1998, The Center.

Bazelon Center for Mental Health Law: *Position statement on involuntary commitment,* Washington, DC, 1999, The Center.

Bogart T, Solomon P: Procedures to share treatment information among mental health providers, consumers and families, *Psychiatr Serv* 50(10):1321, 1999.

Fiesta J: Psychiatric liability: parts 1, 2 and 3, *Nurs Manage* 27(7-9):10, 16,18, 1998.

Gutheil T: A confusion of tongues: competence, insanity, psychiatry, and the law, *Psychiatr Serv* 50(6):767, 1999.

Haggerty L, Hawkins J: Informed consent and the limits of confidentiality, *West J Nurs Res* 22(4):508, 2000.

National Bioethics Advisory Commission: *Research involving persons with mental disorders that may affect decision-making capacity,* Washington, DC, 1998, The Commission.

Spratlen L: Ombudsman: a new role for advanced practice nurses in psychiatric-mental health care, *Perspect Psychiatr Care* 33(3):5, 1997.

Srebnik D, La Fond J: Advance directives for mental health treatment, *Psychiatr Serv* 50(7):919, 1999.

Stuart G, Laraia M: *Principles and practice of psychiatric nursing,* ed 7, St Louis, 2001, Mosby.

Swartz M, Swanson J, Hiday V et al: A randomized controlled trial of outpatient commitment in North Carolina, *Psychiatric Services* 52(3):325, 2001.

Wysoker A: Patient rights: the Americans with Disabilities Act and psychiatric disorders in the workplace, *J Am Psychiatr Nurses Assoc* 6(6):207, 2000.

# Implementing Clinical Practice Standards

## 7

## Nursing Defined

In 1980, *Nursing: A Social Policy Statement* defined nursing as "the diagnosis and treatment of human responses to actual or potential health problems."[1] The 1995 update, *Nursing's Social Policy Statement* added to this definition by acknowledging the following features of contemporary nursing practice[2]:

1. Attention to the full range of human experiences and responses to health and illness without restriction to a problem-focused orientation
2. Integration of objective data with knowledge gained from an understanding of the patient or group's subjective experience
3. Application of scientific knowledge to the processes of diagnosis and treatment
4. Provision of a caring relationship that facilitates health and healing.

## Standards of Psychiatric–Mental Health Clinical Nursing Practice

*Scope and Standards of Psychiatric–Mental Health Clinical Nursing Practice* describes a competent level of professional nursing care and professional performance common to nurses engaged in psychiatric–mental health nursing practice in any setting.[3] These standards apply to nurses who are qualified by education and experience to practice at either the basic level or the advanced level of psychiatric–mental health nursing.

# Standards of Care*

Standards of care pertain to professional nursing activities demonstrated by the nurse throughout the nursing process. These involve assessment, nursing diagnosis, outcome identification, planning, implementation, and evaluation. The nursing process is the foundation of clinical decision making and encompasses all significant action taken by nurses in providing psychiatric–mental health care to all patients.

Figure 7-1 outlines the nursing conditions and nursing behaviors related to each of the psychiatric nursing standards of care.

## Standard I: Assessment

The psychiatric–mental health nurse collects patient health data.

### RATIONALE

The assessment interview—which requires linguistically and culturally effective communication skills, interviewing, behavior observation, database record review, and comprehensive assessment of the patient and relevant systems—enables the psychiatric–mental health nurse to make sound clinical judgments and plan appropriate interventions with the patient.

## Standard II: Diagnosis

The psychiatric–mental health nurse analyzes the assessment data in determining diagnoses.

### RATIONALE

The basis for providing psychiatric–mental health nursing care is the recognition and identification of patterns of response to actual or potential psychiatric illnesses and mental health problems.

## Standard III: Outcome identification

The psychiatric–mental health nurse identifies expected outcomes individualized to the patient.

---

*Reprinted with permission from American Nurses Association: *Scope and standards of psychiatric–mental health clinical nursing practice,* Washington, DC, 2000, The Association.

Figure 7-1
The nursing conditions and behaviors related to the psychiatric nursing standards of care.

**RATIONALE**

Within the context of providing nursing care, the ultimate goal is to influence health outcomes and improve the patient's health issues.

## Standard IV: Planning

The psychiatric–mental health nurse develops a plan of care that prescribes interventions to attain expected outcomes.

**RATIONALE**

A plan of care is used to guide therapeutic interventions systematically, document progress, and achieve the expected patient outcomes.

## Standard V: Implementation

The psychiatric–mental health nurse implements the interventions identified in the plan of care.

**RATIONALE**

In implementing the plan of care, psychiatric–mental health nurses use a wide range of interventions designed to prevent mental and physical illness and promote, maintain, and restore mental and physical health. Psychiatric–mental health nurses select interventions according to their level of practice. At the basic level the nurse may select counseling, milieu therapy, promotion of self-care activities, intake screening and evaluation, psychobiological interventions, health teaching, case management, health promotion and health maintenance, crisis intervention, community-based care, psychiatric home health care, telehealth, and a variety of other approaches to meet the mental health needs of patients. In addition to the intervention options available to the basic-level psychiatric–mental health nurse, at the advanced level the APRN-PMH may provide consultation, engage in psychotherapy, and prescribe pharmacological agents where permitted by state statutes or regulations.

## Standard Va: Counseling

The psychiatric–mental health nurse uses counseling interventions to help patients in improving or regaining their previous coping abilities, fostering mental health, and preventing mental illness and disability.

### Standard Vb: Milieu therapy

The psychiatric–mental health nurse provides, structures, and maintains a therapeutic environment in collaboration with the client and other health care providers.

### Standard Vc: Self-care activities

The psychiatric–mental health nurse structures interventions around the patient's activities of daily living to foster self-care and mental and physical well-being.

### Standard Vd: Psychobiological interventions

The psychiatric–mental health nurse uses knowledge of psychobiological interventions and applies clinical skills to restore the patient's health and prevent further disability.

### Standard Ve: Health teaching

The psychiatric–mental health nurse, through health teaching, assists patients in achieving satisfying, productive, and healthy patterns of living.

### Standard Vf: Case management

The psychiatric–mental health nurse provides case management to coordinate comprehensive health services and ensure continuity of care.

### Standard Vg: Health promotion and health maintenance

The psychiatric–mental health nurse employs strategies and interventions to promote and maintain mental health and prevent mental illness.

## Advanced Practice Interventions Vh-Vj

The following interventions (Vh-Vj) may be performed only by the advanced practice registered nurse in psychiatric–mental health nursing.

### Standard Vh: Psychotherapy

The APRN-PMH uses individual, group, and family psychotherapy, child psychotherapy, and other therapeutic treatments to assist patients in preventing mental illness and disability and in improving mental health status and functional abilities.

## Standard Vi: Prescription of pharmacological agents

The APRN-PMH uses prescriptive authority, procedures, and treatments in accordance with state and federal laws and regulations to treat symptoms of psychiatric illness and improve functional health status.

## Standard Vj: Consultation

The APRN-PMH provides consultation to enhance the abilities of others to provide services for patients and effect change in the system.

## Standard VI: Evaluation

The psychiatric–mental health nurse evaluates the patient's progress in attaining expected outcomes.

**RATIONALE**

Nursing care is a dynamic process involving change in the patient's health status over time, giving rise to the need for data, different diagnoses, and modifications in the plan of care. Therefore evaluation is a continuous process of appraising the effect of nursing interventions and the treatment regimen on the patient's health status and expected health outcomes.

# Standards of Professional Performance*

Standards of professional performance describe a competent level of behavior in the professional nursing role, including activities related to quality of care, performance appraisal, education, collegiality, ethics, collaboration, research, and resource utilization. All psychiatric–mental health nurses are expected to engage in professional role activities appropriate to their education, position, and practice setting. Therefore standards or measurement criteria are used to identify these activities.

## Standard I: Quality of care

The psychiatric–mental health nurse systematically evaluates the quality of care and effectiveness of psychiatric–mental health nursing practice.

---

*Reprinted with permission from American Nurses Association: *Scope and standards of psychiatric–mental health clinical nursing practice,* Washington, DC, 2000, The Association.

## RATIONALE

The dynamic nature of the mental health care environment and the growing body of psychiatric nursing knowledge and research provide both the impetus and the means for the psychiatric–mental health nurse to be competent in clinical practice, to continue to develop professionally, and to improve the quality of patient care.

## Standard II: Performance appraisal

The psychiatric–mental health nurse evaluates his or her own practice in relation to professional practice standards and relevant statutes and regulations.

## RATIONALE

The psychiatric–mental health nurse is accountable to the public for providing competent clinical care and has an inherent responsibility as a professional to evaluate the role and performance of psychiatric–mental health nursing practice according to standards established by the profession and regulatory bodies.

## Standard III: Education

The psychiatric–mental health nurse acquires and maintains current knowledge in nursing practice.

## RATIONALE

The rapid expansion of knowledge pertaining to basic and behavioral sciences, technology, information systems, and research requires a commitment to learning throughout the psychiatric–mental health nurse's professional career. Formal education, continuing education, independent learning activities, and experiential and other learning activities are some of the means the psychiatric–mental health nurse uses to enhance nursing expertise and advance the profession.

## Standard IV: Collegiality

The psychiatric–mental health nurse interacts with and contributes to the professional development of peers, health care providers, and others as colleagues.

## RATIONALE

The psychiatric–mental health nurse is responsible for sharing knowledge, research, and clinical information with colleagues, through formal and informal teaching methods, to enhance professional growth.

## Standard V: Ethics

The psychiatric–mental health nurse's assessments, actions, and recommendations on behalf of patients are determined and implemented in an ethical manner.

### RATIONALE

The public's trust and its right to humane psychiatric–mental health care are upheld by professional nursing practice. Ethical standards describe a code of behaviors to guide professional practice. People with psychiatric–mental health needs are an especially vulnerable population. The foundation of psychiatric–mental health nursing practice is the development of a therapeutic relationship with the patient. Boundaries need to be established to safeguard the patient's well-being.

## Standard VI: Collaboration

The psychiatric–mental health nurse collaborates with the patient, significant others, and health care providers in providing care.

### RATIONALE

Psychiatric–mental health nursing practice requires a coordinated, ongoing interaction between consumers and providers to deliver comprehensive services to the patient and the community. Through the collaborative process, different abilities of health care providers are used to identify problems, communicate, and plan; implement interventions; and evaluate mental health services.

## Standard VII: Research

The psychiatric–mental health nurse contributes to nursing and mental health through the use of research methods and findings.

### RATIONALE

Nurses in psychiatric–mental health nursing are responsible for contributing to the further development of the field of mental health by participating in research. At the basic level of practice the psychiatric–mental health nurse uses research findings to improve clinical care and identifies clinical problems for research study. At the advanced level the psychiatric–mental health nurse engages and/or collaborates with others in the research process to discover, examine, and test knowledge, theories, and creative approaches to practice.

## Standard VIII: Resource use

The psychiatric–mental health nurse considers factors related to safety, effectiveness, and cost in planning and delivering patient care.

### RATIONALE

The patient is entitled to psychiatric–mental health care that is safe, effective, and affordable. As the cost of health care increases, treatment decisions must be made in such a way as to maximize resources and maintain quality of care. The psychiatric–mental health nurse seeks to provide cost-effective quality care by using the most appropriate resources and delegating care to the most appropriate, qualified health care provider.

*your* **INTERNET**
 c o n n e c t i o n

**American Nurses Association:**
www.ana.org

**American Psychiatric Nurses Association:**
www.apna.org

**Canadian Nurses Association:**
www.cna-nurses.ca

**Nursing Net:**
www.nursingnet.org

## References

1. American Nurses Association: *Nursing: a social policy statement,* Kansas City, Mo, 1980, The Association.
2. American Nurses Association: *Nursing's social policy statement,* Kansas City, Mo, 1995, The Association.
3. American Nurses Association: *Scope and standards of psychiatric–mental health clinical nursing practice,* Washington, DC, 2000, The Association.

## Suggested readings

Akhavain P et al: Collaborative practice: a nursing perspective of the psychiatric interdisciplinary treatment team, *Holistic Nurs Pract* 13(2):1, 1999.

American Nurses Association: *Code for nurses with interpretive statements,* Kansas City, Mo, 1985, The Association.

American Nurses Association: *Scope and standards of psychiatric–mental health clinical nursing practice,* Washington, DC, 2000, The Association.

Artnak K, Dimmitt J: Choosing a framework for ethical analysis in advanced practice settings: the case for casuistry, *Arch Psychiatr Nurs* 10:16, 1996.

Baier M et al: Conceptualization and measurement of insight, *Arch Psychiatr Nurs* 12:32, 1998.

Billings C: Professional insights: on peer feedback, *J Am Psychiatr Nurs Assoc* 4(3):103, 1998.

Burdick M, Stuart G, Lewis L: Measuring nursing outcomes in a psychiatric setting, *Issues Ment Health Nurs* 15:137, 1994.

Dombeck M, Brody S: Clinical supervision: a three-way mirror, *Arch Psychiatr Nurs* 9:3, 1995.

Farnam C et al: Health status risk factors of people with severe and persistent mental illness, *J Psychsoc Nurs* 37:16, 1999.

Henson R: Analysis of the concept of mutuality, *Image* 29:77, 1997.

Huang M, Alessi N: Developing trends of the World Wide Web, *Psychiatr Serv* 50(1):31, 1999.

Lamond D, Thompson C: Intuition and analysis in decision making and choice, *J Nurs Scholarship* 32(3):411, 2000.

Lyth G: Clinical supervision: a concept analysis, *J Adv Nurs* 31(3):722, 2000.

Moch S et al: Linking research and practice through discussion, *Image* 29:189, 1997.

Poster E, Dee V, Randell B: The Johnson Behavioral Systems Model as a framework for patient outcome evaluation, *J Am Psychiatr Nurs Assoc* 3:73, 1997.

Stuart G, Laraia M: *Principles and practice of psychiatric nursing,* ed 7, St Louis, 2001, Mosby.

Wilson J, Hobbs H: Therapeutic partnership: a model for clinical practice, *J Psychosoc Nurs* 33:27, 1995.

# Continuum of Psychiatric Care

8

Psychiatric nurses provide treatment throughout the continuum of care. This includes interventions related to primary, secondary, and tertiary prevention.

## Primary Prevention

Primary prevention is biological, social, or psychological intervention that promotes health and well-being or reduces the *incidence* of illness in a community by altering the causative factors before they can do harm.

### Assessment of Preventive Nursing Needs

Assessment of the need for preventive nursing measures includes identification of the following:

1. Risk factors that if present for a person make it more likely that he or she will develop a disorder.
2. Protective factors that improve a person's response to stress.
3. A target population of individuals who are vulnerable to developing mental disorders or who may display maladaptive coping responses to specific stressors or risk factors.

### Planning and Implementation

A national initiative called Healthy People 2010 has been undertaken to promote health and prevent disease in the United States. Specific nursing interventions in primary prevention include health education, environmental change, and support of social systems.

## Health education

Health education involves strengthening individuals and groups through building competence. The assumption is that many maladaptive responses result from a lack of competence. This involves a lack of perceived control over one's life, a low sense of self-efficacy, a lack of effective coping strategies, and the resulting lowered self-esteem. Health education involves the following four levels of intervention:

1. Increasing the individual's or group's awareness of issues and events related to health and illness, such as normal developmental tasks
2. Increasing one's understanding of the dimensions of potential stressors, possible outcomes (both adaptive and maladaptive), and alternative coping responses
3. Increasing one's knowledge of where and how to acquire the needed resources
4. Increasing the individual's or group's problem-solving skills, interpersonal skills, tolerance of stress and frustration, motivation, hope, and self-esteem

## Environmental change

Preventive interventions may be made to modify the individual's or group's immediate environment or the larger social system. These interventions are particularly helpful when the environment has placed new demands on the patient, does not respond to developmental needs, and provides little positive reinforcement. Environmental changes may include the following types:

1. *Economic*—allocating resources for financial aid or assistance in budgeting and managing income
2. *Work*—receiving vocational testing, guidance, education, or retraining that can result in new jobs or careers
3. *Housing*—moving to new quarters, which may mean leaving or returning to family and friends; improving existing housing; gaining or losing family, friends, or roommates
4. *Family*—attending child care facilities, nursery school, grade school, or camp; obtaining access to recreational, social, religious, or community services
5. *Political*—influencing health care structures and procedures; participating in community planning and development; addressing legislative issues

## Support of social systems

Strengthening social supports is a way of buffering or cushioning the effects of a potentially stressful event. The following four types of preventive intervention are possible:

1. Assess communities and neighborhoods to identify problem areas and high-risk groups.
2. Improve linkages between community support systems and formal mental health services.
3. Strengthen existing caregiving networks, including church groups, civic organizations, women's groups, work and neighborhood supports, and self-help groups.
4. Help the individual or group develop, maintain, expand, and use the existing social network.

## Evaluation

The nurse should consider the following points in evaluating primary prevention interventions or programs:

1. *Efficacy.* Does the program or intervention do more good than harm in the opinion of its proponents?
2. *Effectiveness.* Does the intervention do more good than harm to its target population?
3. *Efficiency.* Is the intervention being made available to those who could benefit from it? Is there optimal use of resources?
4. *Length and timing.* Does any evidence indicate the optimal length or timing of the intervention program?
5. *Harmful effects.* Are there data to suggest that the intervention may have harmful effects (e.g., unfavorable consequences of labeling)?
6. *Screening programs.* Is there any information about the program's sensitivity, specificity, and predictive accuracy?
7. *Possible high-risk groups.* Does any evidence suggest that the program would be more efficient if it applied to a specific population at increased risk?
8. *Economic analysis.* What are the results of the cost-benefit and cost-effectiveness analyses?

## Secondary Prevention

Secondary prevention involves reducing the *prevalence* of a disorder. Secondary prevention activities include early case finding, screening, and prompt, effective treatment. Crisis intervention is an important secondary prevention treatment modality.

## Crisis

A crisis is an internal disturbance that results from a stressful event or a perceived threat to the self. A person's usual repertoire of coping mechanisms becomes ineffective in dealing with the threat, and the person experiences a state of disequilibrium and a rise in anxiety. The threat, or precipitating event, can usually be identified.

The goal of crisis intervention is for the person to return to the precrisis level of functioning. Crises are self-limited in time, and the intense conflict they represent can be a period of increased vulnerability, which can stimulate personal growth. What the person does with the crisis determines whether growth or disorganization results.

### Balancing factors

In describing the resolution of a crisis, some important balancing factors need to be considered (Figure 8-1).

Successful resolution of the crisis is more likely if the individual's perception of the event is realistic rather than distorted, if situational supports are available so that others can help solve the problem, and if coping mechanisms are available to help alleviate anxiety.

### Types of crises

1. *Maturational crises.* These are transitional or developmental periods in a person's life during which psychological equilibrium is upset, such as during adolescence, parenthood, marriage, or retirement. Maturational crises require role changes. The nature and extent of the maturational crises can be influenced by the adequacy of role models, interpersonal resources, and the ease of others in accepting the new role.
2. *Situational crises.* These occur when a specific external event upsets an individual's psychological equilibrium or a group's equilibrium. Examples include the loss of a job, divorce, death, school problems, illness, and disasters.

Table 8-1 presents the four phases of human disaster response.

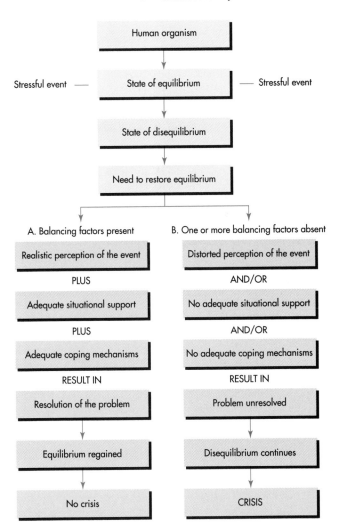

Figure 8-1
**Effect of balancing factors in a stressful event.**
(From Aguilera DC: *Crisis intervention: theory and methodology,* ed 8, St Louis, 1998, Mosby.)

Table 8-1    Four phases of disaster response

| Phase | Response |
|---|---|
| Heroic | Begins at time of impact. A cooperative spirit exists among survivors as they perform acts to save lives. |
| Honeymoon | Begins to appear 2 weeks to 6 months after the disaster. Massive relief efforts are begun. The community works together, with the help of donated resources, to begin community life again. Survivors feel a sense of security. |
| Disillusionment | Lasts from several months to a year. Begins when supportive agencies and services withdraw. A time of anger, resentment, and disappointment. Survivors feel a sense of abandonment. |
| Reconstruction | Lasts for several years. Problem solving improves. Survivors rebuild their community. |

From US Department of Health and Human Services: *Training manual for human service workers in major disasters*, Washington, DC, 1996, US Government Printing Office.

## Assessment

During the assessment phase the nurse must obtain data regarding the nature of the crisis and its effect. The nurse should make the following specific assessments:

1. *Identify the precipitating event,* including the needs that are threatened by the event and the point at which symptoms appeared.
2. *Identify the person's perception of the event,* including the underlying themes and memories associated with the event.
3. *Identify the nature and strength of the person's support system and coping resources,* including family, friends, and significant others who might be of help.
4. *Identify the person's previous strengths and coping mechanisms,* including successful and unsuccessful coping strategies.

## Planning and Implementation

Dynamics underlying the crisis are formulated, alternative solutions to the problem are explored, and steps for achieving the solutions are designated. This process is described in the Patient Education Plan for coping with crisis on page 140. *The expected outcome of nursing care is that the patient will recover from the crisis event and return to a precrisis level of functioning.* A more ambitious expected outcome would be for the patient to recover from the crisis event and attain a higher than precrisis level of functioning with improved quality of life. Four levels of crisis intervention exist, representing a hierarchy from the most basic (level 1) to the most in-depth (level 4):

1. *Environmental manipulation.* These interventions directly change the person's physical or interpersonal situation for the purpose of providing situational support or removing stress.
2. *General support.* This provides individuals with the feeling that the nurse is on their side and will help them. The nurse's demonstration of warmth, acceptance, empathy, and caring results in this type of support.
3. *Generic approach.* This type of crisis intervention is designed to reach individuals at high risk and large numbers of people as soon as possible. It applies a specific method to all people facing a similar crisis, such as assisting disaster victims to work through the grieving process.
4. *Individual approach.* This approach involves the diagnosis and treatment of a specific problem in a specific patient. The individual approach is effective with all types of crises and in a combination of crises or when homicidal or suicidal risk exists.

The techniques of crisis intervention are active, focal, and explorative. They are not interpretive because the goal is quick resolution of an immediate problem. Table 8-2 summarizes crisis intervention techniques. Table 8-3 describes interventions for working with individuals and families with stress resulting from crises.

## Evaluation

1. Has the person returned to the precrisis level of functioning?
2. Have the person's original needs, which were threatened by the precipitating or stressful event, been met?

## Patient Education Plan:  Coping with Crisis

| Content | Instructional Activities | Evaluation |
| --- | --- | --- |
| Describe the crisis event. | Ask about the details of the crisis event, including:<br>1. A timeline of the crisis event<br>2. Who was affected<br>3. The events of the crisis<br>4. Any precipitating events | Patient describes the crisis event in full detail. |
| Explore feelings, thoughts, and behaviors related to the crisis event. | Determine precrisis level of functioning.<br>Discuss patient's perception of the crisis.<br>Determine acute and long-term needs, threats, and challenges. | Patient discusses precrisis level of functioning and perceptions of the crisis.<br>Patient's needs are identified. |
| Identify coping mechanisms. | Ask how stressful events have been handled in the past.<br>Analyze whether these approaches are adaptive or maladaptive for the current crisis event.<br>Suggest additional coping strategies. | Patient identifies adaptive coping mechanisms for the current crisis event. |
| Develop a plan for coping adaptively with the crisis event. | Reinforce adaptive coping mechanisms and health defenses.<br>With patient, construct a coping plan specific for the aftermath of the crisis event. | Patient develops a plan for coping with the crisis event. |
| Assign patient activities from the coping plan. | Review implementation of the coping plan.<br>Help patient generalize coping strategies for use in future crisis events. | Patient reports satisfaction with coping abilities and level of functioning. |

Table 8-2 Techniques of crisis intervention

| Technique | Definition | Example |
|-----------|-----------|---------|
| Catharsis | The release of feelings that take place as the patient talks about emotionally charged areas | "Tell me about how you have been feeling since you lost your job." |
| Clarification | Encouraging patients to express more clearly the relationship between certain events in their life | "I've noticed that after you have an argument with your husband, you become sick and can't leave your bed." |
| Suggestion | Process of influencing individuals so that they accept an idea or belief, particularly the belief that the nurse can help them feel better | "Many other people have found it helpful to talk about this, and I think you will too." |
| Reinforcement of behavior | Giving patients positive responses to adaptive behavior | "That's the first time you were able to defend yourself with your boss, and it went very well. I'm so pleased that you were able to do it." |
| Support of defenses | Encouraging the use of defenses that result in adaptive gratification and discouraging those that result in maladaptive gratification | "Going for a bicycle ride when you were so angry was very helpful, because when you returned, you and your wife were able to talk things through." |
| Raising self-esteem | Helping patients to regain feelings of self-worth | "You are a very strong person to be able to manage the family all this time. I think you will be able to handle this situation too." |
| Exploration of solutions | Examining alternative modes of action geared toward solving the immediate problem | "You seem to know many people in the computer field. Couldn't you contact some of them to see if they might know of available jobs?" |

3. Have the person's maladaptive behaviors or symptoms subsided?
4. Have the person's adaptive coping mechanisms begun to function again?
5. Does the person have a strong support system on which to rely?
6. What has the person learned from this experience that may be helpful in coping with future crises?

Table 8-3    Nursing interventions for crisis events

| Target Areas | Nursing Interventions |
|---|---|
| Basic needs | Provide liaison to social agencies. |
| Physical deficits | Attend to physical emergencies. |
|  | Refer to other health care providers as necessary. |
| Psychological effects |  |
| Shock | Listen attentively to the crisis details. |
| Confusion | Give nurturing support; permit regression. |
| Denial | Permit intermittent denial; identify patient's primary concern. |
| Anxiety | Provide structure; enact antianxiety interventions. |
| Lethargy/heroics | Encourage sublimation and constructive activity. |
| Protective factors |  |
| Coping | Encourage patient's favored, adaptive coping mechanisms; emphasize rationalization, humor, and sublimation. |
| Self-efficacy | Support patient's previous successes and belief in own abilities; dilute irrational self-doubts; emphasize power of expectations to produce results. |
| Support | Add social supports to patient's world; provide professional support; refer for counseling when necessary; help patient generalize new coping strategies. |

Modified from Hardin SB. In McBride AB, Austin JK, editors: *Psychiatric–mental health nursing: integrating the behavioral and biological sciences,* Philadelphia, 1996, WB Saunders.

# Tertiary Prevention

Tertiary prevention activities attempt to reduce the severity of a disorder and its associated *disability*.

## Rehabilitation

Rehabilitation is the process of enabling individuals to return to the highest possible level of functioning. Psychiatric rehabilitation developed from a need to create opportunities for people diagnosed with severe mental illness to live, learn, and work in community environments of their choice. Rehabilitation proposes that those with mental illnesses should be perceived as people with disabilities. Similar to those with physical disabilities, people with psychiatric disabilities need a wide range of services, often for extended periods. Psychiatric rehabilitation uses a person-centered, people-to-people approach that differs from the traditional medical model of care (Table 8-4).

## Assessment of Rehabilitative Nursing Needs

### The individual

1. Identification of the nature and intensity of stressors
2. Exploration of the advantages the patient experiences by being disabled (secondary gain)

Table 8-4   Comparison of psychiatric rehabilitation and traditional medical model of care

| Psychiatric Rehabilitation | Traditional Medical Model |
| --- | --- |
| Focus on wellness and health, not symptoms | Focus on disease/illness and symptoms |
| Based on patient's abilities and functional behavior | Based on patient's disabilities and intrapsychic functioning |
| Caregiving in natural settings | Treatment in institutional settings |
| Adult-to-adult relationship | Expert-to-patient relationship |
| Minimal medications used; minor symptoms tolerated | Medications used until symptoms controlled |
| Case management in partnership with patient | Decision making and treatment choice by physician |
| Emphasis on strengths, self-help, and interdependence | Emphasis on dependence and compliance |

3. Identification of coping resources
4. Assessment of community living skills (Table 8-5)

### The family

1. Analysis of the family structure, including developmental stage, roles, responsibilities, norms, and values
2. Exploration of family attitudes toward the mentally ill member
3. Analysis of the emotional climate around the family
4. Identification of the social supports available to the family, including extended family, friends, financial support, religious involvement, and community contacts
5. Identification of the family's understanding of the patient's problem and the plan of care

Table 8-6 describes the categories and definitions of support needs expressed by family caregivers.

### The community

1. Assessment of existing community agencies that provide services to mentally ill people and their families
2. Identification of gaps in available services or in the effectiveness of existing services

Table 8-7 describes the services needed by patients with serious and persistent mental illness.

## Planning and Implementation

### The individual

1. Mutually determine realistic nurse-patient goals based on the patient's nursing diagnoses.
2. Focus on fostering independence by maximizing the patient's strengths and potential.
3. Facilitate referrals to alternative care programs that assist the patient to function independently or interdependently in the community; may be psychosocial rehabilitation programs or community support programs.
4. Assist the patient to become involved in a social skills training program that uses cognitive and behavioral techniques.
5. Identify resistances to change, if any, and assist the patient to overcome the resistance or find acceptable alternatives.
6. Teach the patient about relevant health care needs, including physical health and mental health. This is discussed in the

Table 8-5   Potential skilled activities needed to achieve goal of psychiatric rehabilitation

| Physical | Emotional | Intellectual |
|---|---|---|
| **Living Skills** | | |
| Personal hygiene | Human relations | Money management |
| Physical fitness | Self-control | Use of community resources |
| Use of public transportation | Selective reward | Goal setting |
| Cooking | Stigma reduction | Problem development |
| Shopping | Problem solving | |
| Cleaning | Conversational skills | |
| Sports participation | | |
| Using recreational facilities | | |
| **Learning Skills** | | |
| Being quiet | Speechmaking | Reading |
| Paying attention | Question asking | Writing |
| Staying seated | Volunteering answers | Arithmetic |
| Observing | Following directions | Study skills |
| Punctuality | Asking for directions | Hobby activities |
| | Listening | Typing |
| **Working Skills** | | |
| Punctuality | Job interviewing | Job qualifying |
| Use of job tools | Job decision making | Job seeking |
| Job strength | Human relations | Specific job tasks |
| Job transportation | Self-control | |
| Specific job tasks | Job keeping | |
| | Specific job tasks | |

From Anthony WA: *Principles of psychiatric rehabilitation,* Baltimore, 1980, University Park Press.

Table 8-6    Categories and definitions of support needs expressed by family caregivers

Emotional Support Categories

| | |
|---|---|
| Acceptance | Absence of stigmatization; acceptance of caregiver despite being related to a mentally ill patient |
| Commitment | Demonstrating to caregiver a commitment to patient's well-being; sharing the burden of caregiving, if only through contact with caregiver |
| Social involvement | Social contacts and companionship for caregiver |
| Affective | Showing caring and love for caregiver, including concern for well-being (with qualities of sympathy, compassion, and occasionally empathy) |
| Mutuality | Reciprocity in supportive exchanges |

Feedback Support Categories

| | |
|---|---|
| Affirmation | Validation of actions, feelings, and decisions associated with caregiving role |
| Listening | Active listening by support person; providing a "sounding board"; allowing for unburdening by caregiver |
| Talking | Opportunity to talk with another person (without the quality of active listening, emotional presence, or the feeling of unburdening) |

From Norbeck J et al: Social support needs of family caregivers of psychiatric patients from three age groups, *Nurs Res* 40:208, 1991.

Patient Education Plan on page 150 for psychiatric patients in rehabilitation programs.

7. Act as the patient's advocate in dealing with significant others and community agencies.
8. Assist the patient to develop a reliable social support network.

## The family

1. Establish a partnership with the family with the goal of assisting the patient.

Table 8-6   Categories and definitions of support needs expressed by family caregivers—cont'd

| Informational or Cognitive Support Categories | |
| --- | --- |
| Illness information | Information about patient's illness, care, or supervision |
| Behavior management | Information about behavior management strategies |
| Coping | Advice about personal coping strategies for caregiver |
| Decision making | Help in decision-making process regarding caregiving issues; offering solutions |
| Perspective | Supportive interactions that give caregiver a new perspective about caregiving or about caregiving situation |
| **Instrumental Support Categories** | |
| Resources | Help in locating resources, negotiating systems, or advocating for needs |
| Respite | Providing time off for caregiver and support for meeting caregiver's needs |
| Care/help | Providing help with actual tasks of caregiving, including physical care assistance and monitoring activities (watching patient's behavior and setting limits) |
| Backup | Help available when needed, including financial help |
| Household | Help with such home activities as repairs, grocery shopping, or housecleaning |

2. Provide the patient and family with psychoeducation about the mental illness and the coping skills that will assist with successful community living (Box 8-1).
3. Provide the family with feedback on the effectiveness of their interactions.
4. Refer the family for formal family therapy if needed.
5. Refer the family to a self-help group.
6. Assist the family to find respite care services.
7. Provide the family with information on available crisis intervention services.

Table 8-7    Comprehensive array of services and opportunities for patients with serious mental illness

| Basic Needs and Opportunities | Special Needs and Opportunities |
| --- | --- |
| Shelter | General Medical Services |
| *Protected (with health, rehabilitative, or social services provided on site)* | Physician assessment and care |
| Hospital | Nursing assessment and care |
| Nursing home | Dentist assessment and care |
| Intermediate care facility | Physical and occupational therapy |
| Crisis facility | Speech and hearing therapy |
| *Semiindependent (linked to services)* | Nutrition counseling |
| Family home | Medication counseling |
| Group home | Home health services |
| Cooperative apartment | |
| Foster care home | Mental Health Services |
| Emergency housing facility | Acute treatment services |
| Other board and care home | Crisis stabilization |
| *Independent (access to services)* | Diagnosis and assessment |
| Apartment | Medication monitoring (psychoactive) |
| Home | Self-medication training |
| | Psychotherapies |
| Food, Clothing, and Household Management | Hospitalization: acute and long-term care |
| Fully provided meals | Habilitation and Rehabilitation |
| Food purchase and preparation assistance | Social and recreational skills development |
| Access to food stamps | Life skills development |
| Homemaker service | Leisure time activities |

From Department of Health and Human Services Steering Committee on the Chronically Mentally Ill: *Toward a national plan for the chronically mentally ill,* Pub No (ADM) 81-1077, Washington, DC, 1981, US Government Printing Office.

## The community

1. Provide education about mental health and mental illness to community groups.
2. Participate in community advocacy groups to encourage the development of comprehensive mental health services.

Table 8-7   Comprehensive array of services and opportunities for patients with serious mental illness—cont'd

| Basic Needs and Opportunities | Special Needs and Opportunities |
| --- | --- |
| Income or Financial Support | Vocational |
| Access to entitlements | Prevocational assessment |
| Employment | counseling |
| | Sheltered work opportunities |
| Meaningful Activities | Transitional employment |
| Work opportunities | Job development and |
| Recreation | placement |
| Education | |
| Religious and spiritual | Social Services |
| Human and social interaction | Family support |
| | Community support assistance |
| Integrative Services | Housing and milieu |
| Patient identification and | management |
| outreach | Legal services |
| Individual assessment and | Entitlement assistance |
| service planning | |
| Case service and resource | |
| management | |
| Advocacy and community | |
| organization | |
| Community information | |
| Education and support | |

3. Foster the development of collaborative networks among community groups involved in or advocating mental health services.
4. Be aware of and involved in the political process at the local, state, and national levels.

Patient Education Plan: Coping with Psychiatric Illness

| Content | Instructional Activities | Evaluation |
| --- | --- | --- |
| Identify and describe common psychiatric diagnoses. | Provide handouts outlining behaviors. Discuss coping behaviors. Assign homework from lay literature. Compare mental illness to physical illness. | Patient recognizes characteristics of the diagnosis. Patient distinguishes between cure and coping. |
| Describe the role of stress in contributing to psychiatric disorders. | Sensitize patient to signs of increased stress. Define stress as a test of coping skills. Teach relaxation exercises. | Patient verbalizes level of stress. Patient performs relaxation exercises and describes a reduction in perceived stress. |
| Assist to gain a sense of control by recognizing personal pattern of signs and symptoms. | Provide feedback when symptomatic behavior occurs. Instruct patient to keep a diary of behaviors and to identify symptoms. | Patient consistently labels symptoms and seeks professional help when necessary. |
| Assist in development of social skills to enable participation in vocational and recreational activities. | Role-play social interaction in a variety of situations. Plan field trips to community activities. Arrange supervised vocational training in real work settings. | Patient participates in progressively more independent social and work activities. |

| Identify and describe community support systems. | Provide a list of community support programs, including self-help groups, mental health care agencies, and social agencies. Invite representatives of programs to speak to patient group. Escort to first agency contact. | Patient selects community programs that offer needed resources. Patient is able to access agency independently. |
| --- | --- | --- |
| Describe and discuss psychoactive medications. | Instruct about actions, side effects, and contraindications to common psychoactive medications. Distribute handouts describing patient's medications. Suggest systems to help patient remember when to take medication and how much. | Patient describes characteristics of prescribed medications. Patient reports effects of prescribed medications. Patient takes medication as prescribed. |

Modified from Buckwalter KC, Kerfoot KM: Teaching patients self care: a critical aspect of psychiatric discharge planning, *J Psychosoc Nurs Ment Health Serv* 20:15, 1982.

---

### Box 8-1    Elements of a Plan for Psychoeducation

- Signs and symptoms
- Natural course of the illness
- Possible etiologies
- Diagnostic tests and measures
- Indicated lifestyle changes
- Treatment options
- Expected treatment outcomes
- Medication effects and side effects
- Therapeutic strategies
- Adaptive coping responses
- Potential compliance problems
- Early warning signs of relapse
- Balancing needs and taking care of self

---

## Evaluation

### Program evaluation

1. Individual program evaluation may include the following:
   - Cost effectiveness
   - Licensure status
   - Accomplishment of stated objectives
   - Patient outcomes
   - Patient or staff satisfaction
2. Commonalities among a group of programs may also be assessed.
3. Programs may be evaluated at a systems level for relevance to community needs and resource utilization.

### Patient evaluation

1. The needs and levels of functioning of individual patients tend to change over time. The nurse must consider this when evaluating patient progress.
2. Evaluation criteria for individual patients must be based on the individual's behavior and treatment goals. Criteria that have been identified for evaluation of patient response to rehabilitation programs include the following:
   - Involvement in community activities, including rehabilitation programs

- Hospitalization recidivism rates
- Ability to find and maintain employment

*your*INTERNET
c o n n e c t i o n

American Institute of Stress:
www.stress.org

American Public Health Association:
www.apha.org

American Red Cross:
www.redcross.org/services/disaster

Crisis, Grief, and Healing:
www.webhealing.com

Healthy People 2010:
web.health.gov/healthypeople

help! Consumer's Guide to Mental Health
Information:
www.iComm.ca/madmagic/help/help.html

International Association of Psychosocial
Rehabilitation Services:
www.iapsrs.org

NAMI: National Alliance for the Mentally Ill:
www.nami.org

National Mental Health Association:
www.nmha.org

## Suggested readings

Adams S et al: Mental health disaster response: nursing interventions across the life span, *J Psychosoc Nurs* 37:11, 1999.

Aguilera D: *Crisis intervention: theory and methodology,* ed 8, St Louis, 1998, Mosby.

Barton R: Psychosocial rehabilitation services in community support systems: a review of outcomes and policy recommendations, *Psychiatr Serv* 50:525, 1999.

Bauer M, McBride L: Psychoeducation: conceptual framework and practical considerations, *J Pract Psychiatry Behav Health* 3:18, 1997.

Donegan K, Palmer-Erbs V: Promoting the importance of work for persons with psychiatric disabilities: the role of the psychiatric nurse, *J Psychosoc Nurs Ment Health Serv* 36:13, 1998.

Gasque-Carter K, Curlee M: The educational needs of families of mentally ill adults: the South Carolina experience, *Psychiatr Serv* 50:520, 1999.

Guo G et al: Assessing the impact of community-based mobile crisis services on preventing hospitalization, *Psychiatric Services* 52:223-228, 2001.

Hamera E et al: Reciprocity between individuals with severe and persistent mental illness and their family members, *J Am Psychiatr Nurs Assoc* 4:182, 1998.

Hoff L, Adamowski K: *Creating excellence in crisis care: a guide to effective training and program designs*, San Francisco, 1998, Jossey-Bass.

Holley H et al: Moving psychiatric patients from hospital to community: views of patients, providers and families, *Psychiatr Serv* 49(4):513, 1998.

Jorm A: Mental health literacy: public knowledge and beliefs about mental disorders, *Br J Psychiatry* 177:396, 2000.

Mrazek P, Haggerty R: *Reducing risks for mental disorders,* Washington, DC, 1994, National Academy Press.

Osterman J, Chemtob C: Emergency intervention for acute traumatic stress, *Psychiatr Serv* 50(6):739, 1999.

Payson A et al: Health teaching needs of clients with serious and persistent mental illness: client and provider perspectives, *J Psychosoc Nurs Ment Health Serv* 36:32, 1998.

Pollio D et al: Content and curriculum in psychoeducation groups for families of persons with severe mental illness, *Psychiatr Serv* 49(6):816, 1998.

Public Health Service: *Healthy people 2010,* Washington, DC, 2000, US Department of Health and Human Services.

Salzer M: Consumer empowerment in mental health organizations: concept, benefits and impediments, *Adm Policy Ment Health* 24:425, 1997.

Saunders J: Family functioning in families providing care for a family member with schizophrenia, *Issues Ment Health Nurs* 20:95, 1999.

Schofield R: Empowerment education for individuals with serious mental illness, *J Psychosoc Nurs* 36(11):35, 1998.

Silverstein S et al: Identifying and addressing cognitive barriers to rehabilitation readiness, *Psychiatr Serv* 49:34, 1998.

Skinner E et al: Met and unmet needs for assistance and quality of life for people with severe and persistent mental disorders, *Ment Health Serv Res* 1(2):109, 1999.

Stuart G, Laraia M: *Principles and practice of psychiatric nursing,* ed 7, St Louis, 2001, Mosby.

Tudor K: *Mental health promotion,* London, 1996, Routledge.

Turnbull G: A review of post-traumatic stress disorder, part II, treatment, *Int J Care Injured* 29(3):169, 1998.

Weaver JD: *Disasters: mental health interventions,* Sarasota, Fla, 1995, Professional Resource Press.

Wilson J, Hobbs H: The family educator: a professional resource for families, *J Psychosoc Nurs Ment Health Serv* 37:22, 1999.

Zealberg J, Hardesty S, Tyson S: Mental health clinicians role in responding to critical incidents in the community, *Psychiatr Serv* 49(3):301, 1998.

Zealberg J, Santos A, Puckett J: Comprehensive emergency mental health care, Dunmore, Pa, 1996, Norton.

# APPLYING PRINCIPLES IN NURSING PRACTICE

# Anxiety Responses and Anxiety Disorders

## Continuum of Anxiety Responses

Anxiety is a diffuse, vague apprehension associated with feelings of uncertainty and helplessness. This emotion has no specific object. It is subjectively experienced and communicated interpersonally. It is different from fear, which is the intellectual appraisal of danger. Anxiety is the emotional response to that appraisal. The capacity to be anxious is necessary for survival, but severe levels of anxiety are incompatible with life (Figure 9-1). Anxiety disorders are the most common psychiatric problems in the United States (Box 9-1).

The levels of anxiety follow:

1. *Mild anxiety* is associated with the tension of daily living; it makes a person alert and increases the person's perceptual field. This anxiety can motivate learning and produce growth and creativity.

2. *Moderate anxiety* allows a person to focus on immediate concerns and block out the periphery. It narrows the person's perceptual field. The person thus experiences selective inattention but can focus on more areas if directed to so do.

3. *Severe anxiety* greatly reduces a person's perceptual field. The person tends to focus on a specific detail and not think about anything else. All behavior is aimed at obtaining relief. The person needs much direction to focus on any other area.

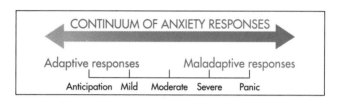

Figure 9-1
Continuum of anxiety responses.

---

### Box 9-1    Prevalence of Anxiety Disorders

- More than 23 million people—approximately one out of every four individuals—in the United States are affected by these debilitating illnesses each year.
- Anxiety disorders cost the United States $46.6 billion in 1990 in direct and indirect costs, almost one third of the total U.S. mental health bill of $148 billion.
- People with panic disorder spend heavily on health services. One survey found that a patient with panic attacks made an average of 37 medical visits a year, compared with five in the general population.
- Less than 25% of people with panic disorders seek help, mainly because they do not realize their physical symptoms (e.g., heart palpitations, chest pains, shortness of breath) are caused by a psychiatric problem.

---

4. *Panic level of anxiety* is associated with awe, dread, and terror. Details are blown out of proportion. Because of experiencing a loss of control, the person is unable to do things even with direction. Panic involves the disorganization of the personality and results in increased motor activity, decreased ability to relate to others, distorted perceptions, and loss of rational thought. This level of anxiety is incompatible with life; if it continues for a long period, exhaustion and death result.

## Assessment

## Behaviors

Anxiety can be expressed directly through physiological and behavioral changes and indirectly through the formation of symptoms or coping mechanisms in an attempt to defend against anxiety. The intensity of the behaviors increases as the level of anxiety increases. Tables 9-1 and 9-2 present the physiological, behavioral, cognitive, and affective responses to anxiety.

## Predisposing Factors

Various theories have been developed to explain the origins of anxiety:

1. In the *psychoanalytical* view, anxiety is the emotional conflict that takes place between two elements of the personality: the id and the superego. The id represents instinctual drives and primitive impulses, whereas the superego reflects conscience and culturally acquired restrictions. The ego, or I, serves to mediate the demands of these two opposing elements, and anxiety functions to warn the ego that it is in danger of being overtaken.

2. In the *interpersonal* view, anxiety arises from the fear of interpersonal disapproval and rejection. It is also related to developmental traumas, such as separations and losses, that lead to specific vulnerabilities. People with low self-esteem are particularly vulnerable to the development of high anxiety.

3. In the *behavioral* view, anxiety is a product of frustration, which is anything that interferes with a person's ability to attain a desired goal. Other behaviorists regard anxiety as a learned drive based on an innate desire to avoid pain. Learning theorists believe that individuals who have been exposed in early life to intense fears are more likely to be predisposed to anxiety in later life. Conflict theorists view anxiety as the clashing of two opposing interests. They believe a reciprocal relationship exists between conflict and anxiety: conflict produces anxiety, and anxiety produces feelings of helplessness, which in turn increase the perceived conflict.

4. *Family studies* show that anxiety disorders typically occur within families. Also, anxiety disorders overlap, as do anxiety disorders and depression.

Table 9-1    Physiological responses to anxiety

| Body System | Responses |
| --- | --- |
| Cardiovascular | Palpitations |
| | Heart "racing" |
| | Increased blood pressure |
| | Faintness* |
| | Actual fainting* |
| | Decreased blood pressure* |
| | Decreased pulse rate* |
| Respiratory | Rapid breathing |
| | Shortness of breath |
| | Pressure on chest |
| | Shallow breathing |
| | Lump in throat |
| | Choking sensation |
| | Gasping |
| Neuromuscular | Increased reflexes |
| | Startle reaction |
| | Eyelid twitching |
| | Insomnia |
| | Tremors |
| | Rigidity |
| | Fidgeting, pacing |
| | Strained face |
| | Generalized weakness |
| | Wobbly legs |
| | Clumsy movement |
| Gastrointestinal | Loss of appetite |
| | Revulsion toward food |
| | Abdominal discomfort |
| | Abdominal pain* |
| | Nausea* |
| | Heartburn* |
| | Diarrhea* |
| Urinary tract | Pressure to urinate* |
| | Frequent urination* |
| Skin | Face flushed |
| | Localized sweating (palms) |
| | Itching |
| | Hot and cold spells |
| | Face pale |
| | Generalized sweating |

*Parasympathetic response.

Table 9-2   Behavioral, cognitive, and affective responses to anxiety

| System | Responses |
|--------|-----------|
| Behavioral | Restlessness |
| | Physical tension |
| | Tremors |
| | Startle reaction |
| | Rapid speech |
| | Lack of coordination |
| | Accident proneness |
| | Interpersonal withdrawal |
| | Inhibition |
| | Flight |
| | Avoidance |
| | Hyperventilation |
| | Hypervigilance |
| Cognitive | Impaired attention |
| | Poor concentration |
| | Forgetfulness |
| | Errors in judgment |
| | Preoccupation |
| | Blocking of thoughts |
| | Decreased perceptual field |
| | Reduced creativity |
| | Diminished productivity |
| | Confusion |
| | Hypervigilance |
| | Self-consciousness |
| | Loss of objectivity |
| | Fear of losing control |
| | Frightening visual images |
| | Fear of injury or death |
| | Flashbacks |
| | Nightmares |

*Continued*

Table 9-2    Behavioral, cognitive, and affective responses to anxiety—cont'd

| System | Responses |
|--------|-----------|
| Affective | Edginess |
| | Impatience |
| | Uneasiness |
| | Tension |
| | Nervousness |
| | Fearfulness |
| | Alarm |
| | Terror |
| | Jitteriness |
| | Jumpiness |
| | Numbness |
| | Guilt |
| | Shame |

5. *Biological studies* show that the brain contains specific receptors for benzodiazepines, drugs that enhance the inhibitory neuroregulator γ-aminobutyric acid (GABA), which plays a major role in biological mechanisms relating to anxiety. In addition, a person's general health and a family history of anxiety have a marked effect on predisposition to anxiety. Anxiety may accompany physical disorders and further reduce a person's capacity to cope with stressors.

## Precipitating Stressors

Precipitating stressors may be derived from internal or external sources. They can be grouped into the following two categories:

1. *Threats to physical integrity* include impending physiological disability or decreased capacity to perform the activities of daily living.
2. *Threats to self-system* suggest harm to the person's identity, self-esteem, and integrated social functioning.

## Appraisal of Stressor

The understanding of anxiety requires integration of many factors, including knowledge from psychoanalytical, interpersonal, behavioral, genetic, and biological perspectives. Appraisal encourages the assessment of patient behaviors and perceptions in developing appropriate nursing interventions. It also suggests a variety of causative factors and stresses the interrelationship among them in explaining the present behavior. Thus a true understanding of anxiety is holistic in nature.

## Coping Resources

The individual can cope with stress and anxiety by mobilizing coping resources in the environment. Such coping resources as economic assets, problem-solving abilities, social supports, and cultural beliefs can help the person integrate stressful experiences and adopt successful coping strategies.

## Coping Mechanisms

When experiencing anxiety, the individual uses various coping mechanisms to try to allay it; the inability to cope with anxiety constructively is a primary cause of pathological behavior. The pattern the person typically uses to cope with mild anxiety tends to remain dominant when anxiety becomes more intense. Mild levels of anxiety are often handled without conscious thought. Moderate and severe levels of anxiety elicit the following two types of coping mechanisms:

1. *Task-oriented reactions* are conscious, action-oriented attempts to meet realistically the demands of the stress situation.
   - *Attack behavior* is used to remove or overcome an obstacle to satisfy a need.
   - *Withdrawal behavior* is used to remove the self either physically or psychologically from the source of the threat.
   - *Compromise behavior* is used to change the person's usual way of operating, substitute goals, or sacrifice aspects of personal needs.
2. *Ego defense mechanisms* help to cope with mild and moderate anxiety. Because they operate on a relatively unconscious level and involve a degree of self-deception and reality distortion, however, they can be maladaptive responses to stress. Table 9-3 summarizes some of the most common ego defense mechanisms.

Table 9-3    Ego defense mechanisms

| Defense Mechanism | Definition | Example |
|---|---|---|
| Compensation | Process by which a person makes up for a self-image deficiency by strongly emphasizing some other feature the person regards as an asset | Mr. L, a 42-year-old businessman, perceives his small physical stature negatively. He tries to overcome this by being aggressive, forceful, and controlling in his business dealings. |
| Denial | Avoidance of disagreeable realities by ignoring or refusing to recognize them; probably simplest and most primitive of all defense mechanisms | Mrs. P has just been told that her breast biopsy indicates a malignancy. When her husband visits her that evening, she says that no one has discussed the laboratory results with her. |
| Displacement | Shift of emotion from a person or object toward which it was originally directed to another usually neutral or less dangerous person or object | Four-year-old Timmy is angry because he has just been punished by his mother for drawing on his bedroom walls. He begins to play "war" with his toy soldiers and has them fight with each other. |
| Dissociation | Separation of any group of mental or behavioral processes from the rest of consciousness or identity | A man brought to the emergency room by the police is unable to explain who he is and where he lives or works. |
| Identification | Process by which a person tries to become like someone the person admires by taking on the other's thoughts, mannerisms, or tastes | Sally, 15 years old, has her hair styled similarly to her young English teacher, whom she admires. |
| Intellectualization | Excessive reasoning or logic used to avoid experiencing disturbing feelings | A woman avoids dealing with her anxiety in shopping malls by explaining that she is saving time and money by not going into them. |

*Continued*

| Introjection | Intense type of identification in which a person incorporates qualities or values of another person or group into own ego structure; one of the earliest mechanisms of children; important in formation of conscience | Eight-year-old Jimmy tells his 3-year-old sister, "Don't scribble in your book of nursery rhymes. Just look at the pretty pictures." |
|---|---|---|
| Isolation | Splitting off of emotional components of a thought, which may be temporary or long term | A second-year medical student dissects a cadaver for her anatomy course without being disturbed by thoughts of death. |
| Projection | Attributing own thoughts or impulses, particularly intolerable wishes, emotional feelings, or motivations, to another person | A young woman who denies she has sexual feelings about a co-worker accuses him of trying to seduce her. |
| Rationalization | Offering a socially acceptable or apparently logical explanation to justify or make acceptable impulses, feelings, behaviors, and motives | John fails an examination and complains that the lectures were not well organized or clearly presented. |
| Reaction formation | Development of conscious attitudes and behavior patterns that are opposite to what a person really feels or would like to do | A married woman who feels attracted to one of her husband's friends treats him rudely. |
| Regression | Retreat to behavior characteristic of an earlier level of development when confronted by stress | Four-year-old Nicole, who has been toilet-trained for more than a year, begins to wet her pants again when her new baby brother is brought home from the hospital. |

Table 9-3 Ego defense mechanisms—cont'd

| Defense Mechanism | Definition | Example |
| --- | --- | --- |
| Repression | Involuntary exclusion of a painful or conflictual thought, impulse, or memory from awareness; the primary ego defense, which other mechanisms tend to reinforce | Mr. T does not recall hitting his wife when she was pregnant. |
| Splitting | Viewing people and situations as either all good or all bad; failure to integrate the positive and negative qualities of the self | A friend tells you that you are the most wonderful person in the world one day, then how much she hates you the next day. |
| Sublimation | Acceptance of a socially approved substitute goal for a drive whose normal channel of expression is blocked | Ed has an impulsive or physically aggressive nature. He tries out for the football team and becomes a star tackle. |
| Suppression | Process often listed as a defense mechanism, but really a conscious analogue of repression; intentional exclusion of material from consciousness; at times may lead to subsequent repression | A young man at work finds he is thinking so much about his date that evening that it is interfering with his work. He decides to put it out of his mind until he leaves the office for the day. |
| Undoing | Act or communication that partially negates a previous one; primitive defense mechanism | Larry makes a passionate declaration of love to Sue on a date. On their next meeting he treats her formally and distantly. |

The formulation of a nursing diagnosis requires that the nurse determine the quality (appropriateness) of the patient's response, the quantity (level) of the patient's anxiety, and the adaptive or maladaptive nature of the coping mechanism used.

The box below presents the primary and related NANDA nursing diagnoses for anxiety responses. A complete nursing

## NANDA Nursing Diagnoses Related to Anxiety Responses

Adjustment, Impaired
*Anxiety
  Breathing pattern, Ineffective
  Communication, Impaired verbal
  Confusion, Acute
*Coping, Ineffective
  Coping, Ineffective community
  Diarrhea
*Fear
  Health maintenance, Ineffective
  Injury, Risk for
  Memory, Impaired
  Nutrition, Imbalanced
  Post-trauma syndrome
  Powerlessness
  Powerlessness, Risk for
  Relocation stress syndrome, Risk for
  Self-esteem, Risk for situational low
  Self-esteem, Situational low
  Sensory perception, Disturbed
  Sleep pattern, Disturbed
  Social interaction, Impaired
  Thought processes, Disturbed
  Urinary elimination, Impaired

*Primary nursing diagnosis for anxiety.
*From North American Nursing Diagnosis Association:* NANDA nursing diagnoses: definitions and classification 2000-2001, *Philadelphia, 2001, The Association.*

assessment would include all maladaptive responses of the patient. Many additional nursing problems would be identified in the way that the patient's anxiety reciprocally influenced other areas of life.

## Related Medical Diagnoses

Many patients experiencing transient or less severe anxiety have no medically diagnosed health problem. However, patients with more severe levels of anxiety most often have neurotic disorders that fall into the category of anxiety disorders in DSM-IV-TR. The box on pages 171-173 describes these disorders.

## Outcome Identification

The expected outcome for patients with maladaptive anxiety responses follows:

*The patient will demonstrate adaptive ways of coping with stress.*

## Planning

Patients need to develop the capacity to tolerate mild anxiety and use it consciously and constructively. In this way the self becomes stronger and more integrated. A Patient Education Plan for teaching the relaxation response is presented on pages 176 and 177.

## Implementation

Empirically validated treatments for some of the medical diagnoses related to anxiety disorders are summarized in Table 9-4.

### Intervening in Severe and Panic Levels of Anxiety

The highest-priority nursing goals should address lowering the patient's severe or panic levels of anxiety, and related nursing interventions should be supportive and protective. See the Nursing Treatment Plan Summary related to severe and panic levels of anxiety.

### Intervening in Moderate Level Anxiety

When a patient's anxiety is reduced to the mild or moderate level, the nurse may implement insight-oriented or reeducative nursing interventions. These interventions involve the patient in a

## DSM-IV-TR Medical Diagnoses Related to Anxiety Responses

| DSM-IV-TR Medical Diagnosis | Essential Features |
| --- | --- |
| Panic disorder without agoraphobia | Recurrent unexpected panic attacks (Box 9-2); at least one of the attacks has been followed by a month or more of (1) persistent concern about having additional attacks, (2) worry about the implications of the attack or its consequences, or (3) a significant change in behavior related to the attacks; also, the absence of agoraphobia. |
| Panic disorder with agoraphobia | Meets the above criteria plus the presence of agoraphobia, which is anxiety about being in places or situations from which escape might be difficult (or embarrassing) or in which help may not be available in the event of having an unexpected or situationally predisposed panic attack. Agoraphobic fears typically involve characteristic clusters of situations that include being outside the home alone; being in a crowd or standing in a line; being on a bridge; and traveling in a bus, train, or car. Agoraphobic situations are avoided, are endured with marked distress or with anxiety about having a panic attack, or require the presence of a companion. |
| Agoraphobia without history of panic disorder | Presence of agoraphobia and has never met criteria for panic disorder. |

*Modified from American Psychiatric Association: Diagnostic and statistical manual of mental disorders, ed 4, text revision (DSM-IV-TR), Washington, DC, 2000, The Association.*
*Continued*

## DSM-IV-TR Medical Diagnoses Related to Anxiety Responses—cont'd

| DSM-IV-TR Diagnosis—cont'd | Essential Features—cont'd |
|---|---|
| Specific phobia | Marked and persistent fear that is excessive or unreasonable, cued by the presence or anticipation of a specific object or situation (e.g., flying, heights, animals, receiving an injection, seeing blood). Exposure to the phobic stimulus almost invariably provokes an immediate anxiety response. The person recognizes that the fear is excessive, and the distress or avoidance interferes with the person's normal routines. |
| Social phobia | Marked and persistent fear of one or more social or performance situations in which the person is exposed to unfamiliar people or to possible scrutiny by others. The individual fears that he or she will act in a way (or show anxiety symptoms) that will be humiliating or embarrassing. Exposure to the feared situation almost invariably provokes anxiety. The person recognizes that the fear is excessive, and the distress or avoidance interferes with the person's normal routine. |
| Obsessive-compulsive disorder | Either obsessions or compulsions (Box 9-3) are recognized as excessive and interfere with the person's normal routine. |

| | |
|---|---|
| Posttraumatic stress disorder | The person has been exposed to a traumatic event in which both the following occurred:<br>1. The person experienced, witnessed, or was confronted with an event or events that involved actual or threatened death or serious injury or a threat to the physical integrity of self or others.<br>2. The person's response involved intense fear, helplessness, or horror. The person reexperiences the traumatic event, avoids stimuli associated with the trauma, and experiences a numbing of general responsiveness. |
| Acute stress disorder | Meets the above criteria for exposure to a traumatic event, and the person experiences three of the following symptoms: sense of detachment, reduced awareness of surroundings, derealization, depersonalization, and dissociated amnesia. |
| Generalized anxiety disorder | Excessive anxiety and worry, occurring more days than not for at least 6 months, about a number of events or activities. The person finds it difficult to control the worry and experiences at least three of the following six symptoms: restlessness or feeling keyed up or on edge, being easily fatigued, difficulty concentrating or mind going blank, irritability, muscle tension, and sleep disturbance. |

*Modified from American Psychiatric Association: Diagnostic and statistical manual of mental disorders, ed 4, text revision (DSM-IV-TR), Washington, DC, 2000, The Association.*

## Box 9-2   Criteria for Panic Attacks

A panic attack is a discrete period of intense fear or
  discomfort in which at least four of the following
  symptoms develop abruptly and reach a peak within
  10 minutes:
1. Palpitations, pounding heart, or accelerated heart rate
2. Sweating
3. Trembling or shaking
4. Sensations of shortness of breath or smothering
5. Feeling of choking
6. Chest pain or discomfort
7. Nausea or abdominal distress
8. Feeling dizzy, unsteady, lightheaded, or faint
9. Derealization (feelings of unreality) or depersonalization (being detached from self)
10. Fear of losing control or going crazy
11. Fear of dying
12. Paresthesias (numbness or tingling sensations)
13. Chills or hot flashes

problem-solving process and are described in the Nursing Treatment Plan Summary for moderate anxiety on pages 180-184.

## Evaluation

1. Have threats to the patient's physical integrity or self-system
   been reduced in nature, number, origin, or timing?
2. Do the patient's behaviors reflect a mild or less severe level
   of anxiety?
3. Have the patient's coping resources been adequately assessed and mobilized?
4. Does the patient recognize his or her own anxiety and have
   insight into feelings?
5. Is the patient using adaptive coping responses?
6. Has the patient learned new adaptive strategies to reduce
   anxiety?
7. Is the patient using mild anxiety to promote personal change
   and growth?

*Text continued on p. 185*

## Box 9-3   Criteria for Obsessions and Compulsions

Obsessions

1. Recurrent and persistent thoughts, impulses, or images are experienced at some time during the disturbance as intrusive and inappropriate and cause marked anxiety or distress.
2. The thoughts, impulses, or images are not simply excessive worries about real-life problems.
3. The person attempts to ignore or suppress such thoughts or impulses or to neutralize them with some other thought or action.
4. The person recognizes that the obsessional thoughts, impulses, or images are a product of his or her own mind.

Compulsions

1. The person feels driven to perform repetitive behaviors (e.g., handwashing, ordering, checking) or mental acts (e.g., praying, counting, repeating words silently) in response to an obsession or according to rigidly applied rules.
2. The behaviors or mental acts are aimed at preventing or reducing distress or preventing some dreaded event or situation; however, these behaviors or mental acts are not connected realistically with what they are designed to neutralize or prevent, or they are clearly excessive.

Patient Education Plan: **Teaching the Relaxation Response**

| Content | Instructional Activities | Evaluation |
|---------|--------------------------|------------|
| Describe characteristics and benefits of relaxation. | Discuss physiological changes associated with relaxation and contrast these with anxiety behaviors. | Patient identifies own responses to anxiety.<br>Patient describes elements of a relaxed state. |
| Teach deep muscle relaxation through sequence of tension-relaxation exercises. | Engage patient in progressive procedure of tensing and relaxing muscles until whole body is relaxed. | Patient can tense and relax all muscle groups.<br>Patient identifies those muscles that become particularly tense. |
| Discuss relaxation procedure of meditation and its components. | Describe elements of meditation and assist patient in using this technique. | Patient selects word or scene with pleasant connotations and engages in relaxed meditation. |

| | | |
|---|---|---|
| Assist in overcoming anxiety-provoking situations through systematic desensitization. | with patient, construct hierarchy of anxiety-provoking situations or scenes. Through imagination or reality, work through these scenes, using relaxation techniques. | Patient identifies and ranks anxiety-provoking situations. Patient exposes self to these situations while remaining relaxed. |
| Allow rehearsing and practical use of relaxation in a safe environment. | Have patient role-play stressful situations with you or other patients. | Patient becomes more comfortable with new behavior in a safe and supportive setting. |
| Encourage patient to use relaxation techniques in life. | Assign use of the relaxation response in everyday experiences as homework. Support success of patient who uses relaxation in life situation. | Patient uses relaxation in real-life situations. Patient is able to regulate anxiety response through use of relaxation techniques. |

Table 9-4 Summarizing the evidence on treatments for anxiety disorders

---

**DISORDER:** Generalized anxiety disorder (GAD)
**TREATMENT:**

- Most treatment outcome studies have shown active treatments to be superior to non-directive approaches, and uniformly superior to no treatment; however, most of these studies failed to demonstrate differential rates of efficacy among active treatments.
- Recent studies suggested cognitive-behavioral therapy (combining relaxation exercises and cognitive therapy), with the goal of bringing the worry process under control, to be most efficacious.
- The benzodiazepines reduced the anxiety and worry symptoms of GAD.
- Buspirone appeared comparable to the benzodiazepines in alleviating GAD symptoms.
- The tricyclic antidepressants showed utility in the treatment of GAD.

**DISORDER:** Obsessive-compulsive disorder (OCD)
**TREATMENT:**

- Cognitive-behavioral therapy involving exposure and ritual prevention methods reduced or eliminated the obsessions and behavioral and mental rituals of OCD.
- Approximately 40% to 60% of OCD patients respond to serotonergic reuptake inhibitors (SRIs), including clomipramine, fluvoxamine, paroxetine, fluoxetine, and sertraline, with mean improvement in obsessions and compulsions of approximately 20% to 40%.

---

Modified from Nathan P, Gorman J: *A guide to treatments that work,* New York, 1998, Oxford University Press.

Table 9-4   Summarizing the evidence on treatments for anxiety disorders—cont'd

**DISORDER:** Panic disorder with and without agoraphobia
**TREATMENT:**

- Situational in vivo exposure substantially reduced symptoms of panic disorder with agoraphobia.
- Cognitive-behavioral treatments that focused on education about the nature of anxiety and panic and provided some form of exposure and coping skills acquisition significantly reduced symptoms of panic disorder without agoraphobia.
- Tricyclic antidepressants and monoamine oxidase inhibitors (MAOIs) reduced the number of panic attacks and also reduced anticipatory anxiety and phobic avoidance, although side effects caused some patients to drop out from clinical trials.
- The benzodiazepines (e.g., Alprazolam) eliminated panic attacks in 55% to 75% of patients.
- More recently, SRIs and selective serotonin reuptake inhibitors (SSRIs) have produced reductions in panic frequency, generalized anxiety, disability, and phobic avoidance.

**DISORDER:** Posttraumatic stress disorder (PTSD)
**TREATMENT:**

- MAOIs reduced intrusive thoughts, improved sleep, and moderated anxiety and depression in PTSD patients.
- Tricyclic antidepressants reduced intrusive thoughts and obsessions and moderated depression in these patients.
- SSRIs markedly reduced intrusive thoughts, avoidance, and sleep problems.
- Exposure therapies (systematic desensitization, flooding, prolonged exposure, and implosive therapy) and, to a lesser extent, anxiety management techniques (utilizing cognitive-behavioral strategies) reduced PTSD symptoms, including anxiety and depression, and increased social functioning.

Nursing Treatment Plan Summary:    Severe and Panic Anxiety Responses

Nursing Diagnosis: Severe/panic level of anxiety
Expected Outcome: Patient will reduce anxiety to a moderate or mild level.

| Short-term Goals | Interventions | Rationale |
| --- | --- | --- |
| Patient will be protected from harm. | Initially accept and support, rather than attack, patient's defenses. | Severe and panic levels of anxiety can be reduced by initially allowing patient to determine amount of stress that can be handled. |
| | Acknowledge reality of the pain associated with patient's present coping mechanisms. | |
| | Do not focus on the phobia, ritual, or physical complaint itself. Give feedback to patient about behavior, stressors and their appraisal, and coping resources. | If patient is unable to release anxiety, tension may mount to the panic level and patient may lose control. |
| | Reinforce idea that physical health is related to emotional health and that this area will need exploration in the future. | At this time, patient has no alternatives for present coping mechanisms. |
| | In time, begin to place limits on patient's maladaptive behavior in a supportive way. | |

| Patient will experience fewer anxiety-provoking situations. | Assume a calm manner with patient. Decrease environmental stimulation. Limit patient's interaction with other patients to minimize contagious aspects of anxiety. Identify and modify anxiety-provoking situations for patient. Administer supportive physical measures, such as warm baths and massages. | Patient's behavior may be modified by altering environment and patient's interaction with it. |
| Patient will engage in a daily schedule of activities. | Initially share an activity with patient to provide support and reinforce socially productive behavior. Provide for physical exercise of some type. Plan a schedule or list of activities that can be carried out daily. Involve family members and other support systems as much as possible. | By encouraging outside activities, nurse limits the time patient has available for destructive coping mechanisms while increasing participation in and enjoyment of other aspects of life. |
| Patient will experience relief from the symptoms of severe anxiety. | Administer medications that help reduce patient's discomfort. Observe for medication side effects and initiate relevant health teaching. | Effect of a therapeutic relationship may be enhanced if chemical control of symptoms allows patient to direct attention to underlying conflicts. |

## Nursing Treatment Plan Summary:  Moderate Anxiety Responses

Nursing Diagnosis: Moderate level of anxiety

Expected Outcome: Patient will demonstrate adaptive ways of coping with stress.

| Short-term Goals | Interventions | Rationale |
| --- | --- | --- |
| Patient will identify and describe feelings of anxiety. | Help patient identify and describe underlying feelings. Link patient's behavior with such feelings. Validate all inferences and assumptions with patient. Use open questions to move from nonthreatening topics to issues of conflict. Vary amount of anxiety to enhance patient's motivation. In time, use supportive confrontation judiciously. | To adopt new coping responses, patient first needs to be aware of feelings and to overcome conscious or unconscious denial and resistance. |

| Patient will identify antecedents of anxiety. | Help patient describe the situations and interactions that immediately precede anxiety. Review patient's appraisal of the stressor, values being threatened, and way in which the conflict developed. Relate patient's present experiences with relevant ones from the past. | Once feelings of anxiety are recognized, patient needs to understand their development, including precipitating stressors, appraisal of the stressor, and available resources. |
| --- | --- | --- |
| Patient will describe adaptive and maladaptive coping responses. | Explore how patient reduced anxiety in the past and what types of actions produced relief. Point out maladaptive and destructive effects of present coping responses. Encourage patient to use adaptive coping responses that were effective in the past. Focus responsibility for change on patient. Actively help patient correlate cause-and-effect relationships while maintaining anxiety within appropriate limits. Assist patient in reappraising value, nature, and meaning of the stressor when appropriate. | New adaptive coping responses can be learned through analyzing coping mechanisms used in the past, reappraising the stressor, using available resources, and accepting responsibility for change. |

*Continued*

## Nursing Treatment Plan Summary: Moderate Anxiety Responses—cont'd

| Short-term Goals | Interventions | Rationale |
|---|---|---|
| Patient will implement two adaptive responses for coping with anxiety. | Help patient identify ways to restructure thoughts, modify behavior, use resources, and test new coping responses. Encourage physical activity to discharge energy. Include significant others as resources and social supports in helping patient learn new coping responses. Teach patient relaxation exercises to increase control and self-reliance and reduce stress. | A person can also cope with stress by regulating the attendant emotional distress through use of stress management techniques. |

*your* **INTERNET**
c o n n e c t i o n

**Anxiety Disorders Association of America:**
www.adaa.org

**The Anxiety Panic Internet Resource:**
www.algy.com/anxiety

**Freedom from Fear:**
freedomfromfear.org

**National Center for PTSD:**
www.ncptsd.org

**OC & Spectrum Disorders Association:**
www.ocdhelp.org

## Suggested readings

American Psychiatric Association: Practice guidelines for the treatment of patients with panic disorder, *Am J Psychiatry* 155(5):1, 1998.

Antai-Otong D: The neurobiology of anxiety disorders: implications for psychiatric nursing practice, *Issues Ment Health Nurs* 21:71, 2000.

Benham E: Coping strategies: a psychoeducational approach to post-traumatic symptomatology, *J Psychosoc Nurs* 6:30, 1995.

Eddy M, Walbroehl G: Recognition and treatment of obsessive-compulsive disorder, *Am Fam Physician* 57(7):1623-1628, 1632-1634, 1998.

Freedy J, Hobfoll S: *Traumatic stress: from theory to practice,* New York, 1995, Plenum Press.

Greist J, Jefferson J: *Panic disorder and agoraphobia: a guide,* Madison, Wisc, 1998, Madison Institute of Medicine.

March J et al: The expert consensus guidelines series: treatment of obsessive-compulsive disorder, *Expert Knowledge Systems,* 1998.

Post-traumatic stress disorder, parts I and II, *Harv Ment Health Lett* 12:1, 13:1, 1996.

Saeed S, Bruce T: Panic disorder: effective treatment options, *Am Fam Physician* 57(10):2405-2412, 2419-2420, 1998.

Simpson H, Fallon B: Obsessive-compulsive disorder: an overview, *J Psychiatr Pract* 6(1):3, 2000.

Simpson H, Kozak M: Cognitive-behavioral therapy for obsessive-compulsive disorder, *J Psychiatr Pract* 6:59, 2000.

Smith S, Sherril K, Colenda C: Assessing and treating anxiety in elderly persons, *Psychiatr Serv* 46:36, 1995.

Stuart G, Laraia M: Panic disorder with agoraphobia. In McBride AB, Austin JK: *Psychiatric–mental health nursing: integrating the behavioral and biological sciences,* Philadelphia, 1996, WB Saunders.

Stuart G, Laraia M: *Principles and practice of psychiatric nursing,* ed 7, St Louis, 2001, Mosby.

Tucker W: Recognition and management of posttraumatic stress disorder: approaches for the practitioner, *J Pract Psychiatr Behav Health,* 4:20, 1998.

Wakefiled M, Pallister R: Cognitive-behavioral approaches to panic disorder, *J Psychosoc Nurs* 35:12, 1997.

Wells A: *Cognitive therapy of anxiety disorders: a practice manual and conceptual guide,* New York, 1997, John Wiley & Sons.

# Psycho-physiological Responses and Somatoform and Sleep Disorders

**10**

## Continuum of Psychophysiological Responses

The degree of interconnection between mind and body has always been of interest to scientists and philosophers. For a long time in the history of medicine, body and mind were viewed as separate. More recently, renewed attention has been given to the interrelationship between these two separate aspects of human functioning. Much of the research has focused on the stress response and the impact of stress, including the effect of psychological stress on physiological functioning, and vice versa.

One of the prominent investigators of the stress response, Hans Selye, described the general adaptation syndrome, a three-stage process of responding to stress, as follows:

1. *The alarm reaction.* This is the immediate response to a stressor that has not been eliminated locally. Adrenocortical response mechanisms are mobilized, resulting in the behaviors associated with the fight-or-flight response.

2. *Stage of resistance.* In this stage there is some resistance to the stressor. The body adapts at a lower than optimal level of functioning, requiring greater than usual expenditure of energy for survival.

Figure 10-1
Continuum of psychophysiological responses.

3. *Stage of exhaustion.* The adaptive mechanisms become worn out and fail in this stage. The negative effect of the stressor spreads to the entire organism. If the stressor is not removed or counteracted, death will ultimately result.

Figure 10-1 illustrates the range of possible psychophysiological responses to stress based on Selye's theory.

## Assessment

### Behaviors

Many behaviors are associated with psychophysiological disorders. Careful assessment is needed to define and treat actual organic problems. This type of illness should never be dismissed as "only psychosomatic" or "all in one's head." Serious psychophysiological disorders can be fatal if not treated appropriately.

#### Physiological

The primary behaviors observed with psychophysiological responses are the physical symptoms. These symptoms lead the person to seek health care. Psychological factors affecting the physical condition may involve any body part. Box 10-1 lists the most common organ systems involved.

#### Psychological

Some people have physical symptoms without any organic impairment. These *somatoform disorders* include the following:

1. *Somatization disorder,* in which the person has many physical complaints
2. *Conversion disorder,* in which a loss or alteration of physical functioning occurs

**Box 10-1   Physical Conditions Affected by Psychological Factors**

Cardiovascular

Migraine
Essential hypertension
Angina
Tension headaches

Musculoskeletal

Rheumatoid arthritis
Low back pain
   (idiopathic)
Gastrointestinal
Anorexia nervosa
Peptic ulcer
Irritable bowel
   syndrome
Colitis
Obesity

Respiratory

Hyperventilation
Asthma

Skin

Neurodermatitis
Eczema
Psoriasis
Pruritus

Genitourinary

Impotence
Frigidity
Premenstrual syndrome

Endocrine

Hyperthyroidism
Diabetes

3. *Hypochondriasis,* the fear or belief that the person has an illness
4. *Body dysmorphic disorder,* in which a person with a normal appearance is concerned about having a physical defect
5. *Pain disorder,* in which psychological factors play an important role in the onset, severity, or maintenance of the pain

## Pain

Pain is increasingly recognized as more than a sensory phenomenon; it is recognized as a complex sensory and emotional experience underlying potential disease. Pain is influenced by behavioral, cognitive, motivational, and cultural processes and thus requires sophisticated assessments and multifaceted treatments for its control. By definition, chronic pain consists of pain of at least 6 months' duration. *Somatoform pain disorder* is a preoccupation with pain without physical disease to account for its intensity. It does not follow a neuroanatomical distribution. A close correlation also may exist between stress and conflict and the initiation or exacerbation of the pain.

## Sleep

Sleep disturbances are common in the general population and among people with psychiatric disorders. Insomnia is the most prevalent sleep disorder. Up to 30% of the population have insomnia and seek help for it. Other sleep disturbances include excessive daytime sleepiness, difficulty sleeping during desired sleep time, and unusual nocturnal events such as nightmares and sleepwalking. The consequences of sleep disorders, sleep deprivation, and sleepiness include reduced productivity, lowered cognitive performance, increased likelihood of accidents, higher risk of morbidity and mortality, and decreased quality of life. Sleep disorders are more common in elderly persons.

Sleep disorders are classified into the following four major groupings:

1. Disorders of initiating or maintaining sleep, also known as **insomnia.** Anxiety and depression are major causes of insomnia.
2. Disorders of excessive somnolence, also known as **hypersomnia.** This category includes narcolepsy, sleep apnea, and nocturnal movement disorders such as restless legs.
3. Disorders of the sleep-wake schedule, characterized by normal sleep but at the wrong time. These are transient disturbances often associated with jet lag and work shift changes. They are usually self-limited and resolve as the body readjusts to a new sleep-wake schedule.
4. Disorders associated with sleep stages, also known as **parasomnia.** This category includes diverse conditions such as sleepwalking, night terrors, nightmares, and enuresis. These sleep problems are often experienced by children and can have a significant effect on functioning and well-being.

## Predisposing Factors

Biopsychosocial factors believed to influence the individual's psychophysiological response to stress include the following:

1. *Biological factors*
   - Emotions have been linked to the arousal of the neuroendocrine system through the release of corticosteroids; the

actions of neurotransmitter systems; and the changes in postsynaptic receptors in response to stress.

- Genetic factors have been shown to influence the prevalence of some psychophysiological disorders.
- Psychoimmunology explores the connection between the mind and the immune system and is discovering biological factors that influence the way the brain protects itself from cells damaged by trauma, disease, or stress.

2. *Psychological factors*
- The type A personality represents the connection of a personality type to a physiological disorder, in this case, heart disease.
- Other investigators have documented a relationship between personality style and physiological disorders such as hypertension and migraine headaches.
- Physical illness may occur with no evidence of organic impairment. In this case, psychological conflicts and anxiety are suspected to predispose a person to respond somatically.

3. *Sociocultural factors*
- The severity of the person's symptoms is influenced by aspects of the social and cultural environment.
- The symptoms shape and structure the person's social world as the illness, by its very presence, initiates a series of changes in the person's environment. The resulting chain of illness-related, interpersonal events then becomes a part of the social course of the person's illness.

## Precipitating Stressors

Psychophysiological illnesses result from an attempt to cope with anxiety. Therefore the stressors related to the psychological responses to anxiety discussed in Chapter 9 also apply to the physiological response. The precipitating stressor may be one overwhelming experience or may seem relatively minor. Interpersonal losses are often associated with the development of physical symptoms. Sometimes a psychophysiological illness results from an accumulation of apparently minor stressful events.

## Appraisal of Stressor

The complex interaction between mind and body may be most evident in psychophysiological responses to stress. These resulting illnesses reinforce the need for an integrated approach to determining etiology and understanding a person's appraisal of stress and its effects. Social and cultural factors play a particularly important role in the expression of adaptive and maladaptive behaviors and must be prime considerations in planning effective, individualized treatment strategies.

## Coping Resources

One of the most important aspects of promoting adaptive psychophysiological responses involves changing health habits. Social support from family, friends, and caregivers is also an important resource.

## Coping Mechanisms

The psychophysiological disorders may be viewed as attempts to cope with the anxiety associated with overwhelming stress. Ego defense mechanisms associated with these disorders include the following:
1. Repression of feelings, conflicts, and unacceptable impulses
2. Denial of psychological problems
3. Compensation
4. Regression

## Nursing Diagnosis

The nursing diagnosis must reflect the complexity of the biopsychosocial interaction, which is the hallmark of psychophysiological disorders. The individual's effort to cope with stress-related anxiety may result in numerous somatic and emotional disorders. Care must be taken to consider all the possible disruptions when formulating a complete nursing diagnosis.

The box on page 193 presents the primary and related NANDA nursing diagnoses for maladaptive psychophysiological responses. A complete nursing assessment would include all maladaptive responses of the patient, and many additional nursing diagnoses would be identified.

## Related Medical Diagnoses

Medical disorders related to psychophysiological responses are classified under the general headings of somatoform disorders,

## NANDA Nursing Diagnoses Related to Maladaptive Psychophysiological Responses

*Adjustment, Impaired
Anxiety
Body Image, Disturbed
Coping, Ineffective
Denial, Ineffective
Family processes, Interrupted
Fear
Health maintenance, Ineffective
Hopelessness
Mobility, Impaired physical
Nutrition, Imbalanced: less than body requirements
*Pain, Chronic
Powerlessness
Powerlessness, Risk for
Self-care deficit
Self-esteem, Risk for situational low
Self-esteem, Situational low
Skin integrity, Impaired
*Sleep pattern, Disturbed
Social interaction, Impaired
Social isolation
Spiritual distress

*Primary nursing diagnosis for maladaptive psychophysiological responses.
*From North American Nursing Diagnosis Association:* NANDA nursing diagnoses: definitions and classification 2000-2001, *Philadelphia, 2001, The Association.*

sleep disorders, and psychological factors affecting medical condition in the DSM-IV-TR. These are described on pages 194 and 195.

## Outcome Identification

The expected outcome when working with a patient with maladaptive psychophysiological responses follows:

*The patient will express feelings verbally rather than through the development of physical symptoms.*

## DSM-IV-TR Medical Diagnoses Related to Maladaptive Psychophysiological Responses

| DSM-IV-TR Diagnosis | Essential Features |
|---|---|
| Somatization disorder | History of many physical complaints beginning before age 30, occurring over several years, and resulting in treatment being sought or significant impairment in social or occupational functioning. The patient must display at least four pain symptoms, two gastrointestinal symptoms, one sexual symptom, and one symptom suggesting a neurological disorder. |
| Conversion disorder | One or more symptoms or deficits affecting voluntary motor or sensory function and suggesting a neurological or general medical condition. Psychological factors are judged to be associated with the symptom or deficit because the initiation or exacerbation of the symptom or deficit is preceded by conflicts or other stressors. The symptom or deficit cannot be fully explained by a neurological or general medical condition and is not a culturally sanctioned behavior or experience. |
| Hypochondriasis | Preoccupation with fears of having, or ideas that one has, a serious disease based on the person's misinterpretation of bodily symptoms. The preoccupation persists for at least 6 months despite appropriate medical evaluation and reassurance. It causes clinically significant distress or impairment in functioning. |
| Body dysmorphic disorder | Preoccupation with an imagined or exaggerated defect in appearance that causes clinically significant distress or impairment in functioning. |

| | |
|---|---|
| Pain disorder | Pain in one or more anatomical sites is predominant focus of the clinical presentation. It is of sufficient severity to warrant clinical attention and causes clinically significant distress or impairment in functioning. Psychological factors are judged to have an important role in the onset, severity, exacerbation, or maintenance of the pain. |
| Primary insomnia | Difficulty initiating or maintaining sleep, or nonrestorative sleep, for at least 1 month that causes clinically significant distress or impairment in functioning. |
| Primary hypersomnia | Excessive sleepiness for at least 1 month, as evidenced by either prolonged sleep episodes or daytime sleep episodes occurring almost daily, that causes clinically significant distress or impairment in functioning. |
| Narcolepsy | Irresistible attacks of refreshing sleep occurring daily over at least 3 months with cataplexy (brief episodes of sudden bilateral loss of muscle tone) and hallucinations or sleep paralysis at the beginning or end of sleep episodes. |
| Breathing-related sleep disorder | Sleep disruption leading to excessive sleepiness or insomnia judged to be caused by sleep apnea or central alveolar hypoventilation syndrome. |
| Circadian rhythm sleep disorder | Persistent or recurrent pattern of sleep disruption leading to excessive sleepiness or insomnia that is caused by a mismatch between the sleep-wake schedule required by a person's environment and the circadian sleep-wake pattern and that causes clinically significant distress or impairment in functioning. |
| Psychological factors affecting medical condition | Presence of a medical condition in which psychological factors influence its cause, interfere with its treatment, constitute additional health risks for the individual, or elicit stress-related physiological responses that precipitate or exacerbate its symptoms. |

*Modified from American Psychiatric Association: Diagnostic and statistical manual of mental disorders, ed 4, text revision (DSM-IV-TR), Washington, DC, 2000, The Association.*

## Planning

A Patient Education Plan for teaching adaptive coping strategies is presented on page 197.

## Implementation

Empirically validated treatments for some of the medical diagnoses related to psychophysiological responses are summarized in Table 10-1.

## Intervening in Psychophysiological Illness

The highest priority for nursing intervention is attending to the patient's physiological needs. This assists the patient to meet basic needs for safety and security. It is also valuable for fostering the development of a trusting relationship. Box 10-2 presents sleep hygiene strategies. A Nursing Treatment Plan Summary for patients with maladaptive psychophysiological responses is presented on pages 200 and 201.

## Evaluation

1. Have threats to the patient's physical integrity or self-system been reduced in nature, origin, or timing?
2. Do the patient's behaviors reflect greater self-awareness and acceptance of emotional experiences?
3. Have the patient's coping resources been adequately assessed and mobilized?
4. Does the patient recognize the level of stress, and does the patient have insight into own feelings?
5. Is the patient using adaptive coping responses?
6. Has the patient learned new adaptive strategies to cope effectively with life stressors?
7. Is the patient using greater self-understanding to promote personal change and growth?

*Text continued on p. 202*

Patient Education Plan:  **Teaching Adaptive Coping Strategies**

| Content | Instructional Activities | Evaluation |
|---|---|---|
| Define and describe stress. | List feelings that indicate stress. Discuss behaviors associated with elevated stress. | Patient identifies behaviors associated with stressful situations. |
| Recognize stressful situations. | Ask patient to describe situations experienced as stressful. Role-play the situation (with videotape if possible). Discuss stress-related behaviors observed and feelings experienced. | Patient identifies stressful experiences. Patient describes own behaviors when stressed. |
| Review common life stressors. | Discuss common elements of stressful experiences. Review the role-played stressful situations. | Patient identifies stressful aspects of life. |
| Identify adaptive and maladaptive coping mechanisms. | Discuss alternative ways to cope with the stressors. Role-play at least one coping mechanism. | Patient identifies and practices adaptive coping mechanisms. |
| Assign use of adaptive strategy to cope with stress. | Provide feedback about effectiveness of the selected coping mechanism. | Patient selects an adaptive coping strategy when experiencing stress. |

Table 10-1    Summarizing the evidence on treatments for psychophysiological responses

---

**DISORDER:** Body dysmorphic disorder
**TREATMENT:**
- Cognitive-behavior therapy helped patients identify and challenge distorted body perceptions and interrupted self-critical thoughts, especially when employed in conjunction with guided exposure and response prevention.

**DISORDER:** Hypochondriasis
**TREATMENT:**
- Cognitive-behavior therapy has proven helpful in correcting the misinformation and exaggerated beliefs, as well as pointing out the cognitive processes maintaining disease fears in hypochondriasis.

**DISORDER:** Pain disorder
**TREATMENT:**
- Individual and group cognitive-behavior therapy reduced pain-related distress and disability. Antidepressants decreased pain intensity.

**DISORDER:** Sleep disorders
**TREATMENT:**
- The benzodiazepines and zolpidem typically reduced sleep onset by 15 to 30 minutes, decreased the number of awakenings to an absolute level of 1 to 3 per night, and increased total sleep time by about 15 to 45 minutes. These pharmacological agents act more reliably than behavioral interventions in the short term.

- Over the long term, behavioral interventions, including stimulus control, sleep restriction, relaxation strategies, and cognitive behavioral therapy, reduced sleep onset, decreased awakenings, and increased total sleep time. These behavioral interventions produced more sustained effects than pharmacological agents.

---

Modified from Nathan P, Gorman J: *A guide to treatments that work,* New York, 1998, Oxford University Press.

## Box 10-2   Sleep Hygiene Strategies

- Set a regular bedtime and wake-up time 7 days a week.
- Exercise daily to aid sleep initiation and maintenance; however, vigorous exercise too close to bedtime may make falling asleep difficult.
- Schedule time to wind down and relax before bed.
- Avoid worrying when trying to fall asleep.
- Guard against nighttime interruptions. Earplugs may help with a noisy partner. Heavy window shades help to screen out light. Create a comfortable bed.
- Maintain a cool temperature in the room. A warm bath or warm drink before bed helps some people fall asleep.
- Excessive hunger or fullness may interfere with sleep. Avoid large meals before bed. If hungry, a light carbohydrate snack may be helpful.
- Avoid caffeinated drinks, excessive fluid intake, stimulating drugs, and excessive alcohol in the evening and before bedtime.
- Excessive napping may make it difficult for some people to fall asleep at night.
- Do not eat, read, work, or watch television in bed. The bed and bedroom should be used only for sleep and sex.
- Maintain a reasonable weight. Excessive weight may result in daytime fatigue and sleep apnea.
- Get out of bed and engage in other activities if not able to fall asleep.

Nursing Treatment Plan Summary:  Maladaptive Psychophysiological Responses

Nursing Diagnosis: Impaired adjustment

Expected Outcome: Patient will express feelings verbally rather than through the development of physical symptoms.

| Short-term Goals | Interventions | Rationale |
| --- | --- | --- |
| Patient will identify areas of stress and conflict and relate feelings, thoughts, and behaviors to them. | Assist patient in identifying stressful situations by reviewing events surrounding the development of physical symptoms. Facilitate the association among thoughts, feelings, and behaviors. | Inability to deal with intrapsychic conflict leads to anxiety and stress, resulting in physiological dysfunction. |
| Patient will describe present defenses and evaluate whether they are adaptive or maladaptive. | Proceed slowly in analyzing defenses. Explore alternative coping behaviors with patient. Teach patient stress management techniques (e.g., relaxation, imagery). | Defenses should not be attacked; rather, nurse should support positive exploration of patient and suggest alternative responses. |

| | | |
|---|---|---|
| Patient will adopt two new coping mechanisms to deal with stress. | Give patient positive feedback for new adaptive behaviors. Actively support patient in testing new coping mechanisms. Enlist support of family and significant others to reinforce change. | Change requires time and positive reinforcement from others. Family members can be particularly important in promoting adaptive responses. |
| Patient will display decreased physical symptoms and greater biological integrity. | Encourage physical activity to reduce stress. Counsel patient on diet and nutrition needs. Review patient's sleep habits and promote good sleep hygiene practices. | Wellness requires a balance between biological and psychosocial needs. Interventions focused on patient's physiological needs can help patient restore biological integrity. |

*your* **INTERNET**
c o n n e c t i o n

Academy of Psychosomatic Medicine:
www.apm.org

American Sleep Disorders Association:
www.asda.org

The Sleep Medicine Home Page:
www.users.cloud9.net/~thorpy

The SLEEP WELL:
www.stanford.edu/~dement

## Suggested readings

Birch S, Hammerschlag R, Berman B: Acupuncture in the treatment of pain, *J Altern Complement Med* 2:101, 1996.

Blumenthal S, Fine T: Sleep abnormalities associated with mental and addictive disorders: implications for research and clinical practice, *J Pract Psychiatry Behav Health* 3:67, 1996.

Buysse DJ, Perlis ME: The evaluation and treatment of insomnia, *J Pract Psychiatry Behav Health* 3:80, 1996.

Demitrack M: Chronic fatigue syndrome and fibromyalgia: dilemmas in diagnosis and clinical management, *Psychiatr Clin North Am* 21(3): 671, 1998.

Eddy M, Walbroehl G: Insomnia, *Am Fam Physician* 59(7):1911-1916, 1918, 1999.

Edinger J, Wohlgemuth W, Radtke R et al: Cognitive behavioral therapy for treatment of chronic primary insomnia, *JAMA* 285:1856-1864, 2001.

Holmes E et al: Development of a sleep management program for people with severe mental illness, *Psychiatr Rehabil J* 19:9, 1995.

Keefe FJ, Goli V: A practical guide to behavioral assessment and treatment of chronic pain, *J Pract Psychiatry Behav Health* 5:151, 1996.

Lowery BJ, Houldin AD: From stressor to illness: the psychobiological-biological connection. In McBride AB, Austin JK, editors: *Psychiatric–mental health nursing: integrating the behavioral and biological sciences,* Philadelphia, 1996, WB Saunders.

National Center on Sleep Disorders Research Working Group: Recognizing problem sleepiness in your patients, *Am Fam Physician* 59(4):937-944, 1999.

Oakley LD, Potter C: *Psychiatric primary care,* St Louis, 1997, Mosby.

Rajput V, Bromley S: Chronic insomnia: a practical review, *Am Fam Physician* 60(5):1431-1438, discussion 1441-1442, 1999.

Selye H: *The stress of life,* New York, 1956, McGraw-Hill.

Stoudemire A: *Psychological factors affecting medical conditions,* Washington, DC, 1995, American Psychiatric Press.

Stuart G, Laraia M: *Principles and practice of psychiatric nursing,* ed 7, St Louis, 2001, Mosby.

Wise T: The worried patient: clinical management of the patient with hypochondriasis, *J Pract Psychiatr Behav Health* 3:223, 1997.

Yantis M: Identifying depression as a symptom of sleep apnea, *J Psychosoc Nurs* 37(10):28, 1999.

# Self-Concept Responses and Dissociative Disorders

## Continuum of Self-Concept Responses

*Self-concept* is defined as all the notions, beliefs, and convictions that constitute an individual's knowledge of self and that influence relationships with others. Self-concept does not exist at birth; it is learned as a result of a person's unique experiences within the self, with significant others, and with worldly realities. Self-concept consists of the following components:

1. *Body image*—the sum of the individual's conscious and unconscious attitudes toward his or her body. It includes present and past perceptions and feelings about size, function, appearance, and potential. Body image is modified continually by new perceptions and experiences.

2. *Self-ideal*—the individual's perception of how he or she should behave based on certain personal standards, aspirations, goals, or values.

3. *Self-esteem*—the individual's judgment of personal worth obtained by analyzing how well one's behavior conforms to self-ideal. High self-esteem is a feeling rooted in unconditional acceptance of self, despite mistakes, defeats, and failures, as an innately worthy and important being.

4. *Role performance*—sets of socially expected behavior patterns associated with an individual's function in various social groups. Ascribed roles are assigned roles over which the person has no choice. Assumed roles are those selected or chosen by the individual.
5. *Personal identity*—the organizing principle of the personality that accounts for the individual's unity, continuity, consistency, and uniqueness. It connotes autonomy and includes perceptions of one's sexuality. Identity formation begins in infancy and proceeds throughout life but is the major task of the adolescent period.

## The Healthy Personality

An individual with a healthy personality experiences the following:
1. Positive and accurate body image
2. Realistic self-ideal
3. Positive self-concept
4. High self-esteem
5. Satisfying role performance
6. Clear sense of identity

The self-concept responses along the health-illness continuum range from the most adaptive state of self-actualization to the more maladaptive states of identity diffusion and depersonalization (Figure 11-1). *Identity diffusion* is an individual's failure to integrate various childhood identifications into a harmonious adult psychosocial personality. *Depersonalization* is a feeling of unreality and alienation from the self. It is associated with the panic level of anxiety and failure in reality testing. The individual has difficulty

Figure 11-1
**Continuum of self-concept responses.**

### Box 11-1    Behaviors Associated with Low Self-Esteem

- Criticism of self and others
- Decreased productivity
- Destructiveness toward others
- Disruptions in relatedness
- Exaggerated sense of self-importance
- Feelings of inadequacy
- Guilt
- Irritability or excessive anger
- Negative feelings about one's body
- Perceived role strain
- Pessimistic view of life
- Physical complaints
- Polarizing view of life
- Rejection of personal capabilities
- Self-destructiveness
- Self-diminution
- Social withdrawal
- Substance abuse
- Withdrawal from reality
- Worrying

distinguishing the self from others, and the person's body has an unreal and strange quality about it.

## Assessment

### Behaviors

Data collection by the nurse should include both objective and observable behaviors and the patient's subjective and internal world. Boxes 11-1 to 11-3 list behaviors related to low self-esteem, identity diffusion, and depersonalization.

### Predisposing Factors

Numerous factors contribute to alterations in an individual's self-concept. These may be divided as follows:

1. *Factors affecting self-esteem* include parental rejection, unrealistic parental expectations, repeated failures, lack of per-

## Box 11-2  Behaviors Associated with Identity Diffusion

- Absence of moral code
- Contradictory personality traits
- Exploitative interpersonal relationships
- Feelings of emptiness
- Fluctuating feelings about self
- Gender confusion
- High degree of anxiety
- Inability to empathize with others
- Lack of authenticity
- Problems with intimacy

## Box 11-3  Behaviors Associated with Depersonalization

### Affective

Feelings of alienation from self
Feelings of insecurity, inferiority, fear, shame
Feelings of unreality
Heightened sense of isolation
Inability to derive pleasure or sense of accomplishment
Lack of sense of inner continuity
Loss of identity

### Perceptual

Auditory and visual hallucinations
Confusion about one's sexuality
Difficulty distinguishing self from others
Disturbed body image
Experiencing world as dreamlike

*Continued*

---

**Box 11-3    Behaviors Associated with Depersonalization—cont'd**

Cognitive

Confusion
Disoriented to time
Distorted thinking
Disturbance of memory
Impaired judgment
Separate personalities within same person

Behavioral

Blunting of affect
Emotional passivity and nonresponsiveness
Incongruent or idiosyncratic communication
Lack of spontaneity and animation
Loss of impulse control
Loss of initiative and decision-making ability
Social withdrawal

---

sonal responsibility, dependency on others, and unrealistic self-ideals.
2. *Factors affecting role performance* are gender role stereotypes, work role demands, and cultural role expectations.
3. *Factors affecting personal identity* include parental distrust, peer pressure, and changes in the social structure.

## Precipitating Stressors

Precipitating stressors may be derived from internal or external sources as follows:
1. *Trauma* such as sexual and psychological abuse or witnessing a life-threatening event
2. *Role strain* associated with expected roles or positions that the person experiences as frustration; the three types of role transitions follow:
   - *Developmental role transitions* are normative changes associated with growth. They include developmental stages in an individual's or family's life and cultural norms, values, and pressures to conform.

- *Situational role transitions* occur with the addition or subtraction of significant others through birth or death.
- *Health-illness role transitions* result from moving from a well state to an illness state. Such transitions may be precipitated by the following:

    Loss of a body part
    Changes in body size, shape, appearance, or function
    Physical changes associated with normal growth and development
    Medical and nursing procedures

## Appraisal of Stressor

Whether the problem in self-concept is precipitated by psychological, sociological, or physiological stressors, the critical element is the patient's perception of the threat.

## Coping Resources

All people, no matter how disturbing their behavior, have some areas of personal strength, which might include the following:

- Sports and outdoor activities
- Hobbies and crafts
- Expressive arts
- Health and self-care
- Education or training
- Work, vocation, job, or position
- Special aptitudes
- Intelligence
- Imagination and creativity
- Interpersonal relationships

## Coping Mechanisms

Coping mechanisms include short-term or long-term coping defenses and the use of ego defense mechanisms to protect the person from facing painful self-perceptions. *Short-term defenses* include the following:

1. Activities that provide temporary escape from the person's identity crisis (e.g., loud rock concerts, hard physical labor, obsessive television watching)
2. Activities that provide temporary substitute identities (e.g., joining social, religious, or political clubs, groups, movements, or gangs)

   3. Activities that serve temporarily to strengthen or heighten a
      diffuse sense of self (e.g., competitive sports, academic
      achievement, popularity contests)
   4. Activities that represent short-term attempts to make an
      identity out of the meaninglessness of life itself (e.g., drug
      abuse)
   *Long-term defenses* include the following:
   1. *Identity foreclosure*—the premature adoption of an identity
      that is desired by significant others without coming to terms
      with one's own desires, aspirations, or potential
   2. *Negative identity*—assumption of an identity that is at
      odds with accepted values and accepted expectations of
      society
   *Ego defense mechanisms* include the use of fantasy, dissociation, isolation, projection, displacement, splitting, turning anger
against self, and acting out.

## Nursing Diagnosis

Problems with self-concept are associated with feelings of anxiety, hostility, and guilt. These often create a circular and self-
propagating process for the individual that ultimately results in
maladaptive coping responses. These responses can be seen in a
variety of people experiencing threats to their physical integrity or
self-system.

   The box on page 211 presents the primary and related NANDA
nursing diagnoses for maladaptive self-concept responses. A complete nursing assessment would include all maladaptive responses
of the patient. Many additional nursing problems would be identified in the way that the patient's self-concept reciprocally influenced other areas of life.

### Related Medical Diagnoses

Because they pertain to a person's basic personality structure and
feelings about the self, the nursing diagnoses related to self-
concept can include a variety of medical disorders. A number of
specific medical diagnoses have dominant features that relate to
one's self-concept. The box on page 212 identifies and describes
these diagnoses.

## NANDA Nursing Diagnoses Related to Maladaptive Self-Concept Responses

Adjustment, Impaired
Anxiety
*Body image, Disturbed
Communication, Impaired verbal
Coping, Ineffective
Hopelessness
Identity, Disturbed personal
Loneliness, Risk for
Powerlessness
Powerlessness, Risk for
*Role performance, Ineffective
Self-care deficit
Self-esteem, Risk for situational low
*Self-esteem, Situational low
Sensory perception, Disturbed
Sexuality patterns, Ineffective
Social interaction, Impaired
Social isolation
Spiritual distress
Thought processes, Disturbed
Violence, Risk for self-directed

*Primary nursing diagnosis for alterations in self-concept.
*From North American Nursing Diagnosis Association:* NANDA nursing diagnoses: definitions and classification 2000-2001, *Philadelphia, 2001, The Association.*

## Outcome Identification

The expected outcome when working with a patient with a maladaptive self-concept response follows:

*The patient will obtain the maximum level of self-actualization to realize one's potential.*

## Planning

A Patient Education Plan for promoting the patient's self-differentiation in the family of origin is presented on page 213.

## DSM-IV-TR Medical Diagnoses Related to Maladaptive Self-Concept Responses

| DSM-IV-TR Diagnosis | Essential Features |
|---|---|
| Identity problem | Uncertainty about multiple issues relating to identity, such as long-term goals, career choice, friendship patterns, sexual orientation and behavior, moral values, and group loyalties. |
| Dissociative amnesia | Predominant disturbance is one or more episodes of inability to recall important personal information, usually of a traumatic or stressful nature, that is too extensive to be explained by ordinary forgetfulness. |
| Dissociative fugue | Predominant disturbance is sudden, unexpected travel away from home or one's customary place of work, with inability to recall one's past. Confusion about personal identity or assumption of a new identity. |
| Dissociative identity disorder (multiple personality disorder) | Presence of two or more distinct identities or personality states (each with its own relatively enduring pattern of perceiving, relating to, and thinking about the environment and self). At least two of these identities or personality states recurrently take control of the person's behavior. Inability to recall important personal information that is too extensive to be explained by ordinary forgetfulness. |
| Depersonalization disorder | Persistent or recurrent experiences of feeling detached from and as if one is an outside observer of one's mental processes or body (e.g., feeling as if one is in a dream). During the depersonalization experience, reality testing remains intact. The depersonalization causes clinically significant distress or impairment in functioning. |

Modified from American Psychiatric Association: Diagnostic and statistical manual of mental disorders, ed 4, text revision (DSM-IV-TR), Washington, DC, 2000, The Association.

Patient Education Plan:   **Improving Family Relationships**

| Content | Instructional Activities | Evaluation |
|---|---|---|
| Define concept of self-differentiation in a person's family of origin. | Discuss differences between high and low levels of self-differentiation. Ask patient to identify level of functioning among family members. | Patient identifies own functioning level in family of origin. |
| Describe characteristics of emotional fusion, emotional cutoff, and triangulation. | Analyze types and patterns of family relationships. Use paper and pencil to diagram family patterns. | Patient describes interactional patterns in own family. Patient identifies own roles and behavior. |
| Discuss role of symptom formation and symptom bearer in a family. | Sensitize patient to family dynamics and manifestations of stress. Encourage family communication. | Patient recognizes family's contribution to stress of individual members. Patient contacts family members. |
| Describe a family genogram and show how it is constructed. | Use a blackboard to map out a family genogram. Assign family genogram. | Patient obtains factual information about family. Patient constructs family genogram. |
| Analyze need for objectivity and responsibility for changing own behavior and not that of others. | Role-play interactions with various family members. Encourage testing out new ways of interacting with family members. | Patient demonstrates higher level of differentiation in family of origin. |

### Implementation

Empirically validated treatments for one of the medical disorders related to self-concept responses are summarized in Table 11-1.

## Intervening in Alterations in Self-Concept

Nursing intervention helps the patient examine his or her cognitive appraisal of the situation and related feelings to help the patient gain insight and then take action to bring about behavioral change. This problem-solving approach requires progressive levels of intervention as follows:

1. Expanded self-awareness
2. Self-exploration
3. Self-evaluation
4. Realistic planning
5. Commitment to action

Tables 11-2 through 11-6 describe specific principles, rationales, and nursing interventions for each progressive level in the sequence. A Nursing Treatment Plan Summary for maladaptive self-concept responses is presented on page 223.

### Evaluation

1. Have threats to the patient's physical integrity or self-system been reduced in nature, number, origin, or timing?
2. Do the patient's behaviors reflect greater self-acceptance, self-worth, and self-approval?
3. Have the patient's coping resources been adequately assessed and mobilized?
4. Has the patient expanded self-awareness and engaged in self-exploration and self-evaluation?

*Text continued on p. 224*

Table 11-1    Summarizing the evidence on treatments for self-concept responses

---

**DISORDER:** Dissociative disorders
**TREATMENT:**

- Psychodynamic psychotherapy, hypnosis, and amytal narcosynthesis are treatments of choice for these conditions based on case reports.

---

Modified from Nathan P, Gorman J: *A guide to treatments that work,* New York, 1998, Oxford University Press.

Table 11-2 Nursing interventions for alterations in self-concept at level 1

| Principle | Rationale | Nursing Interventions |
|---|---|---|
| **Goal: To Expand Patient's Self-Awareness** | | |
| Establish an open, trusting relationship. | Reduce threat that nurse poses to patient; help patient to broaden and accept all aspects of personality. | Offer unconditional acceptance. Listen to patient. Encourage discussion of patient's thoughts and feelings. Respond nonjudgmentally. Convey that patient is a valued person who is responsible for and able to help self. |
| Work with whatever ego strength patient possesses. | Some degree of ego strength, such as capacity for reality testing, self-control, or a degree of ego integration, is needed as a foundation for later nursing care. | Identify patient's ego strength. Use guidelines for patient with limited ego resources: 1. Begin by confirming patient's identity. 2. Provide support measures to reduce panic level of anxiety. 3. Approach patient in nondemanding way. 4. Accept and attempt to clarify any verbal or nonverbal communication. |

*Continued*

Table 11-2   Nursing interventions for alterations in self-concept at level 1—cont'd

| Principle | Rationale | Nursing Interventions |
|---|---|---|
| **Goal: To Expand Patient's Self-Awareness—cont'd** | | |
| | | 5. Prevent patient from isolating self. |
| | | 6. Establish simple routine for patient. |
| | | 7. Set limits on inappropriate behavior. |
| | | 8. Orient patient to reality. |
| | | 9. Reinforce appropriate behavior. |
| | | 10. Gradually increase activities and tasks that provide positive experiences. |
| | | 11. Assist in personal hygiene and grooming. |
| | | 12. Encourage patient in self-care. |
| Maximize patient's participation in therapeutic relationship. | Mutuality is necessary for patient to assume ultimate responsibility for own behavior and maladaptive coping responses. | Gradually increase patient's participation in care decisions. Convey that patient is a responsible individual. |

Table 11-3 Nursing interventions for alterations in self-concept at level 2

| Principle | Rationale | Nursing Interventions |
|---|---|---|
| **Goal: To Expand Patient's Self-Exploration** | | |
| Assist patient to accept own feelings and thoughts. | By showing interest in and accepting patient's feelings and thoughts, nurse helps patient to do the same. | Attend to and encourage patient's expression of emotions, beliefs, behavior, and thoughts—verbally, nonverbally, symbolically, or directly. Use therapeutic communication skills and empathic responses. Note patient's use of logical and illogical thinking and reported and observed emotional responses. |
| Help patient clarify concept of self and relationship to others through self-disclosure. | Self-disclosure and understanding self-perceptions are prerequisites to bringing about future change; this alone may reduce anxiety. | Elicit patient's perception of self-strengths and weaknesses. Assist patient to describe self-ideal. Identify patient's self-criticisms. Help patient to describe beliefs on how he or she relates to other people and events. |

Continued

Table 11-3 Nursing interventions for alterations in self-concept at level 2—cont'd

| Principle | Rationale | Nursing Interventions |
|---|---|---|
| **Goal: To Expand Patient's Self-Exploration—cont'd** | | |
| Be aware of and have control of own feelings. | Self-awareness allows nurse to model authentic behavior and limits potential negative effects of countertransference in relationship. | Be open to own feelings. Accept both positive and negative feelings. Practice therapeutic use of self: 1. Share own feelings with patient. 2. Verbalize how another might have felt. 3. Mirror own perception of patient's feelings. |
| Respond empathically, not sympathetically, emphasizing that power to change lies with patient. | Sympathy can reinforce patient's self-pity; rather, nurse should communicate that patient's life situation is subject to self-control. | Use empathic responses and monitor self for feelings of sympathy or pity. Reaffirm that patient is not helpless or powerless in face of problems. Convey verbally and behaviorally that patient is responsible for own behavior, including choice of maladaptive or adaptive coping responses. Discuss scope of patient's choices, areas of ego strength, and available coping resources. Use support systems of family and groups to facilitate patient's self-exploration. Assist patient in recognizing nature of conflict and maladaptive coping responses. |

Table 11-4   Nursing interventions for alterations in self-concept at level 3

| Principle | Rationale | Nursing Interventions |
|---|---|---|
| **Goal: To Expand Patient's Self-Evaluation** | | |
| Help patient define the problem clearly. | Only after problem is accurately defined can alternative choices be proposed. | Identify relevant stressors and patient's appraisal of them. Clarify that patient's beliefs influence both feelings and behaviors. Mutually identify faulty beliefs, misperceptions, distortions, illusions, and unrealistic goals. Mutually identify areas of strength. Place concepts of success and failure in proper perspective. Explore patient's use of coping resources. |
| Explore patient's adaptive and maladaptive coping responses to the problem. | It is necessary to examine patient's coping choices and evaluate both positive and negative consequences. | Describe to patient how all coping responses are freely chosen and have both positive and negative consequences. Contrast adaptive and maladaptive responses. Mutually identify disadvantages of patient's maladaptive coping responses. Mutually identify advantages, or "payoffs," of patient's maladaptive coping responses. Discuss how these payoffs have perpetuated the maladaptive response. Use variety of therapeutic skills, such as: 1. Facilitative communication 2. Supportive confrontation 3. Role clarification 4. Transference and countertransference reaction in the one-to-one relationship 5. Psychodrama |

Table 11-5  Nursing interventions for alterations in self-concept at level 4

| Principle | Rationale | Nursing Interventions |
|---|---|---|
| **Goal: To Assist Patient in Formulating a Realistic Plan of Action** | | |
| Help patient identify alternative solutions. | Only when all possible alternatives have been evaluated can change be effected. | Help patient understand that only he or she can change self, not others.<br>If patient holds inconsistent perceptions, help patient see how to change the following:<br>1. Beliefs or ideals to bring them closer to reality<br>2. Environment to make it consistent with patient's beliefs<br>If self-concept is not consistent with behavior, help patient see how to change the following:<br>1. Behavior to conform to self-concept<br>2. Beliefs underlying self-concept to include behavior<br>3. Self-ideal<br>Mutually review how patient may better use coping resources. |
| Help patient conceptualize own realistic goals. | Goal setting must include a clear definition of the expected change. | Encourage patient to formulate own (not nurse's) goals.<br>Mutually discuss emotional, practical, and reality-based consequences of each goal.<br>Help patient clearly define the concrete change to be made.<br>Encourage patient to enter new experiences for their growth potential.<br>Use role rehearsal, role modeling, role playing, and visualization when appropriate. |

Table 11-6   Nursing interventions for alterations in self-concept at level 5

| Principle | Rationale | Nursing Interventions |
|---|---|---|
| **Goal: To Assist Patient to Become Committed to Decision and Achieve Own Goals** | | |
| Help patient take necessary action to change maladaptive coping responses and maintain adaptive ones. | Ultimate objective in promoting insights is to have patient replace maladaptive coping responses with more adaptive ones. | Provide opportunity for patient to experience success. Reinforce strengths, skills, and healthy aspects of patient's personality. Help patient gain assistance (vocational, financial, social services). Use groups to enhance patient's self-esteem. Promote patient's self-differentiation in family of origin. Allow patient sufficient time to change. Provide appropriate amount of support and positive reinforcement to help patient maintain progress. |

## Nursing Treatment Plan Summary:  Maladaptive Self-Concept Responses

Nursing Diagnosis: Self-esteem disturbance

Expected Outcome: Patient will obtain the maximal level of self-actualization to realize his or her potential.

| Short-term Goals | Interventions | Rationale |
| --- | --- | --- |
| Patient will establish a therapeutic relationship with nurse. | Confirm patient's identity. Provide supportive measures to decrease panic level of anxiety. Set limits on inappropriate behavior. Work with whatever ego strengths patient possesses. Reinforce adaptive behavior. | Mutuality is necessary for patient to assume responsibility for behavior. Some degree of ego integrity is needed for later interventions. |
| Patient will express feelings, behaviors, and thoughts related to present stressful situations. | Assist patient to express and describe feelings and thoughts. Help patient in identifying strengths and weaknesses, self-ideal, and self-criticisms. Respond empathically, emphasizing that the power to change lies within patient. | Self-disclosure and understanding are necessary to bring about change. Use of sympathy is not therapeutic because it can reinforce patient's self-pity; rather, nurse should communicate that patient is in control. |

| Patient will evaluate the positive and negative consequences of self-concept responses. | Identify relevant stressors and patient's appraisal of them. Clarify faulty beliefs and cognitive distortions. Evaluate advantages and disadvantages of current coping responses. | Only after the problem is defined can alternative choices be examined; then the positive and negative consequences of current patterns must be evaluated. |
| Patient will identify one new goal and two adaptive coping responses. | Encourage patient to formulate a new goal. Help patient clearly define the change to be made. Use role rehearsal, role modeling, and visualization to practice the new behavior. | Only after alternatives have been explored can change be effected. Goal setting specifies nature of the change and suggests possible new behavioral strategies. |
| Patient will implement the new adaptive self-concept responses. | Provide opportunity for patient to experience success. Reinforce strengths, skills, and adaptive coping responses. Allow patient sufficient time to change. Promote group and family involvement. Provide appropriate amount of support and positive reinforcement for patient to maintain progress and growth. | Ultimate goal in promoting patient's insight is to have patient replace the maladaptive coping responses with more adaptive ones. |

5. Is the patient using adaptive coping responses?
6. Has the patient learned new adaptive strategies to enhance the level of self-actualization?
7. Is the patient using greater self-understanding to promote personal change and growth?

*your* **INTERNET**
c o n n e c t i o n

**Dissociative identity disorder/multiple personality disorder:**
home.att.net/~boyym/main.html

## Suggested readings

Applegate M: Multiphasic short-term therapy for dissociative identity disorder, *J Am Psychiatr Nurs Assoc* 3:1, 1997.

Bracken B: *Handbook of self-concept,* New York, 1996, John Wiley & Sons.

Burns D: Focusing on ego strengths, *Arch Psychiatr Nurs* 5:202, 1991.

Brynat D. Kessler J: *Beyond integration: one multiple's journey,* New York, 1996, WW Norton.

Czuchta D, Johnson B: Reconstructing a sense of self in patients with chronic mental illness, *Perspect Psychiatr Care* 34(3):31, 1998.

Dallam S, Manderino M: Peer group supports patients with MPD/DD, *J Psychosoc Nurs* 35:22, 1997.

Godbey J, Hutchinson S: Healing from incest: resurrecting the buried self, *Arch Psychiatr Nurs* 10:304, 1996.

Guralnik O et al: Feeling unreal: cognitive processes in depersonalization, *Am J Psychiatry* 157(1):103, 2000.

Horowitz M et al: Self-regard: a new measure, *Am J Psychiatry* 153:382, 1996.

Kluft R: Current issues in dissociative identity disorder, *J Prac Psychiatry Behav Health* 5:3, 1999.

Mruk C: *Self-esteem: research, theory and practice,* New York, 1999, Springer.

Phillips J: *The magic daughter: a memoir of living with multiple personality disorder,* New York, 1995, Viking.

Price B: Explorations in body image care: Peplau and practical knowledge, *J Psychiatr Ment Health Nurs* 5:179, 1998.

Stuart G, Laraia M: *Principles and practice of psychiatric nursing,* ed 7, St Louis, 2001, Mosby.

Vaillant G: *The wisdom of the ego,* Cambridge, Mass, 1993, Harvard University Press.

# Emotional Responses and Mood Disorders

12

## Continuum of Emotional Responses

*Mood* refers to a prolonged emotional state that influences an individual's whole personality and life functioning. It pertains to a person's prevailing and pervading emotion and is synonymous with the terms *affect, feeling state,* and *emotion.* As with other aspects of the personality, emotions or moods serve an adaptive role for the individual. If the expression of emotions is viewed on a continuum of health and illness, the following relevant parameters become apparent (Figure 12-1):

1. *Emotional responsiveness* involves being affected by and being an active participant in one's internal and external worlds. It implies being open to and aware of one's feelings.

2. *Uncomplicated grief reaction* occurs in response to a loss and implies that a person is facing the reality of the loss and is immersed in the work of grieving.

3. *Suppression of emotions* may be evident as a denial of one's feelings, a detachment from them, or an internalization of all aspects of one's affective world.

4. *Delayed grief reaction* is the persistent absence of any emotional response to a loss. The delay may occur at the start of the mourning process, may become evident later in the process, or both. The delay and rejection of grief may occasionally involve many years.

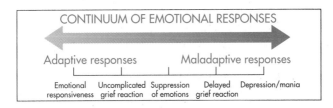

Figure 12-1
Continuum of emotional responses.

5. *Depression,* or melancholia, is an abnormal extension or overelaboration of sadness and grief. It can be used to denote a variety of phenomena, such as a sign, symptom, syndrome, emotional state, reaction, disease, or clinical entity.

6. *Mania* is characterized by an elevated, expansive, or irritable mood. *Hypomania* is used to describe a clinical syndrome similar to but not as severe as that described by the term *mania* or *manic episode.*

Box 12-1 presents facts about depressive and bipolar (manic-depressive) disorders.

## Assessment

### Behaviors

The behaviors associated with depression are varied (Box 12-2). Sadness and slowness may predominate, or states of agitation may occur. The key element to a behavioral assessment is *change*—the individual changes the usual behavioral pattern and responses. The essential feature of mania is a distinct period of intense psychophysiological activation. Box 12-3 lists some behaviors associated with mania.

### Predisposing Factors

Various theories have been proposed to explain severe disturbances of mood. The range of causative factors, which may operate singly or in combination, is evident in the following theories and models:

1. *Genetic factors* have been proposed to account for the transmission of affective disorders through heredity and family history.

---

### Box 12-1    Facts about Mood Disorders

Major Depressive Disorder

- Major depression is among the most common of all clinical problems encountered by primary care practitioners.
- Major depression accounts for more bed days (people off work and in bed) than any other "physical" disorder except cardiovascular disease. Depression is more costly to the economy than chronic respiratory illness, diabetes, arthritis, or hypertension.
- Psychotherapy alone helps some depressed patients, especially those with mild to moderate symptoms.
- Depression can be treated successfully with antidepressant medications in 65% of patients.
- Treatment success rates increase to 85% when alternative or adjunctive medications are used or psychotherapy is combined with medications.

Bipolar (Manic-Depressive) Disorder

- Without modern treatments, patients with bipolar disorder typically spend one fourth their adult life in the hospital and half their life disabled.
- Effective medications (lithium, anticonvulsants), often used in combination with supportive psychotherapy, allow 75% to 80% of manic-depressive patients to lead essentially normal lives.
- These drugs have saved the U.S. economy more than $40 billion since 1970: $13 billion in direct treatment costs and $27 billion in indirect costs.

---

2. *Aggression-turned-inward theory* suggests that depression results from the turning of angry feelings inward against the self.
3. *Object loss theory* refers to the traumatic separation of a person from significant objects of attachment.
4. *Personality organization theory* describes how a negative self-concept and low self-esteem influence a person's belief system and appraisal of stressors.

## Box 12-2   Behaviors Associated with Depression

### Affective

Anger
Anxiety
Apathy
Bitterness
Dejection
Denial of feelings
Despondency
Guilt
Helplessness
Hopelessness
Loneliness
Low self-esteem
Sadness
Sense of worthlessness

### Cognitive

Ambivalence
Confusion
Inability to concentrate
Indecisiveness
Loss of interest and
   motivation
Pessimism
Self-blame
Self-deprecation
Self-destructive thoughts
Uncertainty

### Physiological

Abdominal pain
Anorexia
Backache
Chest pain

### Physiological—cont'd

Constipation
Dizziness
Fatigue
Headache
Impotence
Indigestion
Insomnia
Lassitude
Menstrual changes
Nausea
Overeating
Sexual
   nonresponsiveness
Sleep disturbances
Vomiting
Weight change

### Behavioral

Aggressiveness
Agitation
Alcoholism
Altered activity level
Drug addiction
Intolerance
Irritability
Lack of spontaneity
Overdependency
Poor personal hygiene
Psychomotor retardation
Social isolation
Tearfulness
Underachievement
Withdrawal

---

### Box 12-3  Behaviors Associated with Mania

Affective

Elation or euphoria
Expansiveness
Humor
Inflated self-esteem
Intolerance of criticism
Lack of shame or guilt

Cognitive

Ambition
Denial of realistic
 danger
Distractibility
Flight of ideas
Grandiosity
Illusions
Lack of judgment
Loose associations

Physiological

Dehydration
Inadequate nutrition
Need for little sleep
Weight loss

Behavioral

Aggression
Excessive spending of
 money
Grandiose acts
Hyperactivity
Increased motor activity
Irresponsibility
Irritability or
 argumentativeness
Poor personal grooming
Provocation
Sexual overactivity
Social activity
Verbosity

---

5. *Cognitive model* proposes that depression is a cognitive problem dominated by one's negative evaluation of oneself, one's world, and one's future.

6. *Learned helplessness model* suggests that trauma per se does not produce depression, but rather the belief that one has no control over the important outcomes in one's life; therefore the person refrains from making adaptive responses.

7. *Behavioral model* is derived from the social learning theory framework, which assumes the cause of depression resides in the individual's lack of positively reinforcing interactions with the environment.

8. *Biological model* describes the chemical changes in the body that occur during depressed states, including the deficiency of catecholamines, endocrine dysfunction, hyperse-

cretion of cortisol, neurotransmitter dysregulation, and periodic variations in biological rhythms.

## Precipitating Stressors

Four major sources of stressors can precipitate a disturbance of mood as follows:

1. *Loss of attachment,* real or imagined, includes the loss of love, a person, physical functioning, status, or self-esteem. Because of the actual and symbolic elements involved in the concept of loss, the patient's perceptions take on primary importance.
2. *Major life events* frequently precede a depressive episode and affect a person's current problems and problem-solving abilities.
3. *Role strain* contributes to the development of depression, particularly in women.
4. *Physiological changes* produced by drugs or various physical illnesses (e.g., infections, neoplasms, metabolic imbalances) can precipitate disturbances of mood. Various antihypertensive drugs and the abuse of addictive substances are common precipitating factors. Most chronic, debilitating illnesses are also frequently accompanied by depression. Depression in elderly persons is particularly complex because the diagnosis often involves evaluating for organic brain damage and clinical depression.

## Appraisal of Stressors

Depression results from the interaction among variables at the chemical, experiential, and behavioral levels. The specific form the illness takes depends on the following factors:

1. Genetic vulnerability
2. Developmental events
3. Physiological stressors
4. Psychosocial stressors

This interactive effect underscores the importance of the individual's appraisal of his or her life situation and related stressors.

## Coping Resources

Coping resources include the person's socioeconomic status, family, and interpersonal networks and the secondary organization

---

### Box 12-4    Risk Factors for Depression

Prior episodes of depression
Family history of depression
Prior suicide attempts
Female gender
Age of onset less than 40 years
Postpartum period
Medical comorbidity
Lack of social support
Stressful life events
Personal history of sexual abuse
Current substance abuse

---

provided by the broader social environment. Lack of such personal resources provides additional stress for the individual. Box 12-4 lists the risk factors for depression.

## Coping Mechanisms

A delayed grief reaction reflects the exaggerated use of the defense mechanisms of denial and suppression in an attempt to avoid the intense distress associated with grief. Depression is similar to abortive grieving, using the mechanisms of repression, suppression, denial, and dissociation. Some believe that mania is a mirror image of depression and that, even though the behaviors are dissimilar, the dynamics and coping mechanisms are related.

### Nursing Diagnosis

The diagnosis of mood disturbance depends on an understanding of many interrelated concepts, including anxiety, self-concept, and hostility. An appropriate nursing diagnosis should include the patient's maladaptive coping response and related stressor. The box on page 233 presents the primary and related NANDA nursing diagnoses for maladaptive emotional responses.

## Related Medical Diagnoses

The two major categories of mood or affective disorders identified in DSM-IV-TR, bipolar (manic-depressive) disorders and depres-

## NANDA Nursing Diagnoses Related to Maladaptive Emotional Responses

Anxiety
Communication, Impaired verbal
Coping, Ineffective
Grieving, Anticipatory
*Grieving, Dysfunctional
*Hopelessness
Injury, Risk for
Loneliness, Risk for
Memory, Impaired
Nutrition, Imbalanced
*Powerlessness
Powerlessness, Risk for
Self-care deficit
Self-esteem, Risk for situational low
Self-esteem, Situational low
Sexual dysfunction
Sleep pattern, Disturbed
Social isolation
*Spiritual distress
Suicide, Risk for
Thought processes, Disturbed
Violence, Risk for self-directed

*Primary nursing diagnosis for disturbances in mood.
*From North American Nursing Diagnosis Association:* NANDA nursing diagnoses: definitions and classification 2000-2001, *Philadelphia, 2001, The Association.*

sive (unipolar) disorders, are based on whether manic and depressive episodes are present over time. In the depressive disorder classification, major depression may involve either a single episode or a recurrent depressive illness but without manic attacks. When the patient has one or more manic episodes, with or without a major depressive episode, the category of bipolar disorder is used. The box on page 235 describes medical diagnoses related to mood disorders. Box 12-5 lists diagnostic criteria for major depressive and manic episodes.

## Box 12-5    Diagnostic Criteria for Major Depressive and Manic Episodes

Major Depressive Episode

At least five of the following (including one of the first two) must be present most of the day, almost daily, for at least 2 weeks.

1. **Depressed mood**
2. **Loss of interest or pleasure**
3. Weight loss or gain
4. Insomnia or hypersomnia
5. Psychomotor agitation or retardation
6. Fatigue or loss of energy
7. Feelings of worthlessness
8. Impaired concentration
9. Thoughts of death or suicide

Manic Episode

At least three of the following must be present to a significant degree for at least 1 week.

1. Grandiosity
2. Decreased need for sleep
3. Pressured speech
4. Flight of ideas
5. Distractibility
6. Psychomotor agitation
7. Excessive involvement in pleasurable activities without regard for negative consequences

## Outcome Identification

The expected outcome when working with a patient with a maladaptive emotional response follows:

*The patient will be emotionally responsive and return to preillness level of functioning.*

## Planning

In care planning the nurse's priorities are the reduction and ultimate removal of all the patient's maladaptive emotional responses,

## DSM-IV-TR Medical Diagnoses Related to Maladaptive Emotional Responses

| DSM-IV-TR Diagnosis | Essential Features |
|---|---|
| Bipolar I disorder | Current or past experience of a manic episode, lasting at least 1 week, when the person's mood was abnormally and persistently elevated, expansive, or irritable. The episode is sufficiently severe to cause extreme impairment in social or occupational functioning. Bipolar disorders may be classified as manic (limited to only manic episodes), depressed (history of manic episodes with a current depressive episode), or mixed (both manic and depressive episodes). |
| Bipolar II disorder | Presence or history of one or more major depressive episodes and at least one hypomanic episode. The person has never had a manic episode. |
| Cyclothymic disorder | History of 2 years of hypomania in which the person experienced numerous periods with abnormally elevated, expansive, or irritable moods. These moods did not meet the criteria for a manic episode, and many periods of depressed mood did not meet the criteria of a major depressive episode. |
| Major depressive disorder | Presence of at least five symptoms during the same 2-week period, with one being either depressed mood or loss of interest or pleasure. Other symptoms might include weight loss, insomnia, psychomotor agitation or retardation, fatigue, feelings of worthlessness, diminished ability to think, and recurrent thoughts of death. Major depressions may be classified as a single episode or recurrent. |
| Dysthymic disorder | At least 2 years of a usually depressed mood and at least one of the symptoms mentioned for major depression without meeting the criteria for a major depressive episode. |

*Modified from American Psychiatric Association: Diagnostic and statistical manual of mental disorders, ed 4, text revision (DSM-IV-TR), Washington, DC, 2000, The Association.*

restoration of the patient's occupational and psychosocial functioning, improvement in the patient's quality of life, and minimization of the likelihood of relapse and recurrence. To achieve this, treatment consists of three phases: (1) acute, (2) continuation, and (3) maintenance (Figure 12-2).

## Acute

The goal of acute treatment is to eliminate the symptoms. If patients improve with treatment, they have had a *response.* A successful acute phase treatment brings patients back to an essentially symptom-free state and to a level of functioning comparable to before the illness. This phase usually lasts 6 to 12 weeks, and if patients are symptom free at the end of that time, they are in *remission.*

## Continuation

The goal of continuation treatment is to prevent *relapse,* which is the return of symptoms. The risk of relapse is very high in the first 4 to 6 months after recovery, and one of the greatest mistakes in the treatment of mood disorders is the failure to continue a successful treatment for sufficient time. This phase usually lasts 4 to 9 months.

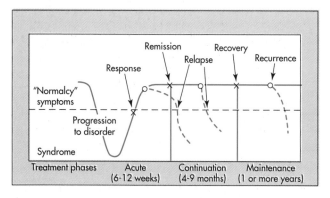

Figure 12-2

**Phases of treatment for patients with mood disorders.**

## Maintenance

The goal of maintenance treatment is to prevent the *recurrence*, or return, of a new episode of illness. This concept is commonly accepted for bipolar illness but is relatively new for major depressive disorders. Several research studies indicate the effectiveness of maintenance therapy in preventing new depressive episodes or lengthening the interval between them. A Patient Education Plan for enhancing social skills is presented on page 238.

### Implementation

Empirically validated treatments for major depressive disorder and bipolar disorder are summarized in Table 12-1.

### Intervening in Depression and Mania

Nursing interventions must reflect the complex nature of the integrative model of mood disturbances and address all maladaptive aspects of a patient's life. Intervening in as many areas as possible should have the greatest effect. A Nursing Treatment Plan Summary for patients with maladaptive emotional responses begins on page 240.

> **NURSE ALERT.** In caring for the patient with a severe mood disorder, the nurse should give highest priority to the potential for suicide. Hospitalization is definitely indicated for the patient at risk for suicide. In the presence of rapidly progressing symptoms and in the absence or rupture of the usual support systems, hospitalization is strongly indicated. Nursing care in this case means protecting patients and assuring them that they will not be allowed to harm themselves. Patients are at particular risk for suicide when they appear to be coming out of depression; they may then have the energy and opportunity to commit suicide. Acute manic states are also life threatening.

### Evaluation

1. Were all possible sources of precipitating stress and the patient's perception of them explored?

*Text continued on p. 245*

## Patient Education Plan: Enhancing Social Skills

| Content | Instructional Activities | Evaluation |
| --- | --- | --- |
| Describe behaviors interfering with social interactions. | Instruct patient on corrective behaviors. | Patient identifies problematic and more facilitative behaviors. |
| Discuss components of social performance relevant to patient's situation. | Model effective interpersonal skills for patient. | Patient describes specific skills to acquire. |
| Analyze how patient could incorporate these specific skills. | Use role playing and guided practice to allow patient to test new behaviors. | Patient shows beginning skill in new social behaviors. |
| Encourage patient to test new skills in other situation. | Give homework assignments for patient to do in natural environment. | Patient discusses ability to complete assigned tasks. |
| Discuss generalization of new skills to other aspects of patient's life and functioning. | Give feedback, encouragement, and praise for newly acquired social skills and their generalization. | Patient is able to integrate new social behaviors in interactions with others. |

**Table 12-1**   Summarizing the evidence on treatments for mood disorders

**DISORDER:** Major depressive disorder (MDD)
**TREATMENT:**

- Tricyclic antidepressants (TCAs), the first antidepressants to be studied extensively, were consistently more efficacious than placebos both in reducing the complex of symptoms of MDD and managing the disorder over the long term.
- Because of their narrow safety margin and significant drug-induced adverse side effects, TCAs have now been largely replaced for the treatment of MDD by selective serotonin re-uptake inhibitors (SSRIs), including fluoxetine, sertraline, and paroxetine and the new compounds, venlafaxine, bupropion, and nefazodone.
- Because of adverse side effects, monoamine oxidase inhibitors (MAOIs) are generally reserved for treatment-refractory MDD patients.
- Interventions using behavior therapy, cognitive-behavior therapy, and interpersonal therapy have all yielded substantial reductions in scores on the two major depression rating scales and in the percentage of patients meeting MDD criteria after treatment; all three treatments have also shown significant maintenance of effect after treatment.

**DISORDER:** Bipolar disorder
**TREATMENT:**

- Although pharmacological interventions are treatments of choice, psychosocial treatments, including psychoeducation and cognitive-behavior therapy for medication and adherence, have also shown promise.
- Lithium reduces the symptoms of acute mania in bipolar I disorder.
- Olanzapine reduces the symptoms of acute mania in bipolar I disorder.
- Valproate has shown effectiveness in reducing the symptoms of acute mania in bipolar I disorder.
- Carbamazepine has demonstrated effectiveness in treating the symptoms of acute mania.
- Lithium has been effective with a substantial percentage of bipolar patients (e.g., 35%-50%) in preventing or reducing the frequency of recurrent affective episodes; however, side effects have interfered with drug compliance.
- Lithium and several antidepressants have also shown moderate effectiveness with acute and chronic bipolar depression.

Nursing Treatment Plan Summary: **Maladaptive Emotional Responses**

**Nursing Diagnosis: Hopelessness**

**Expected Outcome: Patient will be emotionally responsive and return to preillness level of functioning.**

| Short-term Goals | Interventions | Rationale |
|---|---|---|
| Patient's environment will be safe and protective. | Continually evaluate patient's potential for suicide. <br> Hospitalize patient at risk for suicide. <br> Assist patient to move to a new environment when appropriate (e.g., new job, peer group, family setting). | All patients with severe mood disturbances are at high risk for suicide; environmental changes can protect patient, decrease immediate stress, and mobilize additional resources. |
| Patient will establish a therapeutic relationship with nurse. | Use a warm, accepting, empathic approach. <br> Be aware of and in control of own feelings and reactions (e.g., anger, frustration, sympathy). <br> *With depressed patient:* <br> Establish rapport through shared time and supportive companionship. <br> Allow patient time to respond. <br> Personalize care as a way of indicating patient's value as a human being. | Both depressed and manic patients resist becoming involved in a therapeutic alliance; acceptance, persistence, and limit setting are necessary. |

| | | |
|---|---|---|
| Patient will be physiologically stable and able to meet self-care needs. | *With manic patient:*<br>Give simple, truthful responses.<br>Be alert to possible manipulation.<br>Set constructive limits on negative behavior.<br>Use a consistent approach by all health team members.<br>Maintain open communication and sharing of perceptions among team members.<br>Reinforce patient's self-control and positive aspects of patient behavior.<br>Assist patient to meet self-care needs, particularly in areas of nutrition, sleep, and personal hygiene.<br>Encourage patient's independence whenever possible.<br>Administer prescribed medications and somatic treatments. | Physiological changes occur with disturbances of mood; physical care and somatic therapies are required to overcome these problems. |

*Continued*

Nursing Treatment Plan Summary: Maladaptive Emotional Responses—cont'd

| Short-term Goals | Interventions | Rationale |
|---|---|---|
| Patient will be able to recognize and express emotions related to daily events. | Respond empathically with a focus on feelings rather than facts.<br>Acknowledge patient's pain and convey a sense of hope in recovery.<br>Help patient experience feelings and then express them appropriately.<br>Assist patient in adaptive expression of anger. | Patients with severe mood disturbances have difficulty identifying, expressing, and modulating feelings. |
| Patient will evaluate thinking and correct faulty or negative thoughts. | Review patient's conceptualization of the problem but do not necessarily accept conclusions.<br>Identify patient's negative thoughts and help decrease them.<br>Help increase positive thinking.<br>Examine the accuracy of perceptions, logic, and conclusions.<br>Identify misperceptions, distortions, and irrational beliefs.<br>Help patient move from unrealistic to realistic goals.<br>Decrease importance of unattainable goals.<br>Limit amount of patient's negative personal evaluations. | These strategies help increase patient's sense of control over goals and behaviors, enhance self-esteem, and modify negative expectations. |

| | | |
|---|---|---|
| Patient will implement two new behavioral coping strategies. | Assign appropriate action-oriented therapeutic tasks. | Successful behavioral performance counteracts feelings of helplessness and hopelessness. |
| | Encourage activities gradually, escalating them as patient's energy is mobilized. | |
| | Provide a tangible, structured program when appropriate. | |
| | Set goals that are realistic, relevant to patient's needs and interests, and focused on positive activities. | |
| | Focus on present activities, not past or future activities. | |
| | Positively reinforce successful performance. | |
| | Incorporate physical exercise in patient's plan of care. | |

*Continued*

Nursing Treatment Plan Summary: **Maladaptive Emotional Responses—cont'd**

| Short-term Goals | Interventions | Rationale |
| --- | --- | --- |
| Patient will describe rewarding social interactions. | Assess patient's social skills, supports, and interests.<br>Review existing and potential social resources.<br>Instruct and model effective social skills.<br>Use role playing and rehearsal of social interactions.<br>Give feedback and positive reinforcement of effective interpersonal skills.<br>Intervene with families to have them reinforce patient's adaptive emotional responses.<br>Support or engage in family and group therapy when appropriate. | Socialization is an experience incompatible with withdrawal and increases self-esteem through the social reinforcers of approval, acceptance, recognition, and support. |

2. Was the patient appropriately assessed for problems related to self-concept, anger, and interpersonal relationships?

3. Were changes in the patient's usual behavioral patterns and responses explored?

4. Was the patient's personal and family history of previous episodes of depression or elation fully evaluated?

5. Were appropriate precautions taken for possible suicide or self-harm?

6. Was the patient's social network supported as a coping resource?

7. Were the nursing interventions broad in scope and inclusive of the many aspects of the patient's world?

8. Were the patient's transference reactions identified and worked through?

9. Was the nurse aware of personal feelings, conflicts, and ability to confront the range of emotions openly throughout the therapeutic relationship?

10. Is the patient experiencing increased satisfaction and pleasure?

## *your* INTERNET
### connection

**Bipolar Disorders Portal:**
www.pendulum.org

**Depression and Related Affective Disorders Association:**
www.med.jhu.edu/drada

**Depression Screening:**
depression-screening.org

**Dr. Ivan's Depression Central:**
www.psychom.net/depression.central.html

**National Alliance for Research on Schizophrenia and Depression:**
www.mhsource.com/narsad.html

**National Depressive and Manic-Depressive Association:**
www.ndmda.org

**National Foundation for Depressive Illness, Inc.:**
www.depression.org

## Suggested readings

American Psychiatric Association: Practice guideline for the treatment of patients with major depressive disorder, *Am J Psychiatry* 157(4):489, 2000.

Bateman A: Understanding the process of grieving and loss: a critical social thinking perspective, *J Am Psychiatr Nurs Assoc* 5(5):139, 1999.

Beck A et al: *Cognitive therapy of depression,* New York, 1979, Guilford.

Beeber LS: Depression in women. In McBride AB, Austin JK, editors: *Psychiatric–mental health nursing: integrating the behavioral and biological sciences,* Philadelphia, 1996, WB Saunders.

Berlanga C et al: Personality and clinical predictors of recurrence of depression, *Psychiatr Serv* 50(3):376, 1999.

Copeland M: *Living without depression and manic depression: a workbook for maintaining mood stability,* Oakland, Calif, 1994, New Harbinger Publications.

Depression Guideline Panel: *Depression in primary care,* vol 1, *Detection and diagnosis: clinical practice guideline,* No 5, Pub No 93-0550, Rockville, Md, 1993, US Department of Health and Human Services, Public Health Service, Agency for Health Care Policy and Research.

Depression Guideline Panel: *Depression in primary care,* vol 2, *Treatment of major depression: clinical practice guideline,* No 5, Pub No 93-0551, Rockville, Md, 1993, US Department of Health and Human Services, Public Health Service, Agency for Health Care Policy and Research.

Epperson C: Postpartum major depression: detection and treatment, *Am Acad Fam Physicians,* April 15, 1999.

Griffiths K, Christensen H: Quality of web based information on treatment of depression: cross sectional survey, *British Medical Journal* 321:1511, 2000.

Hedaya R: *The antidepressant survival program,* New York, 2000, Crown.

Henry C et al: Antidepressant-induced mania in bipolar patients: identification of risk factors, *J Clin Psychiatry,* 62:249, 2001.

Hilty D et al: A review of bipolar disorder among adults, *Psychiatr Serv* 50(2):201, 1999.

Houston T, Cooper L, Vu H et al: Screening the public for depression through the Internet, *Psychiatric Services,* 52(3):362, 2001.

Jamison K: *An unquiet mind,* New York, 1995, Knopf.

Jozefowski JT: *The phoenix phenomenon: rising from the ashes of grief,* Northvale, NJ, 1999, Jason Aronson.

Kendler K, Thorton L., & Prescott, C. Gender differences in the rates of exposure to stressful life events and sensitivity to their depressogenic effects. *American Journal of Psychiatry,* 158(4):587, 2001.

Manning M: *Undercurrents: a therapist's reckoning with depression,* San Francisco, 1994, HarperCollins.

Masching J: A nurse battling with her own depression, *J Psychosoc Nurs* 34:26, 1996.

McEnany G: Rhythm and blues revisited: biological rhythm disturbances in depression, *J Am Psychiatr Nurs Assoc* 2:15, 1996.

Meredith L, Orlando M, Humphrey N, Camp P, Sherbourne C: Are better ratings of the patient-provider relationship associated with higher quality care for depression? *Medical Care* 39(4):349-360, 2001.

NIH Consensus Development Conference: *Diagnosis and treatment of depression in late life,* Rockville, Md, 1991, US Department of Health and Human Services, Public Health Service, National Institutes of Health.

Pollack L, Cramer R: Perceptions of problems in people hospitalized for bipolar disorder: implications for patient education, *Issues Ment Health Nurs* 21:765, 2000.

Roberts R et al: Does growing old increase the risk for depression? *Am J Psychiatry* 154(10):1384, 1997.

Rosenthal N: *Winter blues: seasonal affective disorder,* New York, 1993, Guilford.

Sebastian L: *Overcoming postpartum depression and anxiety*, Omaha, Neb, 1998, Addicus Books.

Seligman M: *Learned optimism,* New York, 1991, Knopf.

Simmons-Alling S: Bipolar mood disorders: brain, behavior, and nursing. In McBride AB, Austin JK, editors: *Psychiatric–mental health nursing: integrating the behavioral and biological sciences,* Philadelphia, 1996, WB Saunders.

Solomon A: Anatomy of melancholy, *The New Yorker,* January 12, 1998, p 46.

Slater L: *Prozac diary,* New York, 1998, Random House.

Stuart G, Laraia M: *Principles and practice of psychiatric nursing,* ed 7, St Louis, 2001, Mosby.

Suri R, Burt V: The assessment and treatment of postpartum psychiatric disorders, *J Pract Psychiatry Behav Health* 3:67, 1997.

Terman M et al: Seasonal affective disorder and its treatments, *J Pract Psychiatry Behav Health,* September 4:287, 1998.

Webster D, McEnany G: Research and clinical strategies for treatment resistant depression: buyer beware? *J Am Psychiatr Nurses Assoc* 3:17, 1997.

# Self-Protective Responses and Suicidal Behavior

## Continuum of Self-Protective Responses

Self-destructive behavior is any activity that will lead to death if not interrupted. It may be classified as direct or indirect. *Direct self-destructive behavior* includes any form of suicidal activity. The intent is death, and the individual is aware of this as the desired outcome. The behavior is short term in duration. *Indirect self-destructive behavior* includes any activity that is detrimental to a person's physical well-being and that can lead to death. The person is unaware of this potential and usually denies it if confronted. The behavior is usually longer in duration than suicidal behavior. Indirect self-destructive behaviors include the following:

1. Cigarette smoking
2. Reckless driving
3. Gambling
4. Criminal activity
5. Participation in high-risk recreational activities
6. Substance abuse
7. Socially deviant behavior
8. Stress-seeking behavior
9. Eating disorders
10. Noncompliance with medical treatment

A continuum of self-protective responses has self-enhancement as the most adaptive response, with indirect self-destructive be-

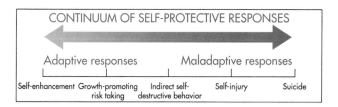

Figure 13-1
Continuum of self-protective responses.

havior, self-injury, and suicide as maladaptive responses (Figure 13-1).

## Assessment

### Behaviors

#### Noncompliance

It has been estimated that half of patients do not comply with their health care treatment plan. People who do not comply with recommended health care activities are generally aware that they have chosen not to care for themselves. Box 13-1 lists the most prominent behaviors associated with noncompliance.

#### Self-injury

Various terms have been used to describe self-injurious behavior: *self-abuse, self-directed aggression, self-harm, self-inflicted injury,* and *self-mutilation.* Self-injury can be defined as the act of deliberating harming one's own body. The injury is done to oneself, without the aid of another person, and the injury is severe enough for tissue damage. Common forms of self-injurious behavior include cutting and burning the skin, banging head and limbs, picking at wounds, and chewing fingers.

#### Suicidal behavior

All suicidal behavior is serious, whatever the intent. In the assessment of suicidal behavior, much emphasis is placed on the lethality of the method threatened or used. Although all suicide threats and attempts must be taken seriously, more vigorous and vigilant atten-

## Box 13-1    Behaviors Associated with Treatment Noncompliance

Awareness of a reason for noncompliance
Minimization of the seriousness of the problem
Chronic illnesses characterized by asymptomatic intervals
Frequent changes in health care providers
Search for miracle cures
Guilt that interferes with obtaining regular care
Concern about control

---

tion is indicated when the person is planning or tries a highly lethal means, such as a gunshot, hanging, or jumping. Less lethal means include carbon monoxide and drug overdose, which allow time for discovery once the suicidal action has begun.

Assessment of the suicidal person also includes whether the person has made a specific plan and whether the means to carry out the plan are available. The most suicidal person is one who plans a violent death, has a specific plan, and has the means readily available.

Suicidal behavior is usually divided into the following three categories:

1. *Suicide threats*—verbal or nonverbal warnings that a person is considering suicide. Suicidal persons may indicate verbally that they will not be around much longer or may communicate nonverbally by giving away prized possessions, revising a will, and so on. These messages should be considered in the context of current life events. The threat represents the person's ambivalence about dying. Lack of a positive response may be interpreted as encouragement to carry out the act.

2. *Suicide attempts*—any self-directed actions taken by the individual that will lead to death if not interrupted.

3. *Completed suicide*—may take place after warning signs have been missed or ignored. Persons who make suicide attempts and who do not really intend to die may do so if they are not discovered in time.

> **NURSE ALERT.**   Directly questioning the patient about sui-
> cidal thought and plans will not result in the patient taking
> suicidal actions. Rather, most people feel relieved to be
> asked about these feelings. One of the most important ques-
> tions to ask suicidal patients is whether they think they can
> control their behavior and refrain from acting on their im-
> pulses. If they cannot do this, immediate psychiatric hospi-
> talization is indicated.

## Predisposing Factors

Five domains of predisposing factors contribute to understanding
self-destructive behavior over the life cycle:

1. *Psychiatric diagnosis*—more than 90% of adults who end
   their lives by suicide have an associated psychiatric illness.
   Three psychiatric disorders that put individuals at particular
   risk for suicide are mood disorders, substance abuse, and
   schizophrenia.
2. *Personality traits*—the three aspects of personality that are
   most closely associated with increased risk of suicide are
   hostility, impulsivity, and depression.
3. *Psychosocial milieu*—recent bereavement, separation or divorce, early loss, and decreased social supports are important factors related to suicide.
4. *Family history*—a family history of suicide is a significant
   risk factor for self-destructive behavior.
5. *Biochemical factors*—data suggest that serotonin-, opiate-,
   and dopamine-mediated processes may be implicated in
   self-destructive behavior.

## Precipitating Stressors

Self-destructive behavior may result from almost any stress the
individual feels is overwhelming. Precipitants are often humiliating life events, such as interpersonal problems, public embar-
rassment, loss of a job, or threat of incarceration. In addition,
knowing someone who attempted or committed suicide or being
exposed to suicide through the media may also make the individual
more vulnerable to self-destructive behavior. Box 13-2 lists factors

---

**Box 13-2**    Factors in the Assessment of the
Self-Destructive Patient

---

Circumstances of an Attempt

Precipitating humiliating life event

Preparatory actions: acquiring a method, putting affairs in
    order, suicidal talk, giving away prized possessions,
    suicidal note

Use of violent method or more lethal drugs/
    poisons

Understanding of lethality of chosen method

Precautions taken against discovery

Presenting Symptoms

Hopelessness

Self-reproach, feelings of failure and unworthiness

Depressed mood

Agitation and restlessness

Persistent insomnia

Weight loss

Slowed speech, fatigue, social withdrawal

Suicidal thoughts and plans

Psychiatric Illness

Previous suicide attempt

Mood disorders

Alcoholism or substance abuse

Conduct disorders and depression in adolescents

---

that the nurse must consider in the assessment of a self-destructive
patient.

## Appraisal of Stressors

Suicide prediction is not possible at any meaningful level. Therefore the nurse must assess each individual for known suicide risk
factors (Box 13-3) and determine the meaning of each of these elements for potential suicidal behavior.

---

**Box 13-2   Factors in the Assessment of the Self-Destructive Patient—cont'd**

Psychiatric Illness—cont'd

Early dementia and confusional states in elderly schizophrenia

Combinations of the above

Psychosocial History

Recently separated, divorced, or bereaved

Living alone

Unemployed, recent job change or loss

Multiple life stresses (move, early loss, breakup of important relationship, school problems, threat of disciplinary crisis)

Chronic medical illness

Excessive drinking or substance abuse

Personality Factors

Impulsivity, aggressivity, hostility

Cognitive rigidity and negativity

Hopelessness

Low self-esteem

Borderline or antisocial disorder

Family History

Family history of suicidal behavior

Family history of mood disorder, alcoholism, or both

---

## Coping Resources

Patients with chronic, painful, or life-threatening illnesses may engage in self-destructive behavior. Frequently these people consciously choose to kill themselves. Quality of life becomes an issue that overrides quantity of life. An ethical dilemma may arise for nurses who become aware of the patient's choice to engage in this behavior. No easy answers are available on how to resolve this conflict. Nurses must do so according to their own belief systems.

### Box 13-3    Suicide Risk Factors

Psychosocial and Clinical

Hopelessness
Caucasian race
Male gender
Advanced age
Living alone

History

Prior suicide attempts
Family history of suicide attempts
Family history of substance abuse

Diagnostic

General medical illness
Psychosis
Substance abuse
Mood disorders

## Coping Mechanisms

Ego defense mechanisms related to indirect self-destructive behavior are (1) denial, the most prominent coping mechanism;
(2) rationalization; (3) intellectualization; and (4) regression. Defense mechanisms should not be challenged without offering alternative means of coping. They may be standing between the person
and suicide.

Suicidal behavior indicates the imminent failure of the coping
mechanisms. A suicidal threat may be one last effort to obtain sufficient help to be able to cope. Completed suicide represents the
failure of the coping and adaptive mechanisms.

## Nursing Diagnosis

The diagnosis of self-destructive behavior must be based on con-
sideration of the seriousness and immediacy of the patient's harmful activity. Patient denial of the self-destructive nature of the behavior must not be allowed to persuade the nurse to underestimate
the need for nursing intervention. The nursing diagnosis is related

## NANDA Nursing Diagnoses Related to Self-Protective Responses

Adjustment, Impaired
Anxiety
Body image, Disturbed
Coping, Ineffective
Denial, Ineffective
Loneliness, Risk for
*Noncompliance (specify)
Self-esteem, Situational low
Self-esteem, Risk for situational low
Self-mutilation
*Self-mutilation, Risk for
Spiritual distress
Suicide, Risk for
*Violence, Risk for self-directed

*Primary nursing diagnosis for self-destructive behavior.
*From North American Nursing Diagnosis Association:* NANDA nursing diagnoses: definitions and classification 2000-2001, *Philadelphia, 2001, The Association.*

to the nurse's observations combined with data collected by other health care providers and the information provided by the patient and significant others.

A complete nursing diagnosis is individualized and related to the total constellation of the patient's behaviors and nursing needs. The box above presents the primary and related NANDA nursing diagnoses for maladaptive self-protective responses.

### Related Medical Diagnoses

Several medical diagnostic classifications include actual or potential self-destructive behavior among the defining criteria. Suicidal behavior is not separately identified as a diagnostic category. Therefore this section includes medical diagnoses in which this type of behavior is listed as possible. (See Chapter 12 for additional descriptions of the mood disorders.) The disorders included in this section are described in the DSM-IV-TR and are identified in the box on page 256.

## DSM-IV-TR Medical Diagnoses Related to Self-Protective Responses

| DSM-IV-TR Diagnosis | Essential Features |
|---|---|
| Bipolar disorder | Presence of a manic episode and no past depressive episodes (see Chapter 12). |
| Major depressive disorder | Presence of at least five symptoms almost daily during the same 2-week period, with one being either depressed mood or loss of interest or pleasure (see Chapter 12). |
| Noncompliance with treatment | Noncompliance with an important aspect of treatment for a mental disorder or a general medical condition. |
| Schizophrenia | Presence of two or more of the following symptoms for a 1-month period: delusions, hallucinations, disorganized speech, disorganized behavior, and negative symptoms (see Chapter 14). |
| Substance use disorders | Presence of substance dependence or substance abuse (see Chapter 17). |

*Modified from American Psychiatric Association: Diagnostic and statistical manual of mental disorders, ed 4, text revision (DSM-IV-TR), Washington, DC, 2000, The Association.*

## Outcome Identification

The expected outcome when working with a patient with maladaptive self-protection responses is as follows:

*The patient will not inflict physical self-injury.*

## Planning

The nursing care plan for the person with self-destructive behavior must focus first on protecting the patient from harm. In addition, the plan must address the factors that contributed to the patient's dangerous behavior. The planning process also involves providing the patient with education about the specific illness. A Patient Education Plan for a patient who is not compliant with medical treatment is presented on page 258.

**NURSE ALERT.** Patients identified as suicidal require special attention from the nurse, who should remember the following guidelines:

1. Take all threats of suicide, verbal or nonverbal, seriously. Report them immediately and institute safety measures.

2. Remove potentially harmful objects from the patient's immediate environment.

3. If the patient is at high risk for suicide, observe constantly, even when the patient is in bed or using the bathroom.

4. Observe carefully when the patient is taking medication. Check the patient's mouth to ensure that pills have been swallowed. Give medication in liquid form if possible.

5. Explain all safety measures to the patient. Communicate caring and concern.

6. Be particularly wary if the patient suddenly becomes calmer and seems at peace. A suicide plan may have been finalized, resulting in relief of anxiety.

Patient Education Plan:  Compliance Counseling

| Content | Instructional Activities | Evaluation |
| --- | --- | --- |
| Assess patient's knowledge of self-care activities. | Ask patient to describe usual lifestyle, diet, exercise, and medication patterns. | Patient describes usual behavior. |
| | Do described behaviors match self-care instruction received in the past? | Patient repeats previous directions. |
| Identify areas in which patient behavior differs from healthy self-care practices. | Describe healthy self-care behavior to patient. Provide written patient education materials. Encourage patient to describe reasons for not performing recommended self-care. | Patient discusses problems with compliance. |
| Discuss alternative approaches to self-care. | Assist patient to identify alternative and more acceptable self-care behaviors. Enable patient to talk about feelings related to illness and treatment. | Patient decides on different approach, shares feelings related to illness. |
| Agree on a reward for compliant behavior. | Ask patient about reward for practicing good self-care. | Patient identifies reward. |
| Reinforce new behavior. | Praise patient for making commitment to healthier lifestyle. | Patient recognizes renewed commitment to self-care. |

## Intervening in Self-Destructive Behavior

The highest-priority nursing interventions are those that protect the patient from immediate danger. In addition, the patient requires assistance in increasing self-esteem and regulating emotions and behaviors. The involvement of family and community support systems is recommended. A Nursing Treatment Plan Summary for patients with maladaptive self-protective responses is presented on pages 260 and 261.

1. Have threats to the patient's physical integrity or self-system been reduced in nature, number, origin, or timing?
2. Do the patient's behaviors reflect concern for his or her own physical, psychological, and social well-being?
3. Have the patient's coping resources been adequately assessed and mobilized?
4. Does the patient describe self and behavior accurately and objectively?
5. Is the patient using adaptive coping responses?
6. Does the patient engage in self-enhancing activities?
7. Is the patient taking reasonable risks that promote personal growth?

## Nursing Treatment Plan Summary:  Maladaptive Self-Protective Responses

**Nursing Diagnosis:** Potential for self-directed violence

**Expected Outcome:** Patient will not inflict physical self-injury.

| Short-term Goals | Interventions | Rationale |
|---|---|---|
| Patient will not engage in self-injury activities. | Observe closely. Remove harmful objects. Provide a safe environment. Provide for basic physiological needs. Contract for safety if appropriate. Monitor medications. | Highest priority is given to life-saving patient care activities. Patient's behavior must be supervised until self-control is adequate for safety. |
| Patient will identify positive aspects of self. | Identify patient's strengths. Encourage patient to participate in activities that patient likes and does well. Encourage good hygiene and grooming. Foster healthy interpersonal relationships. | Self-destructive behavior reflects underlying depression related to low self-esteem and anger directed inward. |

| | | |
|---|---|---|
| Patient will implement two adaptive self-protective responses. | Facilitate awareness, labeling, and expression of feelings. Assist patient to recognize unhealthy coping mechanisms. Identify alternative means of coping. Reward healthy coping behaviors. | Maladaptive coping mechanisms must be replaced with healthy ones to manage stress and anxiety. |
| Patient will identify two social support resources that can be helpful. | Assist significant others to communicate constructively with patient. Promote healthy family relationships. Identify relevant community resources. Initiate referrals to community resources. | Social isolation leads to low self-esteem and depression, perpetuating self-destructive behavior. |
| Patient will be able to describe the treatment plan and its rationale. | Involve patient and significant others in care planning. Explain characteristics of identified health care needs, nursing care needs, medical diagnosis, and recommended treatment and medications. Elicit response to nursing care plan. Modify plan based on patient feedback. | Understanding of and participation in health care planning enhance compliance. |

## Suggested readings

Bloch D: Adolescent suicide as a public health trust, *J Child Adol Psychiatr Nurs* 13(1):26, 1999.

Bultema J: Healing process for the multidisciplinary team: recovering post-inpatient suicide, *J Psychosoc Nurs* 32:19, 1994.

Cardell R, Horton-Deutsch S: A model for assessment of inpatient suicide potential, *Arch Psychiatr Nurs* 8:366, 1994.

Chiles J, Strohsall R: *The suicidal patient: principles of assessment, treatment, and case management,* Washington, DC, 1995, American Psychiatric Press.

Coryell W, Schlesser M: The Dexamethasone suppression test and suicide prediction, *American J of Psychiatry* 158:748-753, 2001.

Dhossche D, Ulusarac A, Syed W: A retrospective study of general hospital patients who commit suicide shortly after being discharged from the hospital, *Archives of Internal Medicine* 161:991-994, 2001.

Goin M: Treating the suicidal patient: the no-suicide contract—who benefits? *J Pract Psychiatry Behav Health* 4:243, 1998.

Green J, Grindel C: Supervision of suicidal patients in adult inpatient psychiatric units in general hospitals, *Psychiatr Serv* 47:859, 1996.

Gupta S et al: Factors associated with suicide attempts among patients with schizophrenia, *Psychiatr Serv* 49(10):1353, 1998.

Hall R et al: Suicide risk assessment: a review of risk factors for suicide in 100 patients who made severe suicide attempts, *Psychosomatics* 40(1):18, 1999.

Jamison K: *Night falls fast,* New York, 1999, Knopf.

Kehrberg C: Self-mutilating behavior, *J Child Adolesc Psychiatr Nurs* 10(3):35, 1997.

Kroll J: Use of no-suicide contracts by psychiatrists in Minnesota, *American Journal of Psychiatry* 157:1684, 2001.

Mann J et al: The neurobiology suicide risk: a review for the clinician, *J Clin Psychiatry* 60(suppl 2):7, 1999.

Oxley S, Meter S: The assessment and management of the suicidal patient, *J Pract Psychiatry Behav Health* 1:327, 1996.

Pawlicki C, Gaumer C: Nursing care of the self-mutilating patient, *Bull Menninger Clin* 57:380, 1993.

Reilly C: Cognitive therapy for the suicidal patient: a case study, *Perspect Psychiatr Care* 34(4):26, 1998.

Shaffer D, Craft L: Methods of adolescent suicide prevention, *J Clin Psychiatry* 60(Suppl 2):70, 1999.

Simpson S, Jamison K: Suicide and mood disorders, *Primary Psychiatry,* p 59, May 1997.

Simpson S, Jamison K: The risk of suicide in patients with bipolar disorders, *J Clin Psychiatry* 60(Suppl 2):53, 1999.

Stuart G, Laraia M: *Principles and practice of psychiatric nursing,* ed 7, St Louis, 2001, Mosby.

Werth J: *Rational suicide? Implications for mental health professionals,* New York, 1996, Taylor & Francis.

Wysoker A: Suicide: risk management strategies, *J Am Psychiatr Nurses Assoc* 5(5):164, 1999.

# Neurobiological Responses and Schizophrenia and Psychotic Disorders

**14**

## Continuum of Neurobiological Responses

The symptoms of psychosis are clustered within five major categories of brain function: cognition, perception, emotion, behavior, and socialization (also referred to as relational). Figure 14-1 presents the continuum of responses related to neurobiological functioning.

### Assessment

### Behaviors

Schizophrenia is a serious, persistent brain disease that results in psychotic behavior, concrete thinking, and difficulties in information processing, interpersonal relationships, and problem solving. Box 14-1 presents information on how schizophrenia affects the individual and society.

#### Related to cognition

Behaviors related to problems in information processing associated with schizophrenia are often referred to as *cognitive deficits*. They include problems with all aspects of memory, attention, form

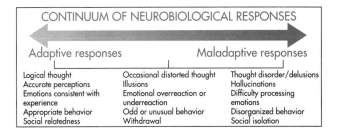

Figure 14-1
Continuum of neurobiological responses.

and content of speech, decision making, and thought content (Box 14-2). Table 14-1 summarizes behaviors related to these problems.

### Related to perception

*Perception* refers to identification and initial interpretation of a stimulus based on information received through the five senses. Box 14-3 summarizes behaviors related to problems with perception. Table 14-2 presents sensory modalities involved in hallucinations.

### Related to emotion

Emotions can be hyperexpressed or hypoexpressed in an incongruent manner. Individuals with schizophrenia typically have problems related to hypoexpression (Box 14-4). These patients also often experience emotions related to the difficulties caused by their illness, such as frustration over barriers to accomplishment of personal goals.

### Related to movement and behavior

Maladaptive neurobiological responses cause behaviors that are odd, unsightly, confusing, difficult to manage, and puzzling to others (Box 14-5).

### Associated with socialization

*Socialization* is the ability to form cooperative and interdependent relationships with others. Box 14-6 summarizes behaviors associated with the relational consequences of maladaptive neurobiological responses.

*Text continued on p. 271*

**Box 14-1    Impact of Schizophrenia on the Individual and Society**

- Approximately 1 in every 100 people in the United States (2.5 million) has schizophrenia, regardless of race, ethnic group, or gender.
- In three of four patients, schizophrenia begins between ages 17 and 25.
- Ninety-five percent of patients with schizophrenia have it for their lifetime.
- The cost of family caregiving and crime-related and welfare-related expenditures resulting from schizophrenia is $33 billion annually in the United States.
- More than 75% of taxpayer dollars spent on treatment of mental illness is used for patients with schizophrenia.
- Patients with schizophrenia occupy 25% of all inpatient hospital beds.
- An estimated one third to one half of homeless people in the United States have schizophrenia.
- Schizophrenia is ranked fourth in the top 10 diseases worldwide in terms of burden of illness. The top three are unipolar depression, alcohol use, and bipolar disorder.
- Schizophrenia is a chronic illness, five times more common than multiple sclerosis, six times more common than insulin-dependent diabetes, 60 times more common than muscular dystrophy, and 80 times more common than Huntington's disease.
- Of patients with schizophrenia, 25% do not respond adequately to traditional antipsychotic medication.
- Approximately 20% to 50% of patients with schizophrenia attempt suicide; 10% succeed.

## Box 14-2   Problems in Cognitive Functioning

Memory

Difficulty retrieving and using stored memory
Impaired short-term/long-term memory

Attention

Difficulty maintaining attention
Poor concentration
Distractibility
Inability to use selective attention

Form and Content of Speech (Formal Thought Disorder)

Loose associations
Tangential/illogical content
Incoherence/word salad/neologism
Circumstantial approach
Pressured/distractible speech
Paucity of speech

Decision Making

Failure to abstract
Indecisiveness
Lack of insight
Impaired concept formation
Impaired judgment
Illogical thinking
Lack of planning and problem-solving skills
Difficulty initiating tasks

Thought Content

Delusions:
    Paranoid
    Grandiose
    Religious
    Somatic
    Nihilistic
    Thought broadcasting
    Thought insertion
    Thought control

Table 14-1    Behaviors related to cognitive problems in schizophrenia

| Cognitive Problems | Behaviors |
|---|---|
| Memory | Forgetfulness |
| | Disinterest |
| | Lack of compliance |
| Attention | Difficulty completing tasks |
| | Difficulty concentrating on work |
| Form and content of speech | Difficulty communicating thoughts and feelings |
| Decision making | Difficulty initiating and completing activities |
| | Concrete thought: |
| | Inability to carry out multistage commands |
| | Problems with time management |
| | Difficulty managing money |
| | Literal interpretation of words and symbols |
| Thought content | Delusions |

## Box 14-3    Behaviors Related to Perceptual Problems Associated with Maladaptive Neurobiological Responses

Hallucinations
Illusions
Sensory integration problems
Poor visceral pain recognition
Problems with stereognosis (recognition of objects by touch)
Problems with graphesthesia (recognition of letters "drawn" on the skin)
Misidentification of faces (including self)

Table 14-2   Sensory modalities involved in hallucinations

| Sense | Characteristics |
| --- | --- |
| Auditory | Hearing noises or sounds, usually in the form of voices. Sounds may range from a simple noise or voice, to a voice talking about the patient, to complete conversations between two or more people about the hallucinating patient. Additional types include audible thoughts, in which the patient hears voices that are speaking what the patient is thinking, and commands that tell the patient to do something, sometimes harmful or dangerous. |
| Visual | Visual stimuli in the form of flashes of light, geometric figures, cartoon figures, and elaborate and complex scenes or visions. Visions can be pleasant or terrifying (e.g., seeing monsters). |
| Olfactory | Putrid, foul, and rancid smells of a repulsive nature, such as blood, urine, or feces. Occasionally the odors can be pleasant. Olfactory hallucinations are typically associated with stroke, tumor, seizures, and the dementias. |
| Gustatory | Putrid, foul, and rancid tastes of a repulsive nature, such as blood, urine, or feces. |
| Tactile | Experiencing pain or discomfort with no apparent stimuli. Feeling electrical sensations coming from the ground, inanimate objects, or other people. |
| Cenesthetic | Feeling body functions, such as blood pulsing through veins and arteries, food digesting, or urine forming. |
| Kinesthetic | Sensation of movement while standing motionless. |

## Box 14-4 Emotional Responses Occurring in Schizophrenia

**Alexithymia**—difficulty naming and describing emotions
**Apathy**—lack of feelings, emotions, interests, or concern
**Anhedonia**—inability or decreased ability to experience pleasure, joy, intimacy, and closeness

## Box 14-5 Abnormal Movements and Behaviors in Schizophrenia

Movements

Catatonia, waxy flexibility, posturing
Extrapyramidal side effects of psychotropic medications
Abnormal eye movements
Grimacing
Apraxia (difficulty carrying out a complex task)
Echopraxia (purposeless imitation of others' movements)
Abnormal gait
Mannerisms

Behaviors

Deterioration in appearance
Aggression/agitation
Repetitive or stereotyped behavior
Avolition (lack of energy and drive)
Lack of persistence at work or school

## Box 14-6 Behaviors Associated with Socialization Resulting from Maladaptive Neurobiological Responses

Social withdrawal and isolation
Low self-esteem
Social inappropriateness
Disinterest in recreational activities
Gender identity confusion
Stigma-related withdrawal by others
Decreased quality of life

1. *Positive Symptoms*
   Delusions
   Hallucinations
   Thought disorders
   Disorganized speech
   Bizarre behavior

2. *Negative Symptoms*
   Flat affect
   Alogia
   Avolition/apathy
   Anhedonia/asociality
   Attention deficit

5. *Social/Occupational Dysfunction*
   Work/activity
   Interpersonal relationships
   Self-care
   Mortality/morbidity

3. *Cognitive Symptoms*
   Impaired attention
   Impaired memory
   Impaired executive functions
      Abstraction
      Concept formation
      Problem solving
      Decision making

4. *Mood Symptoms*
   Dysphoria
   Suicidal ideation
   Hopelessness

Figure 14-2
Core symptom clusters in schizophrenia.

Finally, the symptoms or behaviors related to schizophrenia have been grouped or categorized in various ways. One prominent system groups them into "positive" (additional behaviors) and "negative" (deficit of behaviors) symptoms. Figure 14-2 presents five core symptom clusters that reflect the full impact this illness can have on the individual and society.

## Predisposing Factors

### Biological

Various neurodevelopmental abnormalities associated with maladaptive neurobiological responses are only beginning to be understood, as indicated by the following studies:

1. Brain imaging studies have begun to reveal widespread involvement of the brain in the development of schizophrenia.

Lesions in the frontal, temporal, and limbic areas are related to psychotic behaviors. Enlarged ventricles and decreased cortical mass indicate brain atrophy.

2. Several brain chemicals have been implicated in schizophrenia. Research points most strongly to the following:
   - An excess of the neurotransmitter dopamine
   - An imbalance between dopamine and other neurotransmitters, especially serotonin
   - Problems in the dopamine receptor systems

3. Family studies involving twins and adopted children have suggested a genetic role for schizophrenia. Identical twins, even when raised separately, have a higher co-occurrence of schizophrenia than nonidentical pairs of siblings. Recent genetic research focuses on gene mapping in families with a higher incidence of schizophrenia in first-degree relatives compared with the general population.

### Psychological

Psychodynamic theories for the development of maladaptive neurobiological responses have not been supported by research. Unfortunately, earlier psychological theories led to families being blamed for these disorders. This results in families lacking trust in mental health professionals.

### Sociocultural

Accumulated stress may contribute to the onset of schizophrenia and other psychotic disorders but is not believed to be the primary cause.

## Precipitating Stressors

### Biological

Biological stressors related to maladaptive neurobiological responses include (1) interference in the brain's communication and feedback loop, which regulate information processing; and (2) abnormal gating (nerve communication involving electrolytes) mechanisms in the brain, resulting in inability to attend to stimuli selectively.

## Environmental

A biologically determined threshold for stress tolerance interacts with environmental stressors to determine the occurrence of disturbed behavior.

### Symptom triggers

Triggers are precursors and stimuli that often precede a new episode of illness. Box 14-7 lists common triggers of maladaptive neurobiological responses related to the individual's health, environment, attitudes, and behaviors.

## Appraisal of Stressors

No scientific research indicates that stress causes schizophrenia. However, studies of relapse and symptom exacerbation provide evidence that stress, the person's appraisal of the stressor, and problems with coping may predict the return of symptoms. The *stress diathesis model* states that schizophrenic symptoms develop based on the relationship between the amount of stress a person experiences and an internal stress tolerance threshold. This is an important model because it integrates biological, psychological, and sociocultural factors in explaining the development of schizophrenia.

## Coping Resources

Individual coping resources must be assessed with an understanding of the behavioral results of the brain disorder. Strengths may include such assets as high intelligence or creativity. Parents must actively teach children and young adults coping skills because they cannot usually learn them from observation alone. Family resources may include knowledge about the illness, adequate finances, availability of time and energy, and ability to provide ongoing support.

## Coping Mechanisms

Behaviors that represent efforts to protect the patient from the frightening experiences associated with maladaptive neurobiological responses include the following:

- *Regression,* related to information processing problems and efforts to manage anxiety, leaving little energy for activities of daily living
- *Projection,* as an effort to explain confusing perceptions
- *Withdrawal*

## Box 14-7   Symptom Triggers of Maladaptive Neurobiological Responses

Health

Poor nutrition
Lack of sleep
Out-of-balance circadian rhythms
Fatigue
Infection
Central nervous system drugs
Lack of exercise
Barriers to accessing health care

Environment

Hostile or critical environment
Housing difficulties (unsatisfactory housing)
Pressure to perform (loss of independent living)
Changes in life events and daily patterns of activity
Interpersonal difficulties
Disruptions in interpersonal relationships
Social isolation and lack of social support
Job pressures (poor occupational skills)
Poverty
Lack of transportation (resources)
Stigmatization

Attitudes/Behaviors

"Poor me" (low self-concept)
"It's hopeless" (lack of self-confidence)
"I'm a failure" (loss of motivation to use skills)
"I have no control" (demoralization)
"No one likes me" (unable to meet spiritual needs)
Feeling overpowered by symptoms
Looks and acts different from others of same age and
    culture
Poor social skills
Aggressive behavior
Violent behavior
Poor medication management
Poor symptom management

## Nursing Diagnosis

The following box presents the primary and related NANDA nursing diagnoses for maladaptive neurobiological responses. A complete nursing assessment would include all maladaptive responses, and many additional nursing problems would be identified.

---

### NANDA Nursing Diagnoses Related to Maladaptive Neurobiological Responses

Adjustment, Impaired
Activity intolerance
Anxiety
Caregiver role strain, Risk for
*Communication, Impaired verbal
Conflict, Decisional
Confusion, Acute
Coping, Compromised family, Ineffective, Readiness for enhanced family
Denial, Ineffective
Identity, Disturbed personal
Role performance, Ineffective
Self-care deficit, Bathing/hygiene, Dressing/grooming
Self-esteem, Risk for situational low, Situational low
*Sensory perception, Disturbed
*Social interaction, Impaired
*Social isolation
Suicide, Risk for
Therapeutic regimen management, Effective, Ineffective, Ineffective family
*Thought Processes, Disturbed

---

*Primary nursing diagnosis for maladaptive neurobiological responses.
*From North American Nursing Diagnosis Association:* NANDA nursing diagnoses: definitions and classification 2000-2001, *Philadelphia, 2001, The Association.*

## Related Medical Diagnoses

Maladaptive neurobiological responses are included in the medical diagnostic category of schizophrenia and psychotic disorders. The box on pages 277-279 describes these disorders.

## Outcome Identification

The expected outcome when working with a patient with maladaptive neurobiological responses is:

*The patient will live, learn, and work at the maximum possible level of success, as defined by the individual.*

## Planning

A Family Education Plan for understanding psychosis is presented on pages 280 and 281.

## Implementation

Empirically validated treatments related to schizophrenia are summarized in Table 14-3.

Nursing interventions may include a broad range of psychosocial and psychobiological treatments and are based on the nurse's assessment of the patient's needs and strengths. Significant others are included whenever possible. The major approaches for nursing intervention with patients who have maladaptive neurobiological responses are summarized as follows:

1. *Behavioral strategies.* Table 14-4 presents strategies for nurses working with patients who have psychoses.
2. *Managing delusions.* Box 14-8 presents strategies for working with delusional patients, and Box 14-9 lists barriers to intervention for delusions.
3. *Managing hallucinations.* Box 14-10 outlines strategies for working with patients to help them cope with ongoing hallucinations.
4. *Psychopharmacology.* Antipsychotic medications are described in Chapter 20.
5. *Managing relapse.* Patients and their family members should be informed about how to identify and take action when a relapse is impending. Box 14-11 lists nursing interventions directed toward preventing relapse, and Box 14-12 is a patient guide for potential relapse.

*Text continued on p. 293*

## DSM-IV-TR Medical Diagnoses Related to Maladaptive Neurobiological Responses

| DSM-IV-TR Diagnosis | Essential Features |
|---|---|
| Schizophrenia | At least two of the following, each present for a significant time during a 1-month period:<br>1. Delusions<br>2. Hallucinations<br>3. Disorganized speech<br>4. Grossly disorganized or catatonic behavior<br>5. Negative symptoms (i.e., flat affect, alogia, avolition)<br>For a significant time since the onset of the disturbance, one or more major areas of functioning (e.g., work, interpersonal relations, self-care) are greatly below the level achieved before the onset.<br>Continuous signs of the disturbance persist for at least 6 months. |
| Paranoid type | Preoccupation with one or more delusions or frequent auditory hallucinations. |
| Disorganized type | All the following are prominent: disorganized speech, disorganized behavior, and flat or inappropriate affect; also, does not meet the criteria for catatonic type. |
| Catatonic type | At least two of the following dominate the clinical picture: motor immobility, as evidenced by catalepsy or stupor; excessive motor activity; extreme negativism or mutism; peculiarities of voluntary movement, as evidenced by posturing, stereotyped movements, prominent mannerisms, or prominent grimacing; echolalia; and echopraxia. |

*Modified from American Psychiatric Association: Diagnostic and statistical manual of mental disorders, ed 4, Text Revision (DSM-IV-TR), Washington, DC, 2000, The Association.*
*Continued*

## DSM-IV-TR Medical Diagnoses Related to Maladaptive Neurobiological Responses—cont'd

| DSM-IV-TR Diagnosis | Essential Features |
| --- | --- |
| Undifferentiated type | Symptoms meeting the first general criterion for schizophrenia are present, but criteria for other types are not met. |
| Residual type | Criteria for schizophrenia or any subtype are not met. Continuing evidence of the disturbance is indicated by negative symptoms or attenuated presence of two or more symptoms included in the general criteria. |
| Schizophreniform disorder | Meets criteria for schizophrenia, and an episode lasts at least 1 month but less than 6 months. "With" or "without" good prognostic features is specified based on at least two of the following: onset of prominent psychotic symptoms within 4 weeks of first noticeable change in behavior or functioning; confusion or perplexity at the height of the psychosis; good premorbid social and occupational functioning; and absence of blunted or flat affect. |
| Schizoaffective disorder | Interrupted period of illness, including a major depressive episode or manic episode, concurrent with symptoms of schizophrenia. During the same period of illness, delusions or hallucinations have occurred for at least 2 weeks in the absence of prominent mood symptoms. Symptoms of a mood episode are present during a substantial part of the illness. The condition is not caused by substance abuse or a general medical illness. |

| | |
|---|---|
| Delusional disorder | Nonbizarre delusions (i.e., situations that could occur, such as being followed, being poisoned, or having a disease) lasting at least a month. Has never met criteria for schizophrenia. Apart from the impact of the delusion, functioning and behavior are not greatly affected. |
| Brief psychotic disorder | Presence of at least one of the following: delusions, hallucinations, disorganized speech, and grossly disorganized or catatonic behavior (behaviors are not culturally sanctioned). Duration of 1 day to 1 month, with eventual return to premorbid functioning. Presence (brief reactive psychosis) or absence of marked stressors. |
| Shared psychotic disorder (folie à deux) | A delusion develops in an individual in the context of a close relationship with someone who already has a delusion. The delusions of those involved are similar in content. |

*Modified from American Psychiatric Association: Diagnostic and statistical manual of mental disorders, ed 4, Text Revision (DSM-IV-TR), Washington, DC, 2000, The Association.*

Family Education Plan: Understanding Psychosis

| Content | Instructional Activities | Evaluation |
|---|---|---|
| Describe psychosis. | Introduce participants and leaders. State purpose of group. Define terminology associated with psychosis. | Participant describes the characteristics of psychosis. |
| Identify the causes of psychotic disorders. | Present theories of psychotic disorders. Use audiovisual aids to explain brain anatomy, brain biochemistry, and major neurotransmitters. | Participant discusses the relationship between brain anatomy, brain biochemistry, and major neurotransmitters and the development of psychosis. |
| Define schizophrenia according to symptoms and diagnostic criteria. | Lead a discussion of the diagnostic criteria for schizophrenia. Show a film on schizophrenia. | Participant describes the symptoms and diagnostic criteria for schizophrenia. |
| Describe the relationship between anxiety and psychotic disorders. | Present types and stages of anxiety. Discuss steps in reducing and resolving anxiety. | Participant identifies and describes the stages of anxiety and ways to reduce or resolve it. |
| Analyze the impact of living with hallucinations. | Describe the characteristics of hallucinations. Demonstrate ways to communicate with someone who is hallucinating. | Participant demonstrates effective ways to communicate with a person who has hallucinations. |

| | | |
|---|---|---|
| Analyze the impact of living with delusions. | Describe types of delusions. Demonstrate ways to communicate with someone who has delusions. Discuss interventions for delusions. | Participant demonstrates effective ways to communicate with a person who has delusions. |
| Discuss the use of psychotropic medications and the role of nutrition. | Provide and explain handouts describing the characteristics of psychotropic medications prescribed for schizophrenia. | Participant identifies and describes the characteristics of medications prescribed for self or family member. |
| Describe the characteristics of relapse and the role of compliance with the therapeutic regimen. | Assist participants to describe their own experiences with relapse. Discuss symptom management techniques and the importance of complying with the therapeutic regimen. | Participant describes behaviors that indicate an impending relapse and discusses the importance of symptom management and compliance with the therapeutic regimen. |
| Analyze behaviors that promote wellness. | Discuss the components of wellness. Relate wellness to the elements of symptom management. | Participant analyzes the effect of maintaining a state of wellness on the occurrence of symptoms. |
| Discuss ways to cope adaptively while living with psychosis. | Lead a group discussion focused on the daily problems of living with psychosis and on coping behaviors. Propose ways to create a low-stress environment. | Participant describes ways to modify lifestyle to create a low-stress environment. |

Table 14-3    Summarizing the evidence on treatments for schizophrenia

**DISORDER:** Schizophrenia
**TREATMENT:**

- Conventional antipsychotic medications (e.g., chlorpromazine, fluphenazine, haloperidol, loxapine, perphenazine, trifluoperazine, thiothixene, and thioridazine) markedly reduced the positive symptoms of schizophrenia and significantly decreased the risk of symptomatic relapse and rehospitalization. However, serious neurological side effects made these drugs difficult to tolerate for many patients with schizophrenia.

- More recently, a group of "atypical" antipsychotic drugs (e.g., clozapine, risperidone, olanzapine, quetiapine, ziprasidone) have demonstrated comparable—or better—efficacy with schizophrenic symptoms with significantly less risk of adverse neurological events. These drugs may be especially effective in treating the negative symptoms of schizophrenia.

- Cognitive-behavioral therapy and social learning/token economy programs helped structure, support, and reinforce prosocial behaviors in treatment refractory persons with schizophrenia. Structured, educational family interventions helped maintain gains achieved with medication and customary case management. Social skills training enabled persons with schizophrenia to acquire instrumental and affiliative skills to improve functioning in their communities.

From Nathan P, Gorman J: *A guide to treatments that work,* New York, 1998, Oxford University Press.

Table 14-4  Behavioral strategies for patients with psychosis

| Core Problem | Nursing Interventions |
|---|---|
| Anxiety | Teach patient the symptoms related to anxiety.<br>Assist patient to identify what triggers anxiety.<br>Help patient use symptom management techniques to cope with anxiety.<br>Assess if anxiety is a relapse trigger; if so, devise a plan to reduce anxiety while still in the moderate stage. |
| Depression | Teach patient the symptoms related to depression.<br>Help patient use symptom management techniques to cope with depression.<br>Assess if depression is a relapse trigger; if so, devise a plan to reduce depression while still in a mild stage, because a high correlation exists between depression and ability to perform activities of daily living. |
| Inability to learn from experience | Review both positive and negative experiences.<br>Identify what was and was not successful in helping patient achieve the desired goal.<br>Analyze each experience to determine what went well and what did not. |
| Problems with cause-and-effect reasoning | Help patient sequence events leading to the outcome in each experience.<br>Consider using rehearsal to enact an event before it occurs. |

*Continued*

Table 14-4   Behavioral strategies for patients with psychosis—cont'd

| Core Problem | Nursing Interventions |
|---|---|
| Difficulty assessing passage of time | Teach patient how to use clocks to tell time. |
| | Teach patient to use environmental cues (e.g., sun going down, certain radio program) to orient self to time of day. |
| | Assist patient in creating and maintaining a calendar of scheduled activities. |
| Concrete thinking | Realize patient sees every problem as having one solution. |
| | Teach patient to consider other possible solutions to problems. |
| | Realize patient frequently thinks there is only one way to do a task. |
| | Create alternative methods to approach situations. |
| Difficulty telling background from foreground information | Teach patient to distinguish between important and unimportant information. |
| | Teach patient to focus on only the important information. |
| | Help patient learn to avoid or minimize confusion caused by excess stimulation from noise, large crowds, etc. |
| Slowed information processing | Give patient time to process and respond to information. |
| | Minimize anxiety, which increases information processing difficulties. |
| | Demonstrate genuine interest in trying to understand what patient is saying. |
| | Use clear and simple language when communicating with patient. |

| | |
|---|---|
| Difficulty screening information to share | Teach patient to identify people who patient can talk to about the illness.<br>Teach patient to contact these people when the symptoms are creating problems. |
| Communication difficulties | Let patient know you understand the illness and are a "safe person" to talk with.<br>Use active listening to understand patient.<br>Clarify what patient is trying to convey.<br>Listen for the theme.<br>Seek validation from patient on what is communicated.<br>Help patient with vocabulary as needed.<br>Use the literal meaning of words.<br>Have patient repeat what was heard.<br>Help patient understand the words and phrases used. |
| Problems expressing needs | Assist patient to identify and prioritize needs.<br>Assist patient to express needs in ways that others will understand.<br>Role-play conversations and practice negotiating with others. |
| Low self-concept | Help patient identify and maximize strengths and positive characteristics.<br>Use role play to handle common situations that patients face.<br>Give positive feedback when patient handles a situation well.<br>Help problem-solve a negative situation to determine how it could have been better handled. |
| Forced isolation resulting from stigma | Maximize patient's understanding of the illness.<br>Teach patient to minimize stigmatizing behaviors when possible.<br>Identify comments that are difficult for patient to confront.<br>Teach ways to handle stigma and rude comments.<br>Develop concrete humorous comebacks.<br>Role-play various situations with nurse being the patient. |

*Continued*

Table 14-4   Behavioral strategies for patients with psychosis—cont'd

| Core Problem | Nursing Interventions |
| --- | --- |
| Difficulty with perception and interpretation of sensory stimuli | Review problematic situations with patient. List and assess the thought processes in interpreting events. Help patient reality-test and reframe problematic interpretations. Reinforce positive and productive processes. |
| Poor attention span and difficulty completing tasks | Help patient break tasks into small, sequential steps. Help patient keep focused on a single task, a step at a time. Do not emphasize completing the task. Give directions to patient one step at a time. |
| Inappropriate social behaviors | Identify patient's thought processes that lead to the behavior. Ask patient about the behavior. Help correct inaccurate perceptions. Help patient identify undesirable outcomes of the behavior. Teach appropriate social skills. |
| Difficulty with decision making | Assist patient to decide on desired outcomes. Help patient prioritize goals and categorize them into short term and long term. Help patient establish a timeline for attainment of each goal. Help patient establish small, concrete steps to achieve desired goals. Ensure these small steps are achievable by patient and are congruent with patient's culture and values. |

**Box 14-8    Strategies for Working with Patients with Delusions**

**Place the delusion in a time frame and identify triggers.**
- Identify all the components of the delusion by placing it in time and sequence.
- Identify triggers that may be related to stress or anxiety.
- If delusions are linked to anxiety, teach anxiety management skills.
- Develop a symptom management program.

**Assess the intensity, frequency, and duration of the delusion.**
- Help the patient dispel fleeting delusions in a short time frame.
- Consider temporarily avoiding fixed delusions, or those endured over time, to prevent them from becoming stumbling blocks in the nurse-patient relationship.
- Listen quietly until there is no need to discuss the delusion.

**Identify emotional components of the delusion.**
- Respond to the patient's underlying feelings rather than the illogical nature of the delusions.
- Encourage discussion of the patient's fears, anxiety, and anger without assuming the delusion is right or wrong.

**Observe for evidence of concrete thinking.**
- Determine whether or not the patient takes you literally.
- Determine if you and the patient are using language in the same way.

**Observe speech for symptoms of a thought disorder.**
- Determine if the patient exhibits a thought disorder (e.g., talking in circles, going off on tangents, easily changing subjects, unable to respond to your attempts to redirect).
- Realize that it may not be the appropriate time to point out discrepancies between fact and delusion.

*Continued*

## Box 14-8   Strategies for Working with Patients with Delusions—cont'd

**Observe for the ability to use cause-and-effect reasoning accurately.**
- Determine if the patient can make logical predictions (inductive or deductive) based on past experiences.
- Determine if the patient can conceptualize time.
- Determine if the patient can access and use recent and long-term memory meaningfully.

**Distinguish between description of the experience and facts of the situation.**
- Identify false beliefs about real situations.
- Promote the patient's ability to reality-test.
- Determine if the patient is hallucinating, because this will strengthen the delusion.

**Carefully question the facts as they are presented and their meaning.**
- Talk about the delusion to try to help the patient see it is not true.
- Note that if this step is taken before the previous steps are completed, it may reinforce the delusion.

**Discuss the delusion and its consequences.**
- When intensity of the delusion lessens, discuss the delusion when the patient is ready.
- Discuss the consequences of the delusion.
- Allow the patient to take responsibility for behavior, daily activities, and decision making.
- Encourage the patient's personal responsibility for and participation in wellness and recovery.

**Promote distraction as a way to stop focusing on the delusion.**
- Promote activities that require attention to physical skills and that will help the patient use time constructively.
- Recognize and reinforce healthy and positive aspects of the patient's personality.

**Box 14-9   Barriers to Successful Intervention for Delusions**

1. **Becoming anxious and avoiding the patient**
   This leads to annoyance, anger, a sense of hopelessness and failure, feelings of inadequacy, and potential laughing at or discounting of the patient.

2. **Reinforcing the delusion**
   Do not agree with the delusion, especially to obtain the patient's cooperation.

3. **Attempting to prove the patient is wrong**
   Do not attempt a logical explanation.

4. **Setting unrealistic goals**
   Do not underestimate the power of a delusion and the patient's need for it.

5. **Becoming incorporated into the delusional system**
   This will cause great confusion for the patient and make it impossible to establish the boundaries of the therapeutic relationship.

6. **Failing to clarify confusion surrounding the delusion**
   If the nurse does not clearly understand the complexity and many intricacies of the delusion, the delusion will become more elaborate.

7. **Being inconsistent in intervention**
   The nurse must firmly adhere to the intervention plan. "Try anything" approaches lead to inconsistency, and the patient is less able to identify reality.

8. **Seeing the delusion first and the patient second**
   Avoid using such phrases as, "The person who thinks he's being poisoned."

## Box 14-10 Strategies for Working with Patients with Hallucinations

**Establish a trusting, interpersonal relationship.**
- Remember that if you are anxious or frightened, the patient will be anxious or frightened.
- Be patient, show acceptance, and use active listening skills.

**Assess for symptoms of hallucinations, including duration, intensity, and frequency.**
- Observe for behavioral clues that indicate the presence of hallucinations.
- Observe for clues that identify the level of intensity and duration of the hallucination.
- Help the patient record the number of hallucinations experienced each day.

**Focus on symptoms and ask patient to describe what is happening.**
- Empower the patient by helping to understand the symptoms experienced or demonstrated.
- Help the patient gain control of the hallucinations, seek helpful distractions, and minimize intensity.

**Explore drug and alcohol use.**
- Determine if the patient is using alcohol or drugs (over-the-counter, prescription, or street drugs).
- Determine if these may be responsible for or may exacerbate the hallucinations.

**If the patient asks, simply say you are not experiencing the same stimuli.**
- Respond by letting the patient know what is actually happening in the environment.
- Do not argue with the patient about differences in perceptions.
- When a hallucination occurs, do not leave the patient alone.

**Box 14-10   Strategies for Working with Patients with Hallucinations—cont'd**

**Suggest and reinforce the use of interpersonal relationships as a symptom management technique.**
- Encourage the patient to talk to someone trusted who will give supportive and corrective feedback.
- Assist the patient in mobilizing social supports.

**Help the patient describe and compare current and past hallucinations.**
- Determine if there is a pattern to the patient's hallucinations.
- Encourage the patient to remember when hallucinations first began.
- Pay attention to the content of the hallucination because it may provide clues for predicting behavior.
- Be especially alert for "command" hallucinations that may "compel" the patient to act in a certain way.
- Encourage the patient to describe past and present thoughts, feelings, and actions as they relate to hallucinations.

**Help the patient identify needs that may be reflected in the content of the hallucination.**
- Identify needs that may trigger hallucinations.
- Focus on the patient's unmet needs, and discuss their relationship to the presence of hallucinations.

**Determine the impact of the patient's symptoms on activities of daily living.**
- Provide feedback regarding the patient's general coping responses and activities of daily living.
- Help the patient recognize symptoms, symptom triggers, and symptom management strategies.

---

**Box 14-11    Nursing Interventions to Prevent Relapse**

---

- Identify symptoms that signal relapse.
- Identify symptom triggers.
- Select symptom management techniques.
- Identify coping strategies for symptom triggers.
- Identify support system for future relapse.
- Document action plan in written form and file with key support people.
- Facilitate patient's integration into family and community.

---

---

**Box 14-12    Patient Guide for Handling Potential Relapse**

---

1. **Go to a safe environment** with someone who can assist you if help is needed. This person should be able to monitor behavior that indicates the relapse is becoming worse.
2. **Reduce the stress and demands on you.** This includes reducing stimuli. Some people find a quiet room where they can be alone, perhaps with soft music. Consider using relaxation or distraction techniques. A quiet place where you can talk with a person you trust is often helpful.
3. **Take medications** if this is part of your program. Work with your prescriber to determine if medications may be useful to reduce relapse. Medications are most helpful when used in a safe, quiet environment and with stress reduction techniques.
4. **Talk to a trusted person** about what the voices are saying to you or about the thoughts you are having. The person needs to know ahead of time that you will call if you need help.
5. **Avoid negative people** who make such comments as, "You're thinking crazy" or "Stop that negative talk."

---

6. *Patient and family education.* Patients and their families are much better able to manage the illness if they are provided with information about diagnosis, medications, current research, and community resources.

A Nursing Treatment Plan Summary for the patient with maladaptive neurobiological responses is presented on pages 294-297.

## Evaluation

To evaluate nursing interventions with patients who have maladaptive neurobiological responses, the following questions may be asked:

1. Is the patient able to describe the behaviors that characterize the onset of a relapse?
2. Is the patient able to identify and describe the medications prescribed, the reason for taking them, the frequency of taking them, and the possible side effects?
3. Does the patient participate in relationships with other people at a level that is comfortable for the patient?
4. Is the patient's family aware of the characteristics of the illness and able to participate in a supportive relationship with the patient?
5. Are the patient and family informed about available community resources, such as rehabilitation programs, mental health care providers, educational programs, and support groups, and do they use them?

*Text continued on p. 298*

## Nursing Treatment Plan Summary:  Maladaptive Neurobiological Responses

Nursing Diagnosis: Altered thought processes

Expected Outcome: Patient will live, learn, and work at the maximum possible level of success, as defined by the individual.

| Short-term Goals | Rationale | Interventions |
| --- | --- | --- |
| Patient will participate in brief, regularly scheduled meetings with nurse. | Initiate a nurse-patient relationship contract mutually agreed on by nurse and patient. Schedule brief (5- to 10-minute) frequent contacts with patient. Consistently approach patient at scheduled time. Extend length of sessions gradually based on patient's agreement. | Establishment of a trusting relationship is fundamental to developing open communication. A patient with altered thought processes cannot tolerate extended, intrusive interactions and functions best in a structured environment. |
| Patient will describe delusions and other altered thought processes. | Demonstrate attitude of caring and concern. Validate the meaning of communications with patient. Assist patient to identify the difference between reality and internal thought processes. | Patients are very sensitive to others' responses to their symptoms. A respectful, interested approach enables patient to discuss unusual and frightening thoughts. Identification of reality by a trusted person is helpful. |

| | | |
|---|---|---|
| Patient will identify and describe the effect of brain disease on thought processes. | Provide information about causes of psychoses. Discuss relationship between patient's behaviors and brain function. Involve significant others in educational sessions. | Understanding physiological basis for altered thought processes assists patient to recognize symptoms and to feel in control of the illness. Significant others can provide support and experience less stigma if they are informed about the illness. |
| Patient will identify the signs of impending relapse and describe actions to take to prevent relapse. | Assist patient and significant others to identify behaviors related to altered thought processes that indicate threatened relapse. Identify community resources, and mutually plan actions directed toward prevention of relapse. | Relapse can be predicted if patient and family are alert to warning signs. Early intervention allows patient to be in control of the course of the illness. Family members can be helpful in assisting patient to identify symptoms and in providing support for seeking assistance. |

*Continued*

## Nursing Treatment Plan Summary:    Maladaptive Neurobiological Responses—cont'd

| Short-term Goals | Rationale | Interventions |
| --- | --- | --- |
| Patient will describe symptom management techniques that are helpful in living with altered thought processes. | Describe symptom management techniques that other patients have used. Ask patient to describe techniques used to manage symptoms. Encourage patient to take control of the illness by using symptom management techniques. | Many patients with psychoses continue to have delusions after the acute phase of the illness has passed. They can function better if they learn ways to manage the symptoms. |

Nursing Diagnosis: Social isolation

**Expected Outcome: Patient will live, learn, and work at the maximum possible level of success, as defined by the individual.**

| | | |
| --- | --- | --- |
| Patient will engage in a trusting relationship with nurse. | Initiate a nurse-patient relationship contract mutually agreed on by nurse and patient. Establish mutual goals related to social interaction. Establish trust by consistently meeting the elements of the plan and engaging in open and honest communication. | Patients who have maladaptive neurobiological responses often have difficulty trusting others. Difficulty with information processing causes problems interpreting the communication of others. |

| Patient will discuss personal goals related to social interaction. | Encourage patient to describe current relationship patterns. Discuss past relationship experiences. Identify problems associated with social interaction. Explore goals. | Patient may be unaware of the characteristics of mutually satisfying interpersonal relationships. Honest feedback from nurse can assist patient to identify the reasons for past problems. Knowledge of patient's relationship goals leads to development of realistic behavioral change. |

**Nursing Diagnosis: Social isolation**

**Expected Outcome: Patient will live, learn, and work at the maximal possible level of success, as defined by the individual.**

| Patient will identify behaviors that interfere with social relationships. | Share observations about patient's behavior in social situations. | Identification of problematic behavior helps patient and nurse target changes. |
| Patient will practice alternative social behaviors with nurse. | Discuss possible behavioral changes that will facilitate establishment of social relationships. Role-play alternative behaviors. Provide feedback. | Practice helps patient feel comfortable with new behaviors. Feedback provides reinforcement for successful behavioral change. |
| Patient will select one other person and practice social interaction skills. | Discuss experience of practicing new behavior with another person. Discuss ways of maintaining a relationship. | Patient needs ongoing feedback and support related to maintaining behavioral change. |

*your* **INTERNET**
c o n n e c t i o n

All About Schizophrenia—Mental Health Net:
schizophrenia.mentalhelp.net

Consultant for Pharmacotherapy of Schizophrenia:
mhc.com/Algorithms/Schizophrenia/index.htm

NARSAD: National Alliance for Research on
Schizophrenia and Depression:
www.mhsource.com/narsad.html

The Schizophrenia Home Page:
www.schizophrenia.com

Treatment of Schizophrenia: 1999 Expert Consensus
Guidelines:
www.psychguides.com/gl-
treatment_of_schizophrenia_1999.html

World Fellowship for Schizophrenia and Allied
Disorders:
www.world-schizophrenia.org

## Suggested readings

American Psychiatric Association: Practice guideline for the treatment of patients with schizophrenia, *Am J Psychiatry* 154(Suppl):4, 1997.

Andreason N: A unitary model of schizophrenia, *Arch Gen Psychiatry* 56:781, 1999.

Baier M, Murry R: A descriptive study of insight into illness by persons with schizophrenia, *J Psychosoc Nurs* 37:14, 1999.

Beck A, Rector N: Cognitive therapy of schizophrenia: a new therapy for the new millennium. *American J of Psychotherapy* 54(3):291-300, 2000.

Bustillo J et al: The psychosocial treatment of schizophrenia: an update, *Am J Psychiatry* 158(2):163, 2001.

Chernomas W et al: Perspectives of women living with schizophrenia, *Psychiatric Services* 51(12):1517-1521, 2000.

Corcoran C et al: The neurobiology of the stress cascade and its potential relevance for schizophrenia, *J Psychiatr Pract* 7(1):3, 2001.

Dixon L et al: Services to families of adults with schizophrenia: from treatment recommendations to dissemination, *Psychiatr Serv* 50:233, 1999.

Duzyurek S, Wiener J: Early recognition in schizophrenia: the prodromal stages, *J Pract Psychiatry Behav Health* 7:187, 1999.

Dyck D et al: Management of negative symptoms among patients with schizophrenia attending multiple family groups, *Psychiatr Serv* 551:513, 2000.

Harkavy-Friedman J, Nelson E: Management of the suicidal patient with schizophrenia, *Psychiatr Clin North Am* 20:625, 1997.

Herz M: Early intervention in different phases of schizophrenia, *J Pract Psychiatry Behav Health* 5:197, 1999.

Holmberg S, Kane C: Health and self-care practices of persons with schizophrenia, *Psychiatr Serv* 50:827, 1999.

Jarboe K et al: Diagnosis, neurobiology and treatment of first episode schizophrenia, *J Am Psychiatr Nurses Assoc* 4:S2, 1998.

Jensen LH, Kane CF: Cognitive theory applied to the treatment of delusions of schizophrenia, *Arch Psychiatr Nurs* 6:335, 1996.

Landeen J et al: Factors influencing staff hopefulness in working with people with schizophrenia, *Issues Ment Health Nurs* 17:457, 1996.

Lehman A et al: Translating research into practice: the Schizophrenia Patient Outcomes Research Team (PORT) treatment recommendations, *Schizophr Bull* 24(1):1, 1998.

Lindsay H: Neurodevelopment of schizophrenia revealed, *Clin Psychiatry News* 3:34, 2000.

Lukens E et al: Family psychoeducation in schizophrenia: emerging themes and challenges, *J Pract Psychiatry Behav Health* 5:314, 1999.

McCay E, Ryan K, Amey S: Mitigating engulfment: recovery from a first episode of psychosis, *J Psychosoc Nurs* 34:40, 1996.

McCombs J et al: Antipsychotic drug use patterns and the cost of treating schizophrenia, *Psychiatr Serv* 51:525, 2000.

Moller M, Murphy M: *Recovering from psychosis: a wellness approach,* Nine Mile Falls, Wash, 1998, Psychiatric Rehabilitation Nurses.

Mueser K, Sengupta A, Schooler N et al: Family treatment and medication dosage reduction in schizophrenia: effects on patient social functioning, family attitudes, and burden, *J Consulting and Clinical Psychology* 69:3, 2001.

Olfson M et al: Predicting medication noncompliance after hospital discharge among patients with schizophrenia, *Psychiatr Serv* 51:216, 2000.

Perese EF: Unmet needs of persons with chronic mental illness: relationship to their adaptation to community living, *Issues Ment Health Nurs* 18:19, 1997.

Rose LE: Caring for caregivers: perceptions of social support, *J Psychosoc Nurs* 35:18, 1997.

Ruscher S, deWit R, Mazmanian D: Psychiatric patients' attitudes about medication and factors affecting noncompliance, *Psychiatric Serv* 48:82, 1997.

Stuart G, Laraia M: *Principles and practice of psychiatric nursing,* ed 7, St Louis, 2001, Mosby.

Wuerker A: The family and schizophrenia, *Issues in Mental Health Nursing,* 21:127, 2000.

Yung A et al: Monitoring and care of young people at incipient risk of psychosis, *Schizophr Bull* 22:283, 1996.

# Social Responses and Personality Disorders

15

## Continuum of Social Responses

Humans are socially oriented. To achieve satisfaction with life, they must establish positive interpersonal relationships. In a healthy interpersonal relationship the individuals involved are close to each other while maintaining separate identities. The persons also must establish interdependence, which is a balance of dependence and independence in the relationship. Figure 15-1 presents the continuum of social responses.

## Development of Mature Interpersonal Relationships

The capacity for interpersonal relationships develops throughout the life cycle. Table 15-1 presents the major developmental tasks related to interpersonal growth.

Personality disorders are usually recognizable by adolescence or earlier and continue throughout most of adulthood. They are enduring, inflexible, and maladaptive patterns of response that are severe enough to cause either dysfunctional behavior or profound distress. Personality disorders are relatively common in the United States; an estimated 10% to 18% of the general population have these illnesses. However, only one fifth of these people are receiving treatment. At least some of these disorders are also associated with greater mortality resulting from suicide.

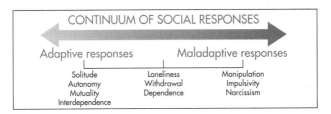

Figure 15-1
**Continuum of social responses.**

Table 15-1 Developmental tasks related to interpersonal growth

| Developmental Stage | Task |
|---|---|
| Infancy | Establish basic trust |
| Toddlerhood | Develop autonomy and beginning of independent behavior |
| Preschool age | Learn to display initiative and a sense of responsibility and conscience |
| School age | Learn competition, cooperation, and compromise |
| Preadolescence | Become intimate with same-sex friend |
| Adolescence | Become intimate with opposite-sex friend and independent from parents |
| Young adulthood | Become interdependent with parents and friends; marry; have children |
| Middle adulthood | Learn to let go |
| Late adulthood | Grieve losses and develop a sense of relatedness to the culture |

## *Assessment*

### Behaviors

The behaviors observed in people with personality disorders are characterized by chronic, maladaptive social responses. The DSM-IV-TR has grouped the personality disorders into three clusters based on descriptive similarities. Table 15-2 presents a specific classification of interpersonal and behavioral characteristics associated with each of the personality disorders. People with

Table 15-2   Classification and features of DSM-IV-TR personality disorders

| Disorder | Features |
| --- | --- |
| **Cluster A: Odd, Eccentric, General Tendency Toward Social and Emotional Withdrawal** | |
| Paranoid | Distrust: persistently suspicious, secretive, withholding, hypervigilant, jealous, envious |
| Schizoid | Social detachment: self-absorbed; restricted emotionality; cold and indifferent; neither desires nor enjoys close relationships; anhedonic, indifferent to others; less disturbed than schizotypal |
| Schizotypal | Interpersonal deficits; cognitive distortions; eccentricities; paranoid; difficulty feeling understood and accepted; odd beliefs, magical thinking, unusual perceptual experiences; social isolation |
| **Cluster B: Overemotional, Dramatic, Erratic, Impulsive** | |
| Antisocial | Disregard for the rights of others; lies; manipulates; exploitative; seductive; repeatedly performs acts that are grounds for arrest |
| Borderline | Instability; impulsivity; hypersensitivity; self-destructive behavior; profound mood shifts; unstable and intense interpersonal relationships |
| Histrionic | Excessive emotionality; attention seeking; superficial and stormy relationships; lively; uncomfortable when not the center of attention |
| Narcissistic | Arrogance; need for admiration; lack of empathy; seductive; socially exploitative; manipulative; grandiose sense of self-importance |

Cluster C: Anxious, Fearful

| | |
|---|---|
| Avoidant | Social inhibition; withdraw from social and occupational situations that involve significant interpersonal contact; longs for relationships; inadequacy; hypersensitivity to negative criticism, rejection, or shame |
| Dependent | Submissive behavior; low self-esteem; dependency in relationships; extreme self-consciousness; urgently and indiscriminately seeks another relationship when close relationship ends; inadequate; helpless |
| Obsessive-compulsive | Unable to express affection; overly cold and rigid; crippling preoccupation with trivial detail, orderliness, perfectionism, and control (i.e., attends to rules, lists, organization, schedules, to the extent that the major point of the activity is lost); superior attitudes. |

Table 15-3    Behaviors related to maladaptive social responses

| Maladaptive Response | Behaviors |
| --- | --- |
| Manipulation | Treats others as objects |
| | Centers relationships around control issues |
| | Is self-oriented or goal oriented, not oriented to others |
| Narcissism | Fragile self-esteem |
| | Constant seeking of praise and admiration |
| | Egocentric attitude |
| | Envy |
| | Rage when others are not supportive |
| Impulsivity | Inability to plan |
| | Inability to learn from experience |
| | Poor judgment |
| | Unreliability |

cluster B personality disorders have unique character features that at times make nursing care complicated and difficult. Frequently occurring maladaptive responses of patients with cluster B personality disorders include manipulation, narcissism, and impulsivity; Table 15-3 lists behaviors related to these responses.

## Predisposing Factors

A variety of factors may lead to maladaptive social responses. Although much research has been done on disorders that affect interpersonal relationships, no specific conclusions exist about their causes. A combination of factors is probably involved, including the following:

1. *Developmental factors.* Any interference with the accomplishment of the developmental tasks listed in Table 15-1 predisposes a person to maladaptive social responses. Disrupted family systems *may* contribute to the development of these responses. Some believe that persons who have these problems were unsuccessful at separating and individuating themselves from their parents. Family norms may discourage relationships outside the family. Family roles are often blurred. Parental alcoholism and child abuse also

predispose the person to maladaptive social responses. Organizations of family members are working with professionals to develop a more accurate picture of the relationship between mental disorder and family stress. This collaborative approach should reduce families being blamed by professionals.

2. *Biological factors.* Genetic factors may contribute to maladaptive social responses. Early evidence suggests involvement of the neurotransmitters in the development of these disorders, but further research is needed.

3. *Sociocultural factors.* Social isolation is a major factor in disturbed relationships. This may result from transiency; norms discouraging approaching others; or the devaluing of less productive members of society, such as elderly, disabled, and chronically ill persons. Isolation may result from the adoption of norms, behaviors, and value systems that differ from those of the majority culture. Unrealistic expectations for relationships is another factor related to these disorders.

## Precipitating Stressors

Precipitating stressors generally involve stressful life events, such as losses, that interfere with the person's ability to relate to others and cause anxiety. They can be grouped into the following two categories:

1. *Sociocultural stressors.* Stress can arise from decreased stability of the family unit and separation from significant others, such as from hospitalization.

2. *Psychological stressors.* Prolonged or extremely intense anxiety coexists with a limited ability to cope. Demands to separate from significant others or failure of others to meet dependency needs may cause high levels of anxiety.

## Appraisal of Stressors

The mature person who can participate in healthy interpersonal relationships is still vulnerable to the effects of psychological stress. A person's appraisal of the stressor is critically important in this regard. The pain of either a single loss or a series of losses can be so great that the person avoids future involvements rather than risk more pain. This response is more likely if the person had difficulty with developmental tasks pertinent to relatedness.

## Coping Resources

Examples of coping resources related to maladaptive social responses include the following:

- Involvement in a broad network of family and friends
- Relationships with pets
- Use of creativity to express interpersonal stress (e.g., art, music, writing)

## Coping Mechanisms

Individuals who have maladaptive social responses use a variety of mechanisms in an effort to cope with anxiety. They relate to two specific types of relationship problems as follows:

1. Coping associated with antisocial personality disorder
   - Projection
   - Splitting
   - Devaluation of others
2. Coping associated with borderline personality disorder
   - Splitting
   - Reaction formation
   - Projection
   - Isolation
   - Idealization of others
   - Devaluation of others
   - Projective identification

## N u r s i n g   D i a g n o s i s

Maladaptive social responses may lead to a range of specific disorders at various levels of severity. The nurse must assess the nature of the patient's disorder and consider the range of behaviors presented.

The box on page 307 presents the primary and related NANDA nursing diagnoses for maladaptive social responses. A complete nursing assessment would include all maladaptive responses of the patient, and many additional nursing problems would be identified.

## NANDA Nursing Diagnoses Related to Maladaptive Social Responses

Adjustment, Impaired
Anxiety
Coping, Compromised family
Coping, Ineffective
Family processes, Interrupted
*Identity, Disturbed personal
Loneliness, Risk for
Role performance, Ineffective
Self-esteem, Risk for situational low
*Self-esteem, Situational low
Self-mutilation
*Self-mutilation, Risk for
*Social interaction, Impaired
Social isolation
Suicide, Risk for
Therapeutic regimen management, Ineffective, Ineffective
   family
Thought processes, Disturbed
*Violence, Risk for other-directed
*Violence, Risk for self-directed

*Primary nursing diagnosis for maladaptive social responses.
*From North American Nursing Diagnosis Association:* NANDA nursing
diagnoses: definitions and classification 2000-2001, *Philadelphia, 2001,
The Association.*

## Related Medical Diagnoses

Many medically diagnosed psychiatric disorders involve problems
with interpersonal relationships. They range in severity from personality disorders to psychoses. The box on pages 308 and 309 describes these disorders.

## DSM-IV-TR Medical Diagnoses Related to Maladaptive Social Responses

| DSM-IV-TR Diagnosis | Essential Features |
| --- | --- |
| Paranoid personality disorder | Pervasive distrust and suspiciousness of others such that their motives are interpreted as malevolent; beginning in early adulthood and present in a variety of contexts. |
| Schizoid personality disorder | Pervasive pattern of detachment from social relationships and a restricted range of expression of emotions in interpersonal settings; beginning in early adulthood and present in a variety of contexts. |
| Schizotypal personality disorder | Pervasive pattern of social and interpersonal deficits marked by acute discomfort with and reduced capacity for close relationships and by cognitive and perceptual distortions and eccentricities of behavior; beginning in early adulthood and present in a variety of contexts. |
| Antisocial personality disorder | Pervasive pattern of disregard for and violation of the rights of others occurring since age 15. |
| Borderline personality disorder | Pervasive pattern of instability in interpersonal relationships, self-image, and affect and marked impulsivity; beginning by early adulthood and present in a variety of contexts. |
| Histrionic personality disorder | Pervasive pattern of excessive emotionality and attention seeking; beginning by early adulthood and present in a variety of contexts. |

| Narcissistic personality disorder | Pervasive pattern of grandiosity (in fantasy or behavior), need for admiration, and lack of empathy; beginning by early adulthood and present in a variety of contexts. |
| Avoidant personality disorder | Pervasive pattern of social inhibition, feelings of inadequacy, and hypersensitivity to negative evaluation; beginning by early adulthood and present in a variety of contexts. |
| Dependent personality disorder | Pervasive and excessive need to be taken care of that leads to submissive and clinging behaviors and fears of separation; beginning by early adulthood and present in a variety of contexts. |
| Obsessive-compulsive personality disorder | Pervasive pattern of preoccupation with orderliness, perfectionism, and mental and interpersonal control, at the expense of flexibility, openness, and efficiency; beginning by early adulthood and present in a variety of contexts. |

*Modified from American Psychiatric Association: Diagnostic and statistical manual of mental disorders, ed 4, text revision (DSM-IV-TR), Washington, DC, 2000, The Association.*

## Outcome Identification

The expected outcome for a patient with maladaptive social responses is as follows:

*The patient will obtain maximal interpersonal satisfaction by establishing and maintaining self-enhancing relationships with others.*

## Planning

A Patient Education Plan for an impulsive patient is presented on page 311.

## Implementation

Empirically validated treatments for some of the medical diagnoses related to personality disorders are summarized in Table 15-4.

The essential elements of nursing intervention with the patient who has maladaptive social responses include the following:

1. Establishing a therapeutic relationship
2. Involving the family to promote and maintain positive change
3. Providing a therapeutic milieu that focuses on realistic expectations, involving the patient in decision making, and processing interactional behaviors in current situations
4. Setting limits and providing structure
5. Protecting the patient from self-harm
6. Focusing on the patient's strengths
7. Implementing contracting and other cognitive-behavioral strategies

A Nursing Treatment Plan Summary for the patient who has maladaptive social responses is presented on pages 313-315.

## Evaluation

The following questions may assist the nurse to evaluate the outcomes of intervention with the patient who has maladaptive social responses:

1. Has the patient become less impulsive, manipulative, or narcissistic?

*Text continued on p. 316*

Patient Education Plan: **Modifying Impulsive Behavior**

| Content | Instructional Activities | Evaluation |
|---|---|---|
| Describe characteristics and consequences of impulsive behavior. | Select a situation in which impulsive behavior occurred. Ask patient to describe what happened. Instruct patient to keep a diary of impulsive actions, including a description of events before and after the incident. | Patient identifies and describes an impulsive incident. Patient maintains a diary of impulsive behaviors. Patient explores the causes and consequences of impulsive behavior. |
| Describe behaviors characteristic of interpersonal anxiety; relate anxiety to impulsive behavior. | Discuss the diary with patient. Assist patient to identify interpersonal anxiety related to impulsive behavior. | Patient connects feelings of interpersonal anxiety with impulsive behavior. |
| Explain stress reduction techniques. | Describe the stress response. Demonstrate relaxation exercises. Assist patient to return the demonstration. | Patient performs relaxation exercises when signs of anxiety appear. |
| Identify alternative responses to anxiety-producing situations. | Using situations from the diary and knowledge of relaxation exercises; assist patient to list possible alternative responses. | Patient identifies at least two alternative responses to each anxiety-producing situation. |
| Practice using alternative responses to anxiety-producing situations. | Role-play each of the identified alternative behaviors. Discuss the feelings associated with impulsive behavior and the alternatives. | Patient describes the relationship between behavior and feelings. Patient selects and performs anxiety-reducing behaviors. |

Table 15-4   Summarizing the evidence on treatments for personality disorders

**DISORDER:** Borderline personality disorder
**TREATMENT:**

- Dialectical behavioral therapy (DBT) produced lower attrition, fewer and less severe episodes of parasuicidal behavior, and fewer days of hospitalization compared with a control condition.
- Noradrenergic agents tended to improve mood but not irritability or dyscontrol, whereas serotonergic agents may act to decrease impulsivity; there are inconsistent data for the utility of antipsychotic and anticonvulsive agents.

**DISORDER:** Mixed personality disorder (excluding Cluster A disorders)
**TREATMENT:**

- An average of 40 weeks of brief dynamic therapy yielded substantial symptomatic improvement at both the end of treatment and after 1.5 years.
- Medications may be useful for several of these disorders, although many methodological problems remain to be worked out.

**DISORDER:** Schizotypal personality disorder (and other Cluster A disorders)
**TREATMENT:**

- Dopamine antagonists may be useful in reducing some of the symptoms of these disorders.

From Nathan P, Gorman J: *A guide to treatments that work,* New York, 1998, Oxford University Press.

## Nursing Treatment Plan Summary:  Maladaptive Social Responses

**Nursing Diagnosis:** Impaired social interaction

**Expected Outcome: Patient will obtain maximal interpersonal satisfaction by establishing and maintaining self-enhancing relationships with others.**

| Short-term Goals | Interventions | Rationale |
| --- | --- | --- |
| Patient will participate in a therapeutic nurse-patient relationship. | Initiate a nurse-patient relationship contract mutually agreed on by patient and nurse. Develop mutual behavioral goals. Maintain consistent behavior by all nursing staff. Communicate honest responses to patient's behavior. Provide honest, immediate feedback about behavioral change. Maintain confidentiality. Demonstrate accessibility. | An atmosphere of trust facilitates open expression of thoughts and feelings; a trusting relationship enables patient to risk sharing feelings; honest responses reinforce openness; staff consistency creates a predictable environment that creates trust. |

*Continued*

Nursing Treatment Plan Summary: Maladaptive Social Responses—cont'd

| Short-term Goals | Interventions | Rationale |
|---|---|---|
| Patient will describe interpersonal strengths and weaknesses. | Provide patient with opportunities to demonstrate strengths (e.g., helping other patients, assuming leadership roles). | Patient with maladaptive social responses is unable to identify accurately interpersonal strengths and weaknesses, leading to fear of closeness and fear of failure. |
| | Assist patient to analyze experiences perceived as failures. | |
| | Communicate acceptance of patient as a person while not accepting maladaptive social behavior. | Nurse must assist patient to separate behavioral incidents from total self-worth and to recognize that patient can be liked even if imperfect. |
| Patient will establish or reestablish one interpersonal relationship that is mutually satisfying and adaptive. | Provide consistent feedback about adaptive and maladaptive social behavior. | Describing and evaluating one's behavior require taking responsibility for the behavior and its consequences. |
| | Encourage patient to describe successful and unsuccessful relationship experiences orally or in a written journal. | Patients need to go beyond understanding or insight to engaging in actual behavioral change. |
| | Assist patient in initiating or resuming a relationship with one other person. | |
| | Review aspects of this relationship with patient. | |
| | Reinforce patient's adaptive social responses. | Nurse must help patient evaluate whether responses are adaptive or maladaptive. Alternatives can then be identified to further the patient's goal achievement. |
| | Evaluate with patient alternatives to maladaptive social responses. | |

Nursing Diagnosis: High risk for self-mutilation

Expected Outcome: Patient will select constructive rather than self-destructive ways of coping with interpersonal anxiety.

| | | |
|---|---|---|
| Patient will not engage in self-mutilation | Develop a contract with patient to notify staff when anxiety is increasing. | When patient is not able to cope with anxiety, protecting patient's safety is nurse's highest priority. |
| | Provide close one-on-one observation of patient when necessary to maintain safety. Remove all potentially dangerous objects from patient and environment. Provide prescribed medications. | A contract helps patient assume responsibility and explore healthier coping responses. |
| Patient will describe self-mutilating episodes. | Assist patient in reviewing these events. Identify cues and triggers that precede self-mutilating behavior. Help patient explore feelings related to these episodes. | Self-mutilation is often a way of relieving extreme anxiety. Structured interpersonal support can help patient review these events. |
| Patient will describe alternatives to self-mutilating behaviors. | Suggest alternative behaviors, such as seeking interpersonal support or engaging in an adaptive anxiety-reducing activity. | Nurse can help patient review the full range of adaptive responses. Supportive but critical evaluation is necessary for behavioral change. |
| Patient will implement one new adaptive response when experiencing high interpersonal anxiety. | Assist patient in selecting new adaptive responses. Reinforce patient's adaptive behavior. Identify positive consequences of the adaptive responses. Discuss ways these may be generalized to other situations. | Nurse should take an active role in setting limits, examining patient behaviors, and reinforcing adaptive actions. These new learned responses can also be reviewed for their applicability to other life events. |

2. Does the patient express satisfaction with the quality of interpersonal relationships?
3. Can the patient participate in close interpersonal relationships?
4. Does the patient verbalize recognition of positive behavioral change?

*your* **INTERNET**
c o n n e c t i o n

**All About Personality Disorders:**
personalitydisorders.mentalhelp.net

**BPD Central Borderline Personality Disorder:**
bpdcentral.com

## Suggested readings

Agronin M, Maletta G: Personality disorders in late life: understanding and overcoming the gap in research, *Am J Geriatr Psychiatry* 8(1):4, 2000.

Black D: *Bad boys, bad men: confronting antisocial personality disorder,* New York, 1999, Oxford University Press.

Blashfield R, Intoccia V: Growth of the literature on the topic of personality disorders, *Am J Psychiatry* 157(3):472, 2000.

Dyckoff D et al: The investigation of behavioral contracting in patients with borderline personality disorder, *J Psychiatr Nurs Assoc* 2:71, 1996.

Grilo C et al: Course and stability of personality disorders, *J Pract Psychiatry Behav Health* 4:61, 1998.

Grinspoon L: Personality disorders, *Harv Ment Health Lett* 16(9):1, 2000.

Hampton M: Dialectical behavior therapy in the treatment of persons with borderline personality disorder, *Arch Psychiatr Nurs* 11:96, 1997.

Kaylor L: Antisocial personality disorder: diagnostic, ethical and treatment issues, *Issues Ment Health Nurs* 20:247, 1999.

Link P: *Clinical assessment and management of severe personality disorders,* Washington, DC, 1996, American Psychiatric Press.

Miller A et al: Dialectical behavior therapy: part II, Clinical application of DBT for patients with multiple problems, *J Pract Psychiatry Behav Health* 4:84, 1998.

Miller B: Characteristics of effective day treatment programming for persons with borderline personality disorder, *Psychiatr Serv* 46:605, 1995.

Nehls N: Being a case manager for persons with borderline personality disorder: perspectives of community mental health center clinicians, *Arch Psychiatr Nurs* 14(1):12, 2000.

Nehls N: Borderline personality disorder: gender stereotypes, stigma and limited system of care, *Issues Ment Health Nursing* 19:97, 1998.

O'Brien L: Inpatient nursing care of patients with borderline personality disorder: a review of the literature, *Aust N Z J Ment Health Nurs* 7:172, 1998.

Perry J et al: Effectiveness of psychotherapy for personality disorders, *Am J Psychiatry* 156:1312, 1999.

Stuart G, Laraia M: *Principles and practice of psychiatric nursing,* ed 7, St Louis, 2001, Mosby.

# Cognitive Responses and Organic Mental Disorders

## Continuum of Cognitive Responses

Maladaptive cognitive responses include inability to make decisions, impaired memory and judgment, disorientation, misperceptions, decreased attention span, and difficulties with logical reasoning. They may occur episodically or be present continuously. Depending on the stressor, the condition may be reversible or characterized by progressive deterioration in functioning. Figure 16-1 illustrates the continuum of cognitive responses.

### Assessment

#### Behaviors

The specific cognitive disorders to be considered include delirium and dementia. Table 16-1 describes the characteristics of delirium and dementia. Depression in elderly people is often misdiagnosed as dementia and is included in Table 16-1 for purposes of comparison.

#### Predisposing Factors

Cognitive responses are generally the result of a biological disruption in the functioning of the central nervous system (CNS). Fac-

Figure 16-1
**Continuum of cognitive responses.**

tors that predispose the individual to developing cognitive disorders include the following:

1. Interference with the supply of oxygen, glucose, and other essential basic nutrients to the brain
   - Arteriosclerotic vascular changes
   - Transient ischemic attacks
   - Cerebral hemorrhage
   - Multiple small brain infarcts
2. Degeneration associated with aging
3. Collection of toxic substances in brain tissue
4. Alzheimer's disease
5. Human immunodeficiency virus (HIV)
6. Chronic liver disease
7. Chronic renal disease
8. Vitamin deficiencies (particularly thiamine)
9. Malnutrition
10. Genetic abnormalities

Major psychiatric disorders, such as schizophrenia, bipolar disorder, anxiety disorders, and depression, may also influence cognitive functioning.

## Precipitating Stressors

Any major assault on the brain is likely to result in a disruption in cognitive functioning. Categories of stressors include the following:

1. Hypoxias
2. Metabolic disorders, including hypothyroidism, hyper-

Table 16-1 Comparison of delirium, depression, and dementia

|  | Delirium | Depression | Dementia |
|---|---|---|---|
| Onset | Rapid (hours to days) | Rapid (weeks to months) | Gradual (years) |
| Course | Wide fluctuations; may continue for weeks if cause not found | May be self-limited or may become chronic without treatment | Chronic; slow but continuous decline |
| Level of consciousness | Fluctuates from hyperalert to difficult to arouse | Normal | Normal |
| Orientation | Patient is disoriented, confused | Patient may seem disoriented | Patient is disoriented, confused |
| Affect | Fluctuating | Sad, depressed, worried, guilty | Labile; apathy in later stages |
| Attention | Always impaired | Difficulty concentrating; patient may check and recheck all actions | May be intact; patient may focus on one thing for long periods |
| Sleep | Always disturbed | Disturbed; excess sleeping or insomnia, especially early morning waking | Usually normal |
| Behavior | Patient is agitated, restless | Patient may be fatigued, apathetic; may occasionally be agitated | Patient may be agitated or apathetic; may wander |
| Speech | Sparse or rapid; patient may be incoherent | Flat, sparse, may have outbursts; understandable | Sparse or rapid; repetitive; patient may be incoherent |

| | | | |
|---|---|---|---|
| Memory | Impaired, especially for recent events | Varies day to day; slow recall; often short-term deficit | Impaired, especially for recent events |
| Cognition | Disordered reasoning | May seem impaired | Disordered reasoning and calculation |
| Thought content | Incoherent, confused; delusions; stereotyped | Negative; hypochondriac, thoughts of death; paranoid | Disorganized, rich content, delusional, paranoid |
| Perception | Misinterpretations, illusions, hallucinations | Distorted; patient may have auditory hallucinations; negative interpretation of people and events | No change |
| Judgment | Poor | Poor | Poor; socially inappropriate behavior |
| Insight | May be present in lucid moments | May be impaired | Absent |
| Performance on mental status exams | Poor but variable; improves during lucid moments and with recovery | Memory impaired; calculation, drawing, following directions usually not impaired; frequent "I don't know" answers | Consistently poor; progressively worsens; patient attempts to answer all questions |

From Holt J: How to help confused patients, *Am J Nurs* 93(8):32, 1993.

thyroidism, hypoglycemia, hypopituitarism, and adrenal disease
3. Toxicity and infection
4. Adverse response to medication
5. Structural changes in the brain, such as tumors or traumas
6. Sensory underload or overload

## Appraisal of Stressors

The specific stressor related to cognitive impairment often cannot be identified, although this is rapidly changing as neuroscientific knowledge increases. In general, when assessing maladaptive cognitive responses, physiological causes are ruled out first, then psychosocial stressors are considered. Even when physiological factors are present, psychosocial stress may further compromise the person's thought process. Thus the person's appraisal of the stressor is critically important.

## Coping Resources

Individual responses include strengths and skills. Caregivers can be supportive and can also provide information about the person's personality characteristics, habits, and routines. Self-help groups can be effective coping resources for caregivers.

## Coping Mechanisms

The way an individual copes emotionally with maladaptive cognitive responses is greatly influenced by past life experience. A person who has developed many coping mechanisms that have been effective in the past is better able to handle the onset of a cognitive problem than a person who already has coping problems. Usual coping mechanisms may be exaggerated as the person tries to adapt to loss of cognitive ability.

Because the basic behavioral disruption in delirium is altered awareness, which reflects a severe biological disturbance in the brain, psychological coping mechanisms are not generally used. For this reason the nurse must protect the patient from harm and substitute for the person's own coping mechanisms by constantly reorienting the patient and reinforcing reality.

Behaviors that may represent attempts by the person with dementia to cope with loss of cognitive ability may include suspiciousness, hostility, joking, depression, seductiveness, and withdrawal. Ego defense mechanisms that may be observed in patients with cognitive impairment include the following:

- Regression
- Denial
- Compensation

## Nursing Diagnosis

Most disorders that result in some degree of cognitive impairment are physiological in origin. Therefore the nurse must consider the patient's physical needs and the psychosocial behavioral problems. A thorough nursing diagnosis reflects all these influences on the patient's behavior. If the patient's cognitive disability interferes with participation in the treatment planning process, it may be necessary to involve a significant other in the formation of the nursing diagnosis.

The box on page 324 presents the primary and related nursing diagnoses for maladaptive cognitive responses. A complete nursing assessment would include all the patient's nursing care needs, and many additional nursing diagnoses would be identified.

### Related Medical Diagnoses

The box on pages 325-327 describes mental disorders that result in maladaptive cognitive responses.

## Outcome Identification

The expected outcome for a patient with maladaptive cognitive responses is as follows:

*The patient will achieve optimal cognitive functioning.*

## Planning

A Family Education Plan for the family of a patient with maladaptive cognitive response is presented on page 328.

## Implementation

### Intervening in Delirium

Nursing interventions for the patient with delirium include the following:

**NURSE ALERT.**    Restraining a delirious patient to maintain an intravenous line may increase agitation. Use restraint only when absolutely necessary, and never leave a restrained delirious patient alone.

1. *Meeting physiological needs*
   - Maintain nutrition and fluid/electrolyte balance.
   - Use nursing measures such as back rub, warm milk, and soothing conversation to promote sleep. Sedatives may be

*Text continued on p. 329*

## NANDA Nursing Diagnoses Related to Maladaptive Cognitive Responses

Anxiety
Communication, Impaired verbal
Confusion, Acute
Confusion, Chronic
Coping, Compromised family
Coping, Ineffective individual
Falls, Risk for
Health maintenance, Ineffective
Home maintenance, Impaired
Injury, Risk for
Memory, Impaired
Mobility, Impaired physical
Role performance, Ineffective
Self-care deficit, Bathing/hygiene, Dressing/grooming, Feeding, Toileting
Sensory perception, Disturbed: visual, auditory, kinesthetic, gustatory, tactile, olfactory
Sleep pattern, Disturbed
Social interaction, Impaired
Social isolation
*Thought processes, Disturbed
Wandering

*Primary nursing diagnosis for maladaptive cognitive responses.
*North American Nursing Diagnosis Association:* NANDA nursing diagnoses: definitions and classification 2000-2001, *Philadelphia, 2001, The Association.*

# DSM-IV-TR Medical Diagnoses Related to Cognitive Responses

| DSM-IV-TR Diagnosis | Essential Features |
|---|---|
| **Delirium (general criteria)** (to be applied to all other categories of delirium) | Disturbed consciousness accompanied by a cognitive change that cannot be accounted for by a dementia. |
| | Impaired ability to focus, sustain, or shift attention. |
| | Cognitive changes, including impaired recent memory, disorientation to time or place, language disturbance, or perceptual disturbance. |
| | Develops over a short time; tends to fluctuate during the course of the day. |
| Delirium caused by a general medical condition | Evidence that the cognitive disturbance is the direct result of a general medical condition. |
| Substance-induced delirium | Evidence of substance intoxication or withdrawal, medication side effects, or toxin exposure judged to be related to the delirium. |
| Delirium with multiple etiologies | Evidence of multiple causes for the delirium. |
| **Dementia (general criteria)** (to be applied to all other categories of dementia) | Development of multiple cognitive deficits, including memory impairment and at least one of the following: aphasia, apraxia, agnosia, or disturbed executive functioning (ability to think abstractly and plan, initiate, sequence, monitor, and stop complex behavior). |
| | Must cause severe impairment in social or occupational functioning. |

*Continued*

## DSM-IV-TR Medical Diagnoses Related to Cognitive Responses—cont'd

| DSM-IV-TR Diagnosis—cont'd | Essential Features—cont'd |
|---|---|
| Dementia of the Alzheimer's type | Gradual onset with continuing cognitive decline. |
| Vascular dementia | All other causes of dementia must be ruled out. Focal neurological signs and symptoms or laboratory evidence of cerebrovascular disease that are judged to be related to the dementia. |
| Dementia caused by other general medical conditions | Evidence that the general medical condition (e.g., HIV, traumatic brain injury, Parkinson's disease, Huntington's disease, Pick's disease, Creutzfeldt-Jakob disease, normal-pressure hydrocephalus, hypothyroidism, brain tumor, vitamin $B_{12}$ deficiency) is etiologically related to the dementia. |
| Substance-induced persisting dementia | Deficits do not occur exclusively during a delirium and persist beyond the usual duration of substance intoxication or withdrawal. Evidence that the deficits are related to persisting effects of substance use (e.g., drug of abuse, medication). |
| Dementia caused by multiple etiologies | Evidence that the dementia has more than one etiology. |

| | |
|---|---|
| Amnestic disorder (general criteria) | Development of memory disorder evidenced by impaired ability to learn new information or to recall previously learned information.<br>Disturbance causes significant impairment in social or occupational functioning and represents a significant decline from a previous level of functioning.<br>Does not occur exclusively during the course of delirium or dementia. |
| Amnestic disorder caused by a general medical condition | Evidence that the disturbance is directly related to a general medical condition (including physical trauma). |
| Substance-induced persisting amnestic disorder | Evidence that the memory disturbance is etiologically related to the persisting effects of substance use (e.g., drug abuse, medication). |

*Modified from American Psychiatric Association:* Diagnostic and statistical manual of mental disorders, *ed 4, text revision (DSM-IV-TR), Washington, DC, 2000, The Association.*

Family Education Plan:    Helping a Family Member with Maladaptive Cognitive Responses

| Content | Instructional Activities | Evaluation |
|---|---|---|
| Explain possible causes of maladaptive cognitive responses. | Describe predisposing factors and precipitating stressors that may lead to impaired cognition; provide printed reference materials. | Family identifies possible causes of patient's disorders. |
| Define and describe orientation to time, place, and person. | Define three spheres of orientation; role-play interpersonal responses to disorientation. | Family identifies disorientation and provides reorientation. |
| Describe relationship of cognitive functioning level to ability to communicate. | Describe impact of maladaptive cognitive responses on communication; demonstrate effective communication techniques; videotape and discuss return demonstration. | Family adjusts communication approaches to patient's ability to interact. |
| Describe effect of maladaptive cognitive responses on self-care behaviors. | Describe usual progression of gain or loss of self-care ability related to nature of disorder; encourage learner to assist in providing care to patient; provide written instructional materials. | Family assists with activities of daily living as required by patient's level of biopsychosocial functioning. |
| Refer to community resources. | Provide a list of community resources; arrange to meet with staff members of selected community programs; visit meetings of selected programs. | Family describes various programs that provide services relevant to patient's and family's needs and will contact appropriate programs when needed. |

contraindicated until the cause of the delirium has been found.

2. *Intervening in perceptual disturbances* (e.g., hallucinations)
   - Keep light on in room to minimize shadows.
   - Ensure safety by placing the patient in a room with security screens and removing excess furniture.
   - Provide one-to-one nursing care if needed to maintain orientation.
   - Reorient frequently to time, place, and person.

3. *Communication*
   - Give clear messages.
   - Avoid giving choices.
   - Use simple, direct statements.

4. *Patient education*
   - Provide information regarding cause of delirium.
   - Teach the patient and family about prescribed treatment.
   - Inform about prevention of future episodes.
   - Refer to community health nursing agency if further education or nursing intervention is required.

## Intervening in Dementia

Empirically validated treatments for dementia are summarized in Table 16-2. Nursing interventions for the patient with dementia include the following:

1. *Orientation*
   - Mark room clearly with the patient's name.
   - Encourage the patient to keep personal possessions in room.

Table 16-2   Summarizing the evidence on treatments for dementia

---

**Disorder:** Dementia
**Treatment:**
- The efficacy of dihydroergotoxine mesylate (Hydergine), one of two drugs currently approved by the FDA for alleviation of the cognitive deterioration of dementia, remains in question.
- Acetylcholinesterase inhibitors (tacrine and donepezil) are the other FDA-approved drugs for this disorder; they have shown modest clinically significant benefit.

From Nathan P, Gorman J: *A guide to treatments that work,* New York, 1998, Oxford University Press.

- Use a night light.
- Provide clocks and calendars.
- Provide newspapers and discuss them with the patient.
- Orient verbally at frequent intervals.
2. *Communication*
   - Introduce yourself.
   - Show unconditional positive regard for the patient.
   - Use clear, concise verbal communication.
   - Modulate voice.
   - Avoid pronouns.
   - Use yes/no questions.
   - Request one thing at a time.
   - Ensure that verbal agrees with nonverbal communication.
   - Learn about the patient's past life.
   - Provide a sense of sheltered freedom.
3. *Reinforcing coping mechanisms*
4. *Decreasing wandering.* Map the patient's behavior to identify conditions under which the behavior occurs, and intervene preventively.
5. *Decreasing agitation*
   - Explain expectations clearly.
   - Offer choices if the patient can handle them.
   - Provide a schedule of activities.
   - Avoid power struggles. If the patient refuses a request, leave and return in a few minutes.
   - Involve the patient in care whenever possible.
6. *Treating pharmacologically.* Tacrine (Cognex) and donepezil (Aricept) delay progression of Alzheimer's disease. Olanzapine (Zyprexa) can control the agitation associated with dementia and Alzheimer's disease.
7. *Involving family members*
8. *Using community resources*

Nursing interventions with patients who have maladaptive cognitive responses are provided in the Nursing Treatment Plan Summary on pages 331 and 332.

## Evaluation

1. Was the assessment complete enough to correctly identify the problem?
2. Were the goals individualized for this patient?

## Nursing Treatment Plan Summary:  Maladaptive Cognitive Responses

Nursing Diagnosis: Altered thought processes

Expected Outcome: Patient will achieve optimal cognitive functioning.

| Short-term Goals | Interventions | Rationale |
|---|---|---|
| Patient will meet basic biological needs. | Maintain adequate nutrition; monitor fluid intake and output; monitor vital signs. Provide opportunities for rest and stimulation. Assist with ambulation if necessary. Assist with hygiene activities as needed. | Basic biological integrity is necessary for survival. Interventions related to survival are given high priority for nursing intervention. Maladaptive cognitive responses usually involve sensory and perceptual disorders that can endanger patient's safety. |
| Patient will be safe from injury. | Assess sensory and perceptual functioning. Provide access to eyeglasses, hearing aids, canes, walkers, etc., if needed. Observe and correct safety hazards (e.g., obstacles, slippery floors, open flames, inadequate lighting). Supervise medications if necessary. Protect from injury during periods of agitation with one-to-one nursing care; use restraints only if absolutely necessary. | |

Continued

## Nursing Treatment Plan Summary: Maladaptive Cognitive Responses—cont'd

| Short-term Goals | Interventions | Rationale |
|---|---|---|
| Patient will experience an optimal level of self-esteem. | Provide reality orientation. Establish a trusting relationship. Encourage independence. Identify interests and skills; provide opportunities to use them. Give honest praise for accomplishments. Use therapeutic communication techniques to help patient communicate thoughts and feelings. | Cognitive impairment is a threat to self-esteem; a positive nurse-patient relationship can assist patient to express fears and feel secure in the environment; recognition of accomplishments also raises self-esteem. |
| Patient will maintain positive interpersonal relationships. | Initiate contact with significant others. Encourage patient to interact with others; involve in group activities. Teach family and patient about nature of the problem and recommended health care plan. Allow significant others to assist in patient care. Meet with significant others regularly and provide them with an opportunity to talk. Involve patient and family in discharge planning. | Caring relationships with others promote a positive self-concept; communication by significant others can often be understood more easily than that of strangers; family and friends can provide help in knowing patient's habits and preferences; involvement of significant others in caregiving often helps them cope with the stress of patient's health problem. |

3. Was enough time allowed for goal achievement?
4. Did the nurse have the skills needed to carry out the identified interventions?
5. Did environmental factors affect goal achievement?
6. Did additional stressors affect the patient's ability to cope?
7. Was the goal achievable for this patient?
8. What alternative approaches could be tried?

## *your*INTERNET connection

Alzheimer's Association:
www.alz.org

Dementia Research Group Intranet:
dementia.ion.ucl.ac.uk

Family Caregiver Alliance:
www.caregiver.org

Practice Guidelines for the Treatment of Patients with Alzheimer's Disease and Other Dementias of Late Life:
www.psych.org/clin_res/pg_dementia_32701.cfm

## Suggested readings

Academic Highlights: New insights into genetics and pathophysiology of Alzheimer's disease: what are the clinical and therapeutic implications, *J Clin Psychiatry* 61(4):307, 2000.

Allen L: Treating agitation without drugs, *Am J Nurs* 99(4):36, 1999.

American Psychiatric Association: Practice guideline for the treatment of patients with delirium, *Am J Psychiatry* 156(5):Suppl, 1999.

Colenda C: Managing agitated dementia patients: a decision analysis approach, *J Pract Psychiatry Behav Health* 3:156, 1997.

Cummings J, Jeste D: Alzheimer's disease and its management in the year 2010, *Psychiatr Serv* 50(9):1173, 1999.

Desai A, Grossberg G: Risk factors and protective factors for Alzheimer's disease, *Clin Geriatr* 7(11):43, 1999.

Draper B: The diagnosis and treatment of depression in dementia, *Psychiatr Serv* 50(9):1151, 1999.

Garand L et al: The biological basis of behavioral symptoms in dementia, *Issues Ment Health Nurs* 21:91, 2000.

Inouye S: A multicomponent intervention to prevent delirium in hospitalized older patients, *New Engl J Med* 340:669, 1999.

Kelley L et al: Family involvement in care for individuals with dementia protocol, *J Gerontol Nurs* 2:13, 2000.

Masand P: Atypical antipsychotics for elderly patients with neurodegenerative disorders and medical conditions, *Psychiatr Ann* 30(3):202, 2000.

Patkar A, Kunkel E: Treating delirium among elderly patients, *Psychiatr Serv* 48:46, 1997.

Rentz CA: Reminiscence: a supportive intervention for the person with Alzheimer's disease, *J Psychosoc Nurs Ment Health Serv* 33:15, 1995.

Strickland T et al: Dementia in minority elderly, *Clin Geriatr* 7(11):83, 1999.

Stuart G, Laraia M: *Principles and practice of psychiatric nursing,* ed 7, St Louis, 2001, Mosby.

Tariot P: Treatment of agitation in dementia, *J Clin Psychiatry* 60(Suppl 8):11, 1999.

# Chemically Mediated Responses and Substance-Related Disorders

# 17

## Continuum of Chemically Mediated Responses

Although there is a continuum from occasional drug or alcohol use to frequent use to abuse and dependence, not everyone who uses substances becomes an abuser, and every abuser does not become dependent. **Substance abuse** refers to continued use even after problems occur. **Substance dependence** indicates a severe condition, usually considered a disease. **Addiction** generally refers to the psychosocial behaviors related to substance dependence. The terms *addiction* and *dependence* are often used interchangeably. **Dual diagnosis** refers to the coexistence of substance abuse and psychiatric disorders within the same person. **Withdrawal symptoms** result from a biological need for the drug. **Tolerance** means that it takes increasing amounts of the substance to produce the expected effect. Withdrawal symptoms and tolerance are signs of **physical dependence.**

Abused substances include alcohol, opiates, prescription medications, psychotomimetics, cocaine, marijuana, and inhalants. A serious and growing problem in substance abuse is the rapidly increasing use of more than one substance simultaneously or sequentially.

Figure 17-1
Continuum of chemically mediated coping responses.

An individual may achieve a state of relaxation, euphoria, stimulation, or altered awareness by various means. Figure 17-1 illustrates the range of these activities.

## Assessment

### Behaviors

Behaviors that indicate the presence of a substance abuse problem can be assessed by using a screening tool. Box 17-1 presents the Brief Drug Abuse Screening Tool (B-DAST), and Box 17-2 presents the CAGE screening tool for alcoholism. Table 17-1 compares blood alcohol levels and observable behaviors. Table 17-2 summarizes the behaviors associated with substance abuse. Individuals who abuse substances face other risks because of their lifestyle. Accidents and violence occur frequently. Self-neglect contributes to physical, mental, and dental disease. Intravenous drug users and their partners are at high risk for infections with bloodborne pathogens, including HIV and hepatitis B virus (HBV). Finally, individuals who are dually diagnosed have both a substance use and a psychiatric disorder. Their substance use (1) may be causing the psychopathology; (2) may be secondary to the psychopathology as they self-medicate with substances to treat the symptoms of their mental disorder, use substances to enhance symptoms, or use substances to counter the side effects of medications they are taking for their psychiatric disorder; or (3) may be coincidental and not related to the mental disorder.

## Box 17-1 Brief Drug Abuse Screening Test (B-DAST)

Instructions: The following questions concern information about your involvement in and abuse of drugs. Drug abuse refers to (1) the use of prescribed or over-the-counter drugs in excess of the directions and (2) any non-medical use of drugs. Carefully read each statement and decide whether your answer is yes or no. Then circle the appropriate response.

| | | |
|---|---|---|
| Yes | No | 1. Have you used drugs other than those required for medical reasons? |
| Yes | No | 2. Have you abused prescription drugs? |
| Yes | No | 3. Do you abuse more than one drug at a time? |
| Yes | No | 4. Can you get through the week without using drugs (other than those required for medical reasons)?* |
| Yes | No | 5. Are you always able to stop using drugs when you want to?* |
| Yes | No | 6. Have you had blackouts or flashbacks as a result of drug use? |
| Yes | No | 7. Do you ever feel bad about your drug abuse? |
| Yes | No | 8. Does your spouse (or parents) ever complain about your involvement with drugs? |
| Yes | No | 9. Has drug abuse ever created problems between you and your spouse? |

*Items 4 and 5 are scored in the "no" or false direction.
From Skinner HA: *The Drug Abuse Screening Test*, Addict Behav 7(4):363, 1982.

*Continued*

**Box 17-1    Brief Drug Abuse Screening Test (B-DAST)—cont'd**

| | | |
|---|---|---|
| Yes | No | 10. Have you ever lost friends because of your use of drugs? |
| Yes | No | 11. Have you ever neglected your family or missed work because of your use of drugs? |
| Yes | No | 12. Have you ever been in trouble at work because of drug abuse? |
| Yes | No | 13. Have you ever lost a job because of drug abuse? |
| Yes | No | 14. Have you ever gotten into fights when under the influence of drugs? |
| Yes | No | 15. Have you ever engaged in illegal activities in order to obtain drugs? |
| Yes | No | 16. Have you ever been arrested for possession of illegal drugs? |
| Yes | No | 17. Have you ever experienced withdrawal symptoms as a result of heavy drug intake? |
| Yes | No | 18. Have you ever had medical problems as a result of your drug use (e.g., memory loss, hepatitis, convulsions, bleeding)? |
| Yes | No | 19. Have you ever gone to anyone for help for a drug problem? |
| Yes | No | 20. Have you ever been involved in a treatment program specifically related to drug use? |

*From Skinner HA: The Drug Abuse Screening Test, Addict Behav 7(4):363, 1982.*

---

### Box 17-2 The CAGE Questionnaire

- Have you ever felt you ought to **C**ut down on your drinking?
- Have people **A**nnoyed you by criticizing your drinking?
- Have you ever felt bad or **G**uilty about your drinking?
- Have you ever had a drink first thing in the morning to steady your nerves or get rid of a hangover (**E**yeopener)?

Scoring: 1 "yes" answer calls for further inquiry.

---

*From Ewing JA: Detecting alcoholism: the CAGE Questionnaire,* JAMA 252:1905, *1984.*

Table 17-1 Comparison of blood alcohol concentrations to behavioral manifestations of intoxication

| Blood Alcohol Level (g/dl) | Behaviors |
|---|---|
| 0.05 to 0.15 | Euphoria, labile mood, cognitive disturbances (decreased concentration, impaired judgment, loss of sexual inhibitions) |
| 0.15 to 0.25 | Slurred speech, staggering gait, diplopia, drowsiness, labile mood with outbursts |
| 0.3 | Stupor, aggressive behavior, incoherent speech, labored breathing, vomiting |
| 0.4 | Coma |
| 0.5 | Severe respiratory depression, death |

From Antai-Otong D: Helping the alcoholic patient recover, *Am J Nurs* 95(8): 22-29, 1995.

## Predisposing Factors

1. *Biological factors*
   - Familial tendency, especially for alcohol abuse
   - Altered alcohol metabolism resulting in an uncomfortable physiological response
   - Variants of the DRD2 gene, which appears to be associated with the transmission of alcoholism

*Text continued on p. 351*

Table 17-2 Characteristics of substances of abuse

| Substance/Common Street Names | Route/Physical Dependence/ Psychological Dependence | Signs and Symptoms | Special Considerations/ Consequence of Use |
|---|---|---|---|
| Depressants | | | |
| **Alcohol** Booze, brew, juice, spirits | Ingestion Yes/yes | *Use* Depression of major brain functions such as mood, cognition, attention, concentration, insight, judgment, memory, affect, emotional rapport in interpersonal relationships; extent of depression is dose dependent and ranges from lethargy through anesthesia and death; psychomotor impairment, increased reaction time, interruption of hand-eye coordination, motor ataxia, nystagmus, decreased rapid eye movement sleep leading to more dreams and sometimes nightmares | Chronic alcohol use leads to serious disruptions in most organ systems: malnutrition and dehydration; vitamin deficiency leading to Wernicke's encephalopathy and alcoholic amnestic syndrome; impaired liver function, including hepatitis and cirrhosis; esophagitis, gastritis, pancreatitis; osteoporosis; anemia; peripheral neuropathy; impaired pulmonary function; cardiomyopathy; myopathy; disrupted immune system; brain damage |
| **Barbiturates** Barbs, beans, black beauties, blue angels, candy, downers, goof balls, G.B., nebbies, reds, sleepers, yellow jackets, yellows | Ingestion, injection Yes/yes | | |
| **Benzodiazepines** Downers | Ingestion, injection Yes/yes | | |

High susceptibility to other dependencies

Dependence on barbiturates and benzodiazepines may develop insidiously; users may underreport actual amount taken because of guilt about multiple prescriptions and abuse

*Overdose*

Unconsciousness, coma, respiratory depression, death

*Withdrawal*

General depressant withdrawal syndrome; tremors, agitation, anxiety, diaphoresis, increased pulse and blood pressure, sleep disturbances, hallucinosis, seizures, delusions, delirium tremens

*High-dose sedative-hypnotic withdrawal:* short-acting sedative hypnotics (including alcohol) symptoms begin several hours to 1 day after the last dose and peak after 24-36 hours

Long-acting sedative hypnotics: symptoms peak after 5-8 days

*Low-dose sedative-hypnotic withdrawal:* usually transient "symptom rebound" effects (anxiety, insomnia) for 1-2 weeks

May have more severe symptoms: perceptual hyperacusis, psychosis, cerebellar dysfunction, seizures)

*Postacute (protracted) withdrawal:* irritability, anxiety, insomnia, mood instability may occur for months

*Continued*

Table 17-2   Characteristics of substances of abuse—cont'd

| Substance/Common Street Names | Route/Physical Dependence/ Psychological Dependence | Signs and Symptoms | Special Considerations/ Consequence of Use |
|---|---|---|---|
| **Stimulants** | | | |
| **Amphetamines** A, AMT, bam, bennies, crystal, diet pills, dolls, eye openers, lid poppers, pep pills, purple hearts, speed, uppers, wake-ups | Ingestion, injection Yes/yes | *Use* Sudden rush of euphoria, abrupt awakening, increased energy, talkativeness, elation; agitation, hyperactivity, irritability, grandiosity, pressured speech; diaphoresis, anorexia, weight loss, insomnia, increased temperature/ blood pressure/pulse, tachycardia, ectopic heart beats, chest pain, urinary retention, constipation, dry mouth *High-dose:* slurred, rapid, incoherent speech; stereotypical movements, ataxic gait, teeth grinding, illogical thought processes, headache, nausea, vomiting | Certain amphetamines prescribed for attention deficit hyperactivity disorder in children because of a paradoxical depressant action; may be used alternately with depressants |
| **Cocaine** Bernice, bernies, big C, blow, C, charlie, coke, dust, girl, | Inhalation, smoking, injection, topical Yes/yes | | Cocaine use may lead to multiple physical problems: destruction of the nasal septum related to snorting; coronary artery vasoconstriction; cerebrovascular accidents; transient ischemic episodes; sudden death related to respiratory arrest and myocardial infarction |

heaven, jay,
lady, nose candy,
nose powder,
snow, sugar,
white lady;
crack = conan,
freebase, rock,
toke, white
cloud, white
tornado

*Toxic psychosis:* paranoid delusions in clear
sensorium; auditory, visual, or tactile
hallucinations; very labile mood, unprovoked
violence

*Overdose*

Seizures, cardiac arrhythmias, coronary artery
spasms, myocardial infarction, marked increase in blood pressure and temperature; can
lead to cardiovascular shock and death

*Withdrawal*

*Acute withdrawal (after periods of frequent
high-dose use):* intense and unpleasant feelings of depression and fatigue, and sometimes
suicidal ideation

Otherwise: milder symptoms of depression,
anxiety, anhedonia, sleep disturbance, increased appetite, and psychomotor
retardation; decrease steadily over several
weeks

Sometimes user stops stimulants purposely to
decrease tolerance, decreasing amount needed
to "get high"

Intravenous use of stimulants
may lead to the serious
physical consequences de-
scribed under Opiates

*Continued*

Table 17-2 Characteristics of substances of abuse—cont'd

| Substance/Common Street Names | Route/Physical Dependence/ Psychological Dependence | Signs and Symptoms | Special Considerations/ Consequence of Use |
|---|---|---|---|
| **Opiates** | | | |
| **Heroin** H, horse, harry, boy, scag, shit, smack, stuff, white junk, white stuff | Injection, ingestion, inhalation Yes/yes | *Use* Euphoria, relaxation, relief from pain, nodding out (apathy, detachment from reality), impaired judgment, drowsiness), constricted pupils, nausea, constipation, slurred speech, respiratory depression | Intravenous use leads to high risk for infection with blood-borne pathogens, such as HIV or hepatitis B; other infections (e.g., skin abscesses, phlebitis, cellulitis, and septic emboli causing pneumonia, pulmonary abscess, or subacute bacterial endocarditis) may occur as a result of lack of asepsis or contaminated substances |
| **Morphine** | Injection Yes/yes | *Overdose* Unconsciousness, coma, respiratory depression, circulatory depression, respiratory arrest, cardiac arrest, death | |
| **Meperidine** | Ingestion, injection Yes/yes | Anoxia can lead to brain abscess | |
| **Codeine** | Ingestion, injection Yes/yes | | |

| | | |
|---|---|---|
| **Opium** | Smoking, ingestion Yes/yes | |
| **Methadone** | Ingestion Yes/yes | *Withdrawal*<br>*Initially:* drug craving, lacrimation, rhinorrhea, yawning, diaphoresis<br>*In 12-72 hours:* sleep disturbances, mydriasis, anorexia, piloerection, irritability, tremor, weakness, nausea, vomiting, diarrhea, chills, fever, muscle spasms (especially in legs), flushing, spontaneous ejaculation, abdominal pain, hypertension, increased rate and depth of respirations<br>*Protracted withdrawal:* hypersensitivity to sensory stimuli, paresthesias, perceptual distortions, muscle pains, twitching tremors, headache, sleep disturbances, tension, irritability, lack of energy, impaired concentration, derealization, depersonalization<br>May last for several months | Chronic use leads to lack of concern about physical well-being, resulting in malnutrition and dehydration; criminal behavior may occur to acquire money for drugs |

*Continued*

Table 17-2 Characteristics of substances of abuse—cont'd

| Substance/Common Street Names | Route/Physical Dependence/ Psychological Dependence | Signs and Symptoms | Special Considerations/ Consequence of Use |
|---|---|---|---|
| Marijuana<br>Acapulco gold, aunt mary, broccoli, dope, grass, grunt, hay, hemp, herb, J, joint, joy stick, killer weed, maryjane, pot, ragweed, reefer, smoke, weed | Smoking ingestion<br><br>No/yes | *Use*<br>Altered state of awareness, relaxation, mild euphoria, reduced inhibition, red eyes, dry mouth, increased appetite, increased pulse, decreased reflexes; panic reaction<br>*Overdose*<br>Toxic psychosis<br>*Withdrawal*<br>No acute symptoms, but irritability and difficulty sleeping may last for a couple of days | Pulmonary problems; interference with reproductive hormones; may cause fetal abnormalities |

**Hallucinogens**

| | | | |
|---|---|---|---|
| Acid, LSD, DMT, mescaline, MDMA (Ecstact) big D, blotter, blue heaven, cap, D, deeda, flash, L, mellow yellows, microdots, paper acid, sugar, ticket, yello | Ingestion, smoking<br>No/no | *Use*<br>Distorted perceptions and hallucinations in presence of a clear sensorium; distortions of time and space, illusions, depersonalization, mystical experiences, heightened sense of awareness; extreme mood lability; tremor, dizziness, piloerection, paresthesias, synesthesia, nausea and vomiting; increased temperature, pulse, blood pressure, and salivation; panic reaction, "bad trip"<br>*Overdose*<br>Rare with LSD; convulsions, hyperthermia, death<br>*Withdrawal*<br>None | Flashbacks may last for several months; permanent psychosis may occur |

*Continued*

Table 17-2   Characteristics of substances of abuse—cont'd

| Substance/Common Street Names | Route/Physical Dependence/ Psychological Dependence | Signs and Symptoms | Special Considerations/ Consequence of Use |
|---|---|---|---|
| **Phencyclidine (PCP)** | | | |
| Angel dust, DOA, dust, elephant, hog, peace pill, supergrass, tic tac | Smoking, ingestion No/no | *Use* Intensely psychotic experience characterized by bizarre perceptions, confusion, disorientation, euphoria, hallucinations, paranoia, grandiosity, agitation; apparent enhancement of strength and endurance, rage reactions; may be agitated and hyperactive with tendency toward violence or catatonic and withdrawn, or vacillate between the two conditions; red, dry skin; dilated pupils, nystagmus, ataxia, hypertension, rigidity, seizures *Overdose* Seizures, coma, death *Withdrawal* None | If flashbacks occur, they are mild and usually not disturbing |

| Inhalants | | | |
|---|---|---|---|
| Gasoline, glue, aerosol sprays, paint thinner, rush, bolt, huffing, bagging, sniffing | Inhalation Yes/Yes | *Use* <br> *Psychological:* belligerence, assaultiveness, apathy, impaired judgment <br> *Physical:* dizziness, nystagmus, incoordination, slurred speech, unsteady gait, depressed reflexes, tremor, blurred vision, euphoria, anorexia <br> *Overdose* <br> Lethargy, stupor/coma, respiratory arrest, cardiac arrhythmia <br> *Withdrawal* <br> Symptoms similar to alcohol withdrawal | Death from inhalants can occur in different ways: <br> Sudden death is caused by cardiac arrhythmia—sometimes this happens the first time the child uses inhalants <br> Suicide may be a result of impaired judgment. Injury: under the influence of inhalants youth feel invulnerable <br> Burns and frostbite can also be caused by these chemicals <br> Permanent cognitive impairment may require an individual to reside in structured setting |

*Continued*

Table 17-2  Characteristics of substances of abuse—cont'd

| Substance/Common Street Names | Route/Physical Dependence/ Psychological Dependence | Signs and Symptoms | Special Considerations/ Consequence of Use |
|---|---|---|---|
| **Nicotine** | | | |
| Cigarettes, cigars, bidis, kreteks, pipe tobacco, snuff, chewing tobacco | Smoking, chewing, buccal  Yes/yes | *Use* Feelings of pleasure, increased alertness, enhanced mental performance; increased heart rate and blood pressure; restricts blood flow to heart muscle  *Overdose* N/A  *Withdrawal* Anger, anxiety, depressed mood, difficulty concentrating, subsiding within 3-4 weeks; increased appetite and craving for nicotine may persist for months | Smoking by pregnant women contributes to low birth weight, increased incidence of stillborn and premature babies |

2. *Psychological factors*
   - Oral-dependent personality types
   - Low self-esteem often related to childhood abuse
   - Overlearned, maladaptive habit
   - Pleasure seeking and pain avoidance
   - Family traits, including lack of stability, lack of positive role models, lack of trust, inability to treat children as individuals, and parental addiction
3. *Sociocultural factors*
   - Availability and social acceptability of drug use
   - Societal ambivalence about or use or abuse of various substances, such as tobacco, alcohol, and marijuana
   - Cultural attitudes, values, norms, and sanctions
   - Nationality, ethnicity, and religion
   - Poverty with associated family instability and limited opportunities

## Precipitating Stressors

### Withdrawal

Table 17-2 presents general behaviors related to withdrawal from substances.

---

**NURSE ALERT.**   A serious and potentially life-threatening alcohol withdrawal disorder is *alcohol withdrawal delirium,* formerly known as *delirium tremens* (DTs). It usually occurs on the second or third day after the last drink has been taken and ends 48 to 72 hours after onset. Behaviors include the following:

1. Tremor
2. Anxiety
3. Paranoid delusions
4. Visual hallucinations
5. Disorientation
6. Elevated temperature
7. Tachycardia
8. Tachypnea
9. Hyperpnea
10. Vomiting
11. Diarrhea
12. Diaphoresis

**NURSE ALERT.**    Another serious behavioral manifestation that may result from alcohol withdrawal is grand mal convulsions. These do not usually recur once alcohol withdrawal is completed.

A person can predict the severity and duration of withdrawal symptoms by using the following three rules of thumb:
1. The longer the time between last use and appearance of withdrawal symptoms, and the longer these symptoms last, the less intense they will be.
2. The longer the half-life of the drug, the longer withdrawal symptoms will last.
3. The longer the half-life of the drug, the less intense the withdrawal symptoms will be.

**NURSE ALERT.**    Substance use during pregnancy can result in the development of fetal alcohol syndrome or the birth of an addicted infant. Women should be encouraged to remain drug and alcohol free during pregnancy.

## Appraisal of Stressors

The reasons why a person initiates use of substances may include curiosity, desire to be grown up, desire to rebel against authority, peer pressure, desire to ease the pains of living, or desire to feel good. If the substance brings about the desired effects, use is likely to continue. As amount and frequency of substance use increase, so do the perceived stressors that provide a reason for more use. If substance use becomes associated with relief from emotional and social pain in the person's mind, the appraisal of these stressors will lead to more substance use. Perceiving the substance as the answer to these problems, the individual fails to develop healthier coping mechanisms. Gradually it takes more and more of the substance to achieve the same effect.

## Coping Resources

Coping resources enable the person who abuses substances to survive and include the following:

- Effective communication and assertiveness skills
- Strong social support systems
- Alternative pleasurable activities
- Stress reduction techniques
- Vocational skills
- Motivation to change behavior

## Coping Mechanisms

Substance abuse represents an unsuccessful attempt to cope. Healthier defense mechanisms and other adaptive behaviors are either inadequate or have not been developed. Ego defense mechanisms typically used by substance abusers include the following:

1. Denial of the problem
2. Rationalization
3. Projection of responsibility for the behavior
4. Minimization of the amount of alcohol or drug used

## Nursing Diagnosis

The nurse should be aware that individuals who have substance abuse problems also tend to develop multiple physical problems, particularly if the substance abuse problem is severe. The complete plan of nursing care would include diagnosis of all the patient's nursing care needs. For the purposes of this discussion, nursing diagnoses are limited to those more specifically related to substance abuse. The box on page 354 presents the primary and related NANDA nursing diagnoses for maladaptive chemically mediated responses.

## Related Medical Diagnoses

Medical diagnoses related to maladaptive chemically mediated responses are based on the specific substance involved. The box on page 355 describes these diagnoses.

## NANDA Nursing Diagnoses Related to Maladaptive Chemically Mediated Responses

Biological Responses

Growth and development, Delayed (also psychosocial)
Infection, Risk for
Injury, Risk for
Nutrition, Imbalanced
Self-care deficit
*Sensory perception, Disturbed
Sexual dysfunction
Sleep pattern, Disturbed

Cognitive Responses

Knowledge, Deficient
Noncompliance
Therapeutic regimen management, Ineffective, Ineffective
   family
*Thought processes, Disturbed

Psychosocial Responses

Anxiety
Communication, Impaired verbal
*Coping, Ineffective
*Family processes: alcoholism, Dysfunctional
Parenting, Impaired
Self-esteem, Chronic low
Social isolation
Violence, Risk for other-directed, Risk for self-directed

Spiritual Responses

Grieving, Dysfunctional
Hopelessness (also psychosocial)
Powerlessness
Spiritual distress

*Primary nursing diagnosis for chemically mediated response.
*From North American Nursing Diagnosis Association:* NANDA nursing diagnoses:
definitions and classification 2000-2001, *Philadelphia, 2001, The Association*

## DSM-IV-TR Medical Diagnoses Related to Maladaptive Chemically Mediated Responses

| DSM-IV-TR Diagnosis | Essential Features* |
|---|---|
| Substance dependence | Maladaptive pattern of substance use, characterized by any three of the following within 12 months: tolerance; withdrawal; using more of the substance or using for longer than planned; persistent desire but unsuccessful efforts to cut down or control use; much time spent in efforts to obtain, use, or recover from use; interference with social, occupational, or recreational activities; continued use despite knowledge of use-related recurrent physical or psychological problems. |
| Substance abuse | Maladaptive pattern of substance use, characterized by one or more of the following within 12 months: recurrent use resulting in failure to meet role obligations, recurrent use in physically hazardous situations, recurrent use-related legal problems, continued use despite persistent or recurrent use-related social or interpersonal problems. Has never met the criteria for dependence for the class of substance. |

*A single set of essential features has been developed for substance dependence and for substance abuse. The essential features of intoxication and withdrawal vary according to the substance and are listed in Table 17-2.

*Modified from American Psychiatric Association: Diagnostic and statistical manual of mental disorders, ed 4, text revision (DSM-IV-TR), Washington, DC, 2000, The Association.*

## Outcome Identification

The expected outcome for a patient with substance-related with-drawal follows:

*The patient will overcome addiction safely and with a minimum of discomfort.*

The expected outcome for a patient with substance-related de-pendence follows:

*The patient will abstain from using all mood-altering chemicals.*

## Planning

A Patient Education Plan for prevention of substance abuse is presented on page 357.

## Implementation

**NURSE ALERT.**   Withdrawal from dependence on alcohol or drugs may result in life-threatening physical symptoms. The nurse should be familiar with the withdrawal symptoms presented in Table 17-2 and provide appropriate supportive interventions. Any unexpected behaviors or unanticipated worsening of the patient's condition should be reported to the physician promptly.

**NURSE ALERT.**   Unanticipated serious physiological dis-tress in a patient who is a known or suspected substance abuser may be a sign of overdose. The nurse should be fa-miliar with the behaviors associated with overdose of fre-quently abused substances, as described in Table 17-2. If overdose is suspected, the physician should be notified immediately.

## Patient Education Plan:  Preventing Substance Abuse

| Content | Instructional Activities | Evaluation |
|---|---|---|
| Elicit perceptions of substance use. | Lead group discussion about chemical use and experience with it. Correct misperceptions. | Patient describes accurate information about substance use. |
| Demonstrate negative effects of substance abuse. | Show films of physical and psychological effects of substance abuse. Provide written materials. | Patient identifies and describes physical and psychological effects of substance abuse. |
| Provide interaction with peer who has abused chemicals. | Initiate small group discussion with peer group member who has abused substances and quit because of negative experiences. | Patient compares and contrasts advantages and disadvantages of using mind-altering substances. |
| Obtain agreement to abstain from use of mind-altering substances. | Discuss future plans for refusing abused chemicals if offered. | Patient verbally agrees to abstain from using mind-altering substances. |

## Biological Interventions

### Intervening in withdrawal

Substances with potentially life-threatening courses of withdrawal include alcohol, barbiturates, and benzodiazepines. Withdrawal from opiates and stimulants can be extremely uncomfortable but is generally not dangerous, although a patient may become suicidal during the acute phase of cocaine withdrawal. Withdrawal from the general depressants, opiates, and stimulants is treated by gradual tapering of a drug in the same classification and treatment with symptom-specific medication. No identified acute withdrawal pattern is associated with marijuana, hallucinogens, or PCP.

### Intervening in toxic psychosis

Acute toxic psychosis may result from ingestion of hallucinogens or PCP. Hallucinogen users need interpersonal intervention with constant reassurance. PCP users respond poorly to interpersonal stimulation and need to be kept in a quiet, protected environment. These patients may be terrified by the disturbances in perception that result from use of these drugs. They may act impulsively out of fear and harm themselves. Adequate staff should be available to manage this impulse behavior.

### Intervening to maintain abstinence

Maintaining abstinence from abused substances is one of the most difficult issues in working with patients who have substance-related disorders. In treatment for addictions, mild levels of anxiety and depression can generate motivation for change. Therefore these symptoms should not be treated with medication unless they significantly interfere with the patient's functioning and participation in the treatment plan. However, a number of pharmacological therapies can help patients decrease cravings and maintain abstinence: (1) disulfiram (Antabuse); (2) naltrexone (Trexan); (3) nalmefene; (4) opiate agonists, including methadone and LAAM; and (5) calcium acetylhomotaurinate (Acamprosate).

> **NURSE ALERT.**   Disulfiram sensitizes alcoholic patients to alcohol. Ingestion of alcohol while taking disulfiram can lead to serious physical symptoms, possibly resulting in death. Symptoms include severe headache, nausea and vom-

iting, flushing, hypotension, tachycardia, dyspnea, diaphoresis, chest pain, palpitations, dizziness, and confusion. It can also lead to respiratory and cardiac collapse, unconsciousness, convulsions, and death.

The patient must be educated about the potential consequences of drinking while taking this drug. Patient education should also include the provision of a written list of alcohol-containing preparations to be avoided, including cough medicines, rubbing compounds, vinegars, aftershave lotions, and some mouthwashes. Drinking must be avoided for 14 days after disulfiram has been taken.

**NURSE ALERT.** Naltrexone is the first drug approved by the FDA for the treatment of alcohol dependence in more than 40 years. It blocks the euphoric effects of alcohol in the brain and promises new hope for substance abusers.

**NURSE ALERT.** Nalmefene is a newer opioid antagonist that is structurally similar to naltrexone but with a number of pharmacological advances for the treatment of alcohol dependence. These include no dose-dependent association with toxic effects to the liver, greater oral bioavailability, longer duration of antagonist action, and more complete binding with opioid receptor subtypes that are thought to reinforce drinking. It has found to be effective in preventing relapse to heavy drinking and has few side effects.

**NURSE ALERT.** Acamprosate is a new drug to help prevent relapse in alcoholism. It has no sedative, antianxiety, muscle relaxant, or antidepressant properties and produces no withdrawal symptoms. Acamprosate appears to work by lowering the activity of receptors for the excitatory neurotransmitter glutamate.

## Psychological and Social Interventions

Motivational counseling is one of the newer approaches to treatment. Five basic principles are used with this approach:

- *Express empathy through reflective listening.* This communicates respect for and acceptance of patients and their feelings. It also establishes a safe and open environment that helps in examining issues and exploring personal reasons for change.
- *Develop discrepancy between patients' goals or values and their current behavior.* Focus the patient's attention on how current behavior differs from behavior described as ideal or desired.
- *Avoid argument and direct confrontation.* Trying to convince a patient that a problem exists or that change is needed could precipitate even more resistance. Arguments can rapidly degenerate into a power struggle and do not enhance motivation for beneficial change.
- *Roll with resistance.* Resistance is a signal that the patient views the situation differently. There are four types of resistance: arguing, interrupting, denying, or ignoring. The clinician's job is to ask questions in a way that helps the patient to understand and work through resistance.
- *Support self-efficacy.* This requires the clinician to recognize the patient's strengths and bring these to the forefront whenever possible. It involves supporting hope, optimism, and the feasibility of accomplishing change.

Cognitive-behavioral approaches are aimed at improving self-control and social skills in order to reduce drinking. Self-control strategies include goal-setting, self-monitoring, functional analysis of drinking antecedents, and learning alternative coping skills.

Social skills training focuses on learning skills for forming and maintaining interpersonal relationships, assertiveness, and drink refusal.

Contingency management is another behavioral approach that has been successfully applied in many substance abuse treatment programs. In this strategy, rewards (often in the form of vouchers that can be exchanged for desired items) are given for adaptive behavior (such as compliance with treatment or negative urine tests).

Behavioral contracting is also a useful approach. It involves creating a written agreement with the patient that specifies targeted patient behavior and consequences.

Other social interventions can include efforts to assist the person to find non–drug-using social supports in the community. Family counseling and self-help groups such as Alcoholics Anonymous (AA) may be particularly helpful.

Nursing interventions with the substance-abusing patient are summarized in the Nursing Treatment Plan Summary on pages 362-365.

## Interventions with Dually Diagnosed Patients

The dually diagnosed patient needs treatment for both disorders. The best treatment is an integrated one that combines pharmacological, psychosocial, and supportive services. Because both mental illness and substance abuse are chronic, relapsing conditions, the course of treatment can be expected to take considerable time. Table 17-3 describes stages of treatment and related goals and interventions for working with the dually diagnosed patient.

> **NURSE ALERT.**   Because most abused drugs cross the placental barrier, women should be counseled about the possible effects of substance use during pregnancy. The safest pregnancy is one in which the mother is totally drug and alcohol free, with one exception: for pregnant women addicted to heroin, methadone maintenance is safer for the fetus than acute opiate detoxification.

## Evaluation

The evaluation of substance abuse treatment is based on accomplishment of the expected outcomes and short-term goals. The following can be used as evaluation criteria for the treatment of alcoholic patients; they apply to abusers of other drugs as well:

1. Has the patient been able to progress significantly toward achieving the stated goals?
2. Can the patient usually communicate without being defensive?
3. Is the patient able to react appropriately, managing the demands of daily life without use of a drug?
4. Is the patient actively involved in a variety of activities, using external social and activity resources?

*Text continued on p. 367*

## Nursing Treatment Plan Summary:    Maladaptive Chemically Mediated Responses

Nursing Diagnosis: Ineffective individual coping

Expected Outcome: Patient will abstain from using all mood-altering chemicals.

| Short-term Goals | Interventions | Rationale |
|---|---|---|
| Patient will substitute healthy coping responses for substance-abusing behavior. | Confront patient with substance-abusing behavior and its consequences. | Motivation for change is related to recognition of a problem that is upsetting to the individual. |
| | Assist patient to identify substance abuse problem. | Identification of predisposing factors and precipitating stressors must precede planning for more adaptive behavioral responses. |
| | Involve patient in describing situations that lead to substance-abusing behavior. | |
| | Consistently offer support and the expectation that patient does have the strength to overcome the problem. | |
| Patient will assume responsibility for behavior. | Encourage patient to agree to participate in a treatment program. | Denial and rationalization are dysfunctional coping mechanisms that can interfere with recovery. |
| | Develop with patient a written contract for behavioral change that is signed by patient and nurse. | Personal commitment enhances the likelihood of successful abstinence. |
| | Assist patient to identify and adopt healthier coping responses. | |

| Patient will identify and use social support systems. | Identify and assess social support systems available to patient. | Substance abusers are often dependent and socially isolated people who use drugs to gain confidence in social situations. |
| | Provide support to significant others. | Substance-abusing behavior alienates significant others, thus increasing the person's isolation. |
| | Educate patient and significant others about the substance abuse problem and available resources. | It is difficult to manipulate people who have participated in the same behaviors. |
| | Refer patient to appropriate resources and provide support until patient is involved in the program. | Social support systems must be readily available over time and acceptable to patient. |

*Continued*

## Nursing Treatment Plan Summary:   Maladaptive Chemically Mediated Responses—cont'd

**Nursing Diagnosis:** Altered thought processes

**Expected Outcome: Patient will overcome addiction safely and with a minimum of discomfort.**

| Short-term Goals | Interventions | Rationale |
| --- | --- | --- |
| Patient will withdraw from dependence on the abused substance. | Provide supportive physical care: vital signs, nutrition, hydration, seizure precautions. Administer medication according to detoxification schedule. | Detoxification of the physically dependent person can be dangerous and is always uncomfortable. Patient's physical safety must receive high priority for nursing intervention. |
| Patient will be oriented to time, place, person, and situation. | Assess orientation frequently; orient patient if needed; place a clock and calendar where patient can see them. | Cognitive function is usually affected by addiction; disorientation is frightening. |
| Patient will report symptoms of withdrawal. | Observe carefully for withdrawal symptoms and report suspected withdrawal immediately. | Withdrawal symptoms provide powerful motivation for continued substance abuse; judgment may be impaired by substance use. |

| | | |
|---|---|---|
| Patient will correctly interpret environmental stimuli. | Explain all nursing interventions; assign consistent staff; keep soft light on in room; avoid loud noises; encourage trusted family and friends to stay with patient. | Sensory and perceptual alterations related to use of drugs or alcohol are frightening; consistency reduces need to interpret stimuli. |
| Patient will recognize and talk about hallucinations or delusions. | Observe for response to internal stimuli; encourage patient to describe hallucinations or delusions; explain relationship of these experiences to withdrawal from addictive substances. | Assisting patient to identify delusional or hallucinatory experiences and relate them to withdrawal is reassuring. |

Table 17-3 Treatment stages, goals, and interventions for dually diagnosed patients

| Treatment Stage | Suggested Goals and Interventions |
|---|---|
| Engagement | **Goal:** Development of working relationship between patient and nurse<br>**Interventions:** Intervene in crises; assist with practical living problems; establish rapport with family members; demonstrate caring and support; listen actively. |
| Persuasion | **Goal:** Patient acceptance of having a substance abuse problem and the need for active change strategies<br>**Interventions:** Help to analyze pros and cons of substance use; educate patient and family; arrange peer group discussions; expose patient to "double-trouble" self-help groups; adjust medication; persuade patient of need to comply with medication regimen. |
| Active treatment | **Goal:** Abstinence from substance use and compliance with medication regimen<br>**Interventions:** Assist to change thinking patterns, friends, habits, behaviors, and living situations as necessary to support goals; teach social skills; encourage to develop positive social supports through double-trouble self-help groups; enlist family support of changes; monitor urine and breath for substances; offer disulfiram. |
| Relapse prevention | **Goal:** Absence or minimization of return to substance abuse<br>**Interventions:** Reinforce abstinence, compliance, and behavioral changes; identify risk factors and help to practice preventive strategies; encourage continued involvement in double-trouble groups; continued laboratory monitoring. |

5. Does the patient use internal resources to be consistently productive at work and involved in meaningful interpersonal relationships?

---

*your* **INTERNET**
c o n n e c t i o n

**Children of Alcoholics Foundation:**
www.coaf.org

**Drughelp:**
www.drughelp.org

**International Nurses Society on Drug Addictions:**
www.intnsa.org

**National Clearinghouse on Alcohol and Drug Information:**
www.health.org

**National Council on Alcoholism and Drug Dependence:**
www.ncadd.org

**National Institute on Alcoholism and Alcohol Abuse:**
www.niaaa.nih.gov

**National Institute on Drug Abuse:**
www.nida.nih.gov

**Nurses in Recovery:**
www.addictions.org/recoveryworks

**Substance Abuse & Mental Health Services Administration:**
www.samhsa.gov

---

## Suggested readings

Alao A et al: Psychiatric complications of cannabis, *J Pract Psychiatry Behav Health* 5:275, 1999.

American Nurses' Association and National Nurses Society on Addictions: *Standards of addictions nursing practice with selected diagnoses and criteria,* Kansas City, Mo, 1988, The Association.

American Psychiatric Association: Practice guideline for the treatment of patients with substance use disorders: alcohol, cocaine, opioids, *Am J Psychiatry* 152:11, 1995.

American Psychiatric Association: Practice guideline for the treatment of patients with nicotine dependence, *Am J Psychiatry* 153(suppl):1, 1996.

Cataldo J, Talley S: Helping our clients with smoking cessation, *Amer J of Psych Nurs* 7(1):26, 2001.

Finfgeld D: Resolving alcohol problems using an online self-help approach, *J Psychosoc Nurs* 38(2):33, 2000.

Finke L, Williams J, Stanley R: Nurses referred to a peer assistance program for alcohol and drug problems, *Arch Psychiatr Nurs* 10:319, 1996.

Garbutt J et al: Pharmacological treatment of alcohol dependence: a review of the evidence, *JAMA* 281:1318, 1999.

Humphreys K, Moos R, Cohen C: Social and community resources and long-term recovery from treated and untreated alcoholism, *J Stud Alcohol* 5:231, 1997.

Irvin J et al: Efficacy of relapse prevention: a meta-analytic review, *J Consult Clin Psychol* 67:563, 1999.

Marcus M: An interdisciplinary team model for substance abuse prevention in communities, *J Professional Nurs* 16(3):158, 2000.

Mayo-Smith M et al: Pharmacological management of alcohol withdrawal: a meta-analysis and evidence-based practice guideline, *JAMA* 278:144, 1998.

McCabe S: Rapid detox: understanding new treatment approaches for the addicted patient, *Perspect Psychiatr Care* 36(4):113-120, 2000.

Miele G, Trautman K, Hasin D: Assessing comorbid mental and substance-use disorders: a guide for clinical practice, *J Pract Psychiatry Behav Health* 2:272, 1996.

Miller N, Gold M: Management of withdrawal syndromes and relapse prevention in drug and alcohol dependence, *Am Fam Physician* 58(1):139-146, 1998.

Mueser K et al: Integrated mental health and substance abuse treatment for severe psychiatric disorders, *J Pract Psychiatry Behav Health* 4:129, 1998.

Mynatt S: A model of contributing risk factors to chemical dependency in nurses, *J Psychosoc Nurs* 34:13, 1996.

Nagle MA, D'Avanzo CE: *Addictions and substance abuse: strategies for advanced practice nursing,* Upper Saddle River, NJ, 2001, Prentice-Hall, Inc.

National Institute on Drug Abuse: *Summary of findings from the 1998 National household survey on drug abuse,* Rockville, Md, 1999, The Institute.

Nehlig A: Are we dependent upon coffee and caffeine? A review on human and animal data, *Neurosci Biobehav Rev* 23:563, 1999.

Nestler E, Aghajanian G: Molecular and cellular basis of addiction, *Science* 278:58, 1997.

Ott P et al: *Sourcebook on substance abuse: etiology, epidemiology, assessment, and treatment,* Boston, 1999, Allyn and Bacon.

Pollack L, Stuebben G: Addiction education groups for inpatients with dual diagnoses, *J Am Psychiatr Nurses Assoc* 4:121, 1998.

Rigler S: Alcoholism in the elderly, *Am Fam Physician* 61(6):1710-1716, 1883-1884, 1887-1888, 2000.

Schneider Institute for Health Policy, Brandeis University: *Substance abuse the nation's number one health problem,* Princeton, NJ, 2001, Robert Wood Johnson Foundation.

Stuart G, Laraia M: *Principles and practice of psychiatric nursing,* ed 7, St Louis, 2001, Mosby.

Walters G: Behavioral self-control training for problem drinkers: a meta-analysis of randomized control studies, *Behav Ther* 31:135-149, 2000.

Washington O: Using brief therapeutic interventions to create change in self-efficiency and personal control of chemically dependent women, *Archives of Psychiatric Nursing* 1:32, 2001.

# Eating Regulation Responses and Eating Disorders

18

## Continuum of Eating Regulation Responses

As a pattern of self-regulation, properly controlled eating contributes to psychological, biological, and sociocultural health and well-being. Adaptive eating responses are characterized by balanced eating patterns, appropriate caloric intake, and body weight that is appropriate for height and frame. Illnesses associated with maladaptive eating regulation responses include anorexia nervosa, bulimia nervosa, and binge eating disorder (Figure 18-1). These disorders can cause biological changes, including altered metabolic rates, profound malnutrition, and possibly death.

### Prevalence

#### Anorexia nervosa

Anorexia nervosa occurs in approximately 0.5% to 3.7% of the female population, with onset often between ages 13 and 20. An estimated 1 in 10 to 20 people with anorexia is male.

#### Bulimia nervosa

Bulimia is more common than anorexia, with estimates of 1% to 4% of the female population and a prevalence of 4% to 15% of female high school and college students. The age of onset is

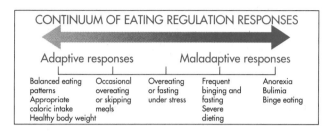

Figure 18-1
Continuum of eating regulation responses.

typically age 15 to 18. An estimated 1 in 10 people with bulimia is male.

## Assessment

Patients with maladaptive eating regulation responses must receive a comprehensive nursing assessment, including complete biological, psychological, and sociocultural evaluation. A full physical examination should be performed, with particular attention to vital signs, weight for height, skin, cardiovascular system, and evidence of laxative or diuretic abuse and vomiting. A dental examination may be indicated, and it is useful to assess growth, sexual development, and general physical development indicators. A psychiatric history, substance abuse history, and family assessment are also needed.

### Behaviors

Box 18-1 lists key features of anorexia nervosa and bulimia nervosa.

#### Binge eating

Binge eating is the rapid consumption of large quantities of food in a discrete period although no agreement exists on exactly how many calories constitute a binge. Emphasis on the individual's perception of loss of control and perceived excessive caloric intake is more important to the nursing assessment than the total number of calories consumed during a binge. Therefore the nurse must carefully assess exactly what each person means by a binge.

**Box 18-1    Key Features of Anorexia Nervosa and Bulimia Nervosa**

Anorexia Nervosa (Without Binging or Purging)

Rare vomiting or diuretic/laxative abuse

More severe weight loss

Slightly younger

More introverted

Hunger denied

Eating behavior may be considered normal and source of esteem

Sexually inactive

Obsessional and perfectionist features predominate

Death from starvation (or suicide in chronically ill patients)

Amenorrhea

More favorable prognosis

Fewer behavioral abnormalities (increase with severity)

Bulimia Nervosa

Frequent vomiting or diuretic/laxative abuse

Less weight loss

Slightly older

More extroverted

Hunger experienced

Eating behavior considered foreign and source of distress

More sexually active

Avoidant, dependent, or borderline features and obsessional features

Death from hypokalemia or suicide

Menses irregular or absent

Less favorable prognosis

Stealing, drug and alcohol abuse, self-mutilation, and other behavioral problems

### Fasting or restricting

People with anorexia often do not consume more than 500 to 700 calories a day and may ingest as few as 200, but they consider their intake adequate for their energy needs. Some individuals with anorexia may not eat for days at a time. Despite these restrictions, many anorexic people are preoccupied or obsessed with food and may do much of the family cooking.

### Purging

Individuals with eating disorders may use a variety of purging behaviors, including excessive exercise, over-the-counter and prescription diuretics, diet pills, laxatives, and steroids. Many patients engage in more than one purging behavior.

### Medical and psychiatric complications

Almost every person with maladaptive eating regulation responses has some type of associated physical problem because all body systems are affected. Many patients seeking treatment for eating disorders also have evidence of other psychiatric disorders, such as depression, obsessive-compulsive disorder, substance abuse disorders, and personality disorders.

## Predisposing Factors

### Biological

It is generally recognized that eating disorders are familial. First-degree female relatives of people with eating disorders are at higher risk than the general population. Concordance rates for eating disorders in monozygotic twins is 52% and in dizygotic twins 11%. A higher risk for other eating disorders and for depression also is seen in first-degree relatives of people with eating disorders, suggesting common etiological factors.

Biological models of the etiology of eating disorders focus on the appetite regulation center in the hypothalamus, which controls specific neurochemical mechanisms for feeding and satiety. Serotonin is thought to be involved in the pathophysiology of eating disorders although these biological models are still in the developmental stage.

### Environmental

A variety of environmental factors may predispose an individual to the development of an eating disorder. Early histories of patients with eating disorders are often complicated by medical and surgical illnesses, separations, family deaths, and conflicted family environments. Sexual abuse has been reported in 20% to 50% of patients with bulimia, but this rate may be similar to that found in patients with other psychiatric disorders.

### Psychological

Most patients with eating disorders exhibit clusters of psychological symptoms, such as rigidity, ritualism, meticulousness, perfectionism, exactness, symmetry, greater risk avoidance and restraint, and poor impulse control. Early separation and individuation conflicts, a pervasive sense of ineffectiveness and helplessness, difficulty interpreting feelings and tolerating intense emotional states, and fear of biological or psychological maturity may predispose an individual to an eating disorder.

### Sociocultural

In cultures where plumpness is either accepted or valued, eating disorders are rare. Also, the sociocultural environment for adolescents and young women in the United States places great emphasis on thinness and control over one's body as a yardstick for self-evaluation.

Psychosocial predisposing factors for the development of eating disorders are summarized in Box 18-2.

## Precipitating Stressors

Individuals with the previous predisposing factors are especially vulnerable to environmental pressures or life stressors, such as the loss of a significant other, interpersonal rejection, and failure.

## Appraisal of Stressors

In addition to a positive correlation existing between stress and the severity of eating disorders, the person's appraisal of the stress appears to play an important role, affecting both the treatment course and the treatment outcome.

## Coping Resources

One of the most important aspects of the assessment of these patients is the level of their motivation to change their behavior. Patients may be asked to identify the advantages and disadvantages of giving up the behavior. This information can be used to evaluate

## Box 18-2   Psychosocial Predisposing Factors for the Development of Eating Disorders

Personal Factors

Weight
Puberty/maturation
Restrained eating/dieting
Body image dissatisfaction
Problems regulating affect
Depression
Perfectionism
Low self-esteem
Stress
Low resiliency/confidence
Poor coping skills
Alcohol and substance use
Sexual/physical abuse
Dating

Family Factors

Parental attitudes
Family functioning
Socioeconomic status

Peers

Attitudes about weight
Behaviors
Teasing

Culture

Media influences

Activities

Gymnastics
Professional dance
Modeling

*From Taylor C, Altman T: Priorities in prevention research for eating disorders,* Psychopharm Bull *33(3):413, 1997.*

a patient's insight, identify coping resources, and stimulate therapeutic issues for further discussion.

## Coping Mechanisms

Anorectic patients most frequently use the defense mechanism of denial in a severely maladaptive way, and they usually do not seek help on their own. The defense mechanisms used by bulimic patients include avoidance, denial, isolation of affect, and intellectualization.

### Nursing Diagnosis

The box on page 377 presents the primary and related NANDA nursing diagnoses for maladaptive eating regulation responses. A complete nursing assessment would include all maladaptive responses of the patient. Additional nursing problems resulting from the eating disorder should also be identified.

## Related Medical Diagnoses

The box on page 378 identifies the medical diagnoses related to maladaptive eating regulation responses and their essential features.

### Outcome Identification

The expected outcome for the patient with maladaptive eating regulation responses is as follows:

*The patient will restore healthy eating patterns and normalize physiological parameters related to body weight and nutrition.*

### Planning

Important considerations in the planning phase of the nursing process are the choice of an inpatient, outpatient, or partial hospitalization treatment setting and the formulation of a nurse-patient contract. Box 18-3 presents clinical criteria for hospitalizing a patient with an eating disorder and is followed by a Family Education Plan for preventing childhood eating problems on pages 380 and 381.

## NANDA Nursing Diagnoses Related to Maladaptive Eating Regulation Responses

\*Anxiety
\*Body image, Disturbed
  Conflict, Decisional
  Coping, Ineffective individual
  Denial, Ineffective
  Family processes, Interrupted
  Fatigue
\*Fluid volume, Deficient
  Growth and development, Delayed
  Hopelessness
  Identity, Disturbed personal
  Injury, Risk for
\*Nutrition, Imbalanced
\*Powerlessness
  Powerlessness, Risk for
  Role performance, Ineffective
\*Self-esteem, Situational low
  Self-esteem, Risk for situational low
  Self-mutilation
\*Self-mutilation, Risk for
  Sexual dysfunction
  Social interaction, Impaired
  Thought processes, Disturbed

\*Primary nursing diagnosis for eating problems.
*From North American Nursing Diagnosis Association:* NANDA nursing diagnoses: definitions and classification 2000-2001, *Philadelphia, 2001, The Association.*

### *Implementation*

Empirically validated treatments for bulimia nervosa are summarized in Table 18-1.

Nursing care for a patient with an eating disorder includes the following areas of intervention:

1. Nutritional stabilization
2. Exercise monitoring

## DSM-IV-TR Medical Diagnoses Related to Maladaptive Eating Regulation Responses

| DSM-IV-TR Diagnosis | Essential Features |
| --- | --- |
| Anorexia nervosa | Intense fear of gaining weight, even when underweight. A disturbance in the way the body is experienced and a refusal to maintain body weight above a minimal normal weight for age and height lead to a body weight 15% below expected. In females there is also the absence of at least three consecutive menstrual cycles. |
| Bulimia nervosa | Recurrent episodes of binge eating with a feeling of lack of control over the eating behavior and persistent overconcern with body shape and weight. The individual also regularly engages in self-induced vomiting, use of laxatives, or rigorous dieting and fasting to counteract the effects of binge eating. |
| Binge eating disorder | Recurrent episodes of binging that are a cause of distress, with a feeling of lack of control over the eating behavior but without behaviors used to prevent weight gain. |

*Modified from American Psychiatric Association: Diagnostic and statistical manual of mental disorders, ed 4, text revision (DSM-IV-TR), Washington, DC, 2000, The Association.*

3. Cognitive behavioral interventions
4. Body image interventions
5. Family involvement
6. Group therapies
7. Medication

A Nursing Treatment Plan Summary for patients with maladaptive eating regulation responses is presented on pages 383-385.

---

## Box 18-3    Clinical Criteria for Hospitalization of Patients with an Eating Disorder

Medical

Need for extensive diagnostic evaluation

Weight loss greater than 25% of body weight over 3 months

Heart rate less than 40 beats/min or greater than 110 beats/min

Temperature less than 97.0° F

Systolic blood pressure less than 70 mm Hg or marked orthostatic hypotension greater than 20 mm Hg/min standing

Serum potassium less than 2.5 mEq/L despite oral potassium replacement

Severe dehydration or vomiting blood

Concurrent somatic illnesses (such as infection)

Psychiatric

Risk of suicide or self-mutilation

Severe depression

Substance abuse

Psychosis

Family crisis

Failure to comply with treatment contract or poor motivation

Inadequate response to outpatient treatment

Family Education Plan:   **Preventing Childhood Eating Problems**

| Content | Instructional Activities | Evaluation |
| --- | --- | --- |
| Describe self-demand feeding and its importance in healthy eating behaviors. | Explore current feeding practices of parents and understanding of healthy eating.<br>Provide information to enhance knowledge of healthy eating behaviors. | Parents identify healthy eating behaviors and self-demand feeding and begin to explore how their relationship with food influences their children's eating. |
| Describe physiological and psychological signs of hunger and satiety, the meaning of both, and differences between both types. | Explore parents' own signs of hunger and satiety and also have parents describe their children's signs. | Parents keep a hunger diary to record physical and psychological signs of hunger and satiety for themselves and their children. |
| Describe danger of psychological hunger. | Explain the use of a hunger diary, which is a daily journal regarding signs of hunger. | Parents can distinguish between psychological and physical hunger. |

| | | |
|---|---|---|
| Explore myths about feeding, e.g., "cleaning the plate" and "eating because other children are starving." | Describe the importance of allowing children to determine their feeding needs and the relationship of healthy eating to children's ability to differentiate between physical and psychological signs of hunger and satiety. Give homework assignment for each parent to interview three other adults about their current eating practices and memories of eating. | Parents complete homework assignment, discuss interview experiences, and describe how perpetuating myths about feeding can harm their children. |
| Implement self-demand feeding at particular developmental stages of children. | Review the stages that children experience with eating and the potential problems they may have at each stage. | Parents discuss the developmental stages of their children and plan for implementing self-demand feeding. |
| Discuss parental experiences related to implementing self-demand feeding. | Review parents' expectations and experiences with implementing self-demand feeding. | Parents relate any problem with self-demand feeding. Nurse evaluates family for further education and plans for follow-up if necessary. |

Table 18-1　Summarizing the evidence on treatments for bulimia nervosa

---

**DISORDER:** Bulimia nervosa
**TREATMENT:**

- Several different classes of antidepressant drugs produced significant, short-term reductions in binge eating and purging.
- Cognitive-behavioral therapy (CBT) was most effective in eliminating the core features of the illness; roughly half the patients receiving CBT reduced binge eating and purging; long-term maintenance of improvement was good.

---

From Nathan P, Gorman J: *A guide to treatments that work,* New York, 1998, Oxford University Press.

## *Evaluation*

1. Have normal eating patterns been restored?
2. Have the biological and psychological sequelae of malnutrition been corrected?
3. Have the associated sociocultural and behavioral problems been resolved so that relapse does not occur?

## Nursing Treatment Plan Summary:   Maladaptive Eating Regulation Responses

Nursing Diagnosis: Altered nutrition

Expected Outcome: Patient will restore healthy eating patterns and normalize physiological parameters related to body weight and nutrition.

| Short-term Goals | Interventions | Rationale |
| --- | --- | --- |
| Patient will engage in treatment and acknowledge having an eating disorder. | Help patient identify maladaptive eating responses. Discuss positive and negative consequences of maladaptive eating responses. Contract with patient to engage in treatment. | First step of treatment is for patient to acknowledge the illness and see the need for help. |
| Patient will be able to describe a balanced diet based on the five food groups. | Complete a nutritional assessment, including eating-related behaviors and preferences. Teach, clarify, and reinforce knowledge of proper nutrition. | Knowledge of healthy nutrition is essential to establishing and maintaining adaptive eating responses. |
| Patient's nutritional status will be stabilized by a specified target date. | Monitor physiological status for signs of compromised nutrition. Administer medications and somatic treatments for management of symptoms. Monitor and evaluate patient's response to somatic treatments. Implement nursing activities as specified in the program contract and protocol. | Weight stabilization must be a central and early goal for the nutritionally compromised patient. Medications may assist the appetite regulation center and neurochemical responses to feeding and satiety. |

*Continued*

### Nursing Treatment Plan Summary:  Maladaptive Eating Regulation Responses—cont'd

| Short-term Goals | Interventions | Rationale |
| --- | --- | --- |
| Patient will participate daily in a balanced exercise program. | Review established exercise routines. Modify exercise patterns, focusing on physical fitness rather than weight reduction. Reinforce new exercise and fitness behaviors. | Focus of a balanced exercise program should be on physical fitness rather than calorie reduction to lose weight. |

Nursing Diagnosis: Body image disturbance

Expected Outcome: Patient will express clear and accurate descriptions of body size, body boundaries, and ideal weight.

| Short-term Goals | Interventions | Rationale |
| --- | --- | --- |
| Patient will correct body image distortions. | Modify body image misperceptions through cognitive and behavioral strategies. Use dance and movement therapies to enhance the integration of mind and body. Employ imagery and relaxation interventions to decrease anxiety related to body perceptions. | Body image distortions involve perceptions, attitudes, and behaviors that place so much emphasis on appearance that they define self-worth. |

| Goal | Intervention | Rationale |
| --- | --- | --- |
| Patient will modify cognitive distortions about body weight, shape, and eating responses. | Assist patient in identifying:<br>1. Cues that trigger problematic eating responses and body image concerns<br>2. Thoughts, feelings, and assumptions associated with the specific cues<br>3. Connections between these thoughts, feelings, and assumptions and eating regulation responses<br>4. Consequences resulting from the eating responses | Cognitive distortions result in lowered self-esteem. Behavioral change occurs as a result of increased awareness of feelings and faulty cognitions. |
| Patient will identify social support systems that reinforce accurate body perceptions and adaptive eating responses. | Include family members in the evaluation and treatment planning process.<br>Assess family as a system and impact of the eating disorder on family functioning.<br>Initiate group therapy to mobilize social support and reinforce adaptive responses. | Patients with eating disorders benefit from involvement of family members and supportive group work. |

*your* INTERNET
   c o n n e c t i o n

   Academy for Eating Disorders:
   www.aedweb.org

   American Anorexia Bulimia Association:
   www.aabainc.org

   Eating Disorders Awareness and Prevention:
   www.edap.org

   Eating Disorder Referral and Information Center:
   www.edreferral.com

   European Council on Eating Disorders:
   www.psyctc.org/eat_d/eced

   Family Resources for Education on Eating
   Disorders:
   cpcug.org/user/rpike/freed.html

   National Eating Disorder Organization:
   www.kidsource.com/nedo

## Suggested readings

American Psychiatric Association: Practice guidelines: practice guidelines for eating disorders, *Am J Psychiatry* 157:1, 2000.

Barber N: The slender ideal and eating disorders: an interdisciplinary "telescope" model, *Int J Eat Disord* 23:295, 1998.

Brewerton TD: Toward a unified theory of serotonin dysregulation in eating and related disorders, *Psychoneuroendocrinology* 20:6, 1995.

Brink P et al: Childhood memories about food: the successful dieters project, *J Child Adolesc Psychiatr Nurs* 12(1):17, 1999.

Cash T, Deagle E: The nature and extent of body-image disturbances in anorexia nervosa and bulimia nervosa: a meta-analysis, *Int J Eat Disord* 22:107, 1997.

Chally P: An eating disorders prevention program, *JCAPN* 11(2):51, 1998.

Erickson B, Yager J: The assessment and treatment of bulimia nervosa, *J Pract Psychiatry Behav Health* 4:76, 1998.

Fairburn C et al: A cognitive behavioural theory of anorexia nervosa, *Behav Res Ther* 37:1, 1999.

Garner D, Garfinkel P: *Handbook of treatment for eating disorders,* New York, 1997, Guilford Publications.

Grilo C: The assessment and treatment of binge eating disorder, *J Pract Psychiatry Behav Health* 4:191, 1998.

Grilo C: Self-help and guided self-help treatments for bulimia nervosa and binge eating disorder, *J Psychiatr Pract* 6:18, 2000.

Keel P et al: Long-term outcome of bulimia nervosa, *Arch Gen Psychiatry* 56:63, 1999.

McGilley B, Pryor T: Assessment and treatment of bulimia nervosa, *Am Fam Physician* 57(11):2743-2750, 1998.

Orbanic S: Understanding bulimia: signs, symptoms and the human experience, *AJN* 101(3):35-42, 2001.

Stein K: The self-schema model: a theoretical approach to the self-concept in eating disorders, *Arch Psychiatr Nurs* 2:96, 1996.

Stuart G, Laraia M: *Principles and practice of psychiatric nursing,* ed 7, St Louis, 2001, Mosby.

Vitrosek K et al: Enhancing motivation for change in treatment-resistant eating disorders, *Clin Psychol Rev* 18(4):391, 1998.

White J, Litovitz G: A comparison of inpatient and outpatient women with eating disorders, *Arch Psychiatr Nurs* 12(4):181, 1998.

Whittal M et al: Review: medication and cognitive behavior therapy control symptoms of bulimia nervosa, *Behav Ther* 30:117, 1999.

Wilson G et al: Psychological versus pharmacological treatments of bulimia nervosa: predictors and processes of change, *J Consult Clin Psychol* 67(4):451, 1999.

Wiederman MW, Pryor TL: Overcoming anorexia nervosa, *J Pract Psychiatry Behav Health* 2:5, 1996.

# Sexual Responses and Sexual Disorders

19

## Continuum of Sexual Responses

*Sexuality* is broadly defined as a desire for contact, warmth, tenderness, or love. It includes looking and talking; handholding, kissing, or self-pleasuring; and the production of mutual orgasm. Sexuality is a part of a person's total sense of self. Four aspects of sexuality are:

1. *Genetic identity,* which is a person's chromosomal gender
2. *Gender identity,* which is a person's perception of his or her own maleness or femaleness
3. *Gender role,* which is made up of the cultural role attributes of one's gender, such as expectations regarding behavior, cognitions, occupations, values, and emotional responses
4. *Sexual orientation*, which is the gender to which one is romantically attracted

Experts in the area of sexuality do not agree on what types of sexual behaviors are "normal." Expressions of sexuality can be viewed on a continuum ranging from adaptive to maladaptive (Figure 19-1). The most adaptive sexual responses are seen as behaviors that meet the following criteria:

1. Between two consenting adults
2. Mutually satisfying to the individuals involved
3. Not psychologically or physically harmful to either party
4. Lacking in force or coercion
5. Conducted in private

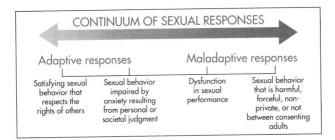

Figure 19-1
Continuum of sexual responses.

Maladaptive sexual responses include behaviors that do not meet one or more of these criteria.

Caution must be used when attempting to label sexual behaviors as adaptive or maladaptive. For instance, sexual behavior can meet the criteria but still be unsatisfactory for an individual if altered by the impact of what society dictates as acceptable and unacceptable behavior.

## Assessment

### Self-Awareness of the Nurse

The most critical element in being able to counsel patients competently about sexuality is nurses' awareness of their own feelings and values. Nurses' level of self-awareness has a direct impact on their ability to intervene effectively with patients.

### Behaviors

Many modes of sexual expression exists. In 1948 Kinsey examined sexual preference using a 7-point rating scale (Figure 19-2) in which 0 represented exclusively heterosexual experiences, 6 represented exclusively homosexual experiences, and 2, 3, or 4 indicated bisexuality. He suggested that most individuals are not exclusively heterosexual or homosexual. The following are definitions of common terms:

1. *Heterosexual*—a person who is sexually attracted to members of the opposite sex
2. *Homosexual*—a person who is sexually attracted to members of the same sex

3. *Bisexual*—a person who is sexually attracted to people of both sexes

4. *Transvestite*—a person who dresses in the clothes of the opposite sex

5. *Transsexual*—a person who is genetically an anatomical male or female but who expresses, with strong conviction, that he or she has the mind of the opposite sex and seeks to change his or her sex legally and through hormonal and surgical sex reassignment

## Predisposing Factors

At present, no one theory can adequately explain the process of sexual development or the factors predisposing a person to mal-

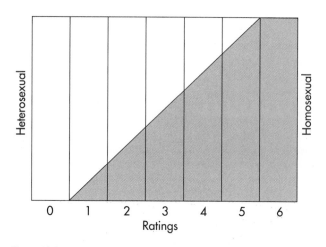

Figure 19-2
Heterosexual-homosexual rating scale. Definitions of the ratings are as follows: *0,* Entirely heterosexual; *1,* largely heterosexual but with incidental homosexual history; *2,* largely heterosexual but with a distinct homosexual history; *3,* equally heterosexual and homosexual; *4,* largely homosexual but with distinct heterosexual history; *5,* largely homosexual but with incidental heterosexual history; *6,* entirely homosexual.
(From Kinsey AC, Pomeroy WB, Martin AC: *Sexual behavior in the human female,* Philadelphia, 1953, WB Saunders.)

adaptive sexual responses. Several theories have been postulated as follows:

1. *Biological factors.* These are initially responsible for the development of gender, that is, whether a person is genetically male or female. The person's somatotype includes chromosomes, hormones, internal and external genitalia, and gonads.

2. *Psychoanalytical view.* Freud viewed sexuality as one of the key forces of human life. He was the first theorist to believe that sexuality was developed before the onset of puberty and that a person's choice of sexual expression depended on an interplay of heredity, biology, and social factors. He proposed that the development of sexuality was specifically related to the development of object relations during the psychosocial stages of development.

3. *Behavioral view.* This perspective views sexual behavior as a measurable response, with both physiological and psychological components, to a learned stimulus or reinforcement event. The treatment of sexual problems involves processes to change behavior through direct intervention without the need to identify underlying causes or psychodynamics.

## Precipitating Stressors

Sexual identity cannot be separated from a person's self-concept or body image. Therefore, when changes occur in the person's body or emotions, sexual responses change as well. Specific threats include the following:

1. Physical illness and injury
2. Psychiatric illness
3. Medications
4. HIV, acquired immunodeficiency syndrome (AIDS)
5. The aging process

## Appraisal of Stressors

Feelings about oneself as a sexual being change throughout the life cycle and are greatly influenced by a person's appraisal of the stressful situation.

## Coping Resources

Coping resources may include the individual's knowledge about sexuality, positive sexual experiences in the past, supportive individuals including the person's sexual partner, and social or cultural norms that encourage healthy expression.

## Coping Mechanisms

Numerous coping mechanisms may be used in the expression of a person's sexual response, including the following:

1. *Fantasy* may be used to enhance sexual experiences.
2. *Denial* may be used to refuse to recognize sexual conflicts or dissatisfactions.
3. *Rationalization* may be used to justify or make acceptable otherwise unacceptable sexual impulses, feelings, behaviors, or motives.
4. *Withdrawal* may be used to cope with unresolved feelings about becoming vulnerable and with the resulting ambivalent feelings about intimacy.

## Nursing Diagnosis

The primary NANDA nursing diagnoses are altered sexuality patterns, which include lack of sexual satisfaction and conflicts involving sex roles and values, and sexual dysfunction, which includes actual physical limitations. The box on page 393 presents the primary and related NANDA diagnoses for variations in sexual response.

## Related Medical Diagnoses

Many people who experience transient variations in sexual response have no medically diagnosed health problem. Patients with more severe or persistent problems are classified in one of three basic categories of DSM-IV-TR: gender identity disorders, paraphilias, and sexual dysfunctions. The box on pages 394 and 395 describes the specific medical diagnoses in each of these diagnostic classes.

## Outcome Identification

The expected outcome for patients with maladaptive sexual responses is as follows:

*The patient will obtain the maximal level of adaptive sexual responses to enhance or maintain health.*

## NANDA Nursing Diagnoses Related to Variations in Sexual Response

Anxiety
Body image, Disturbed
Conflict, Decisional
Fear
Grieving, Dysfunctional
Health maintenance, Ineffective
Health-seeking behaviors
Identity, Disturbed personal
Loneliness, Risk for
Pain, Chronic
Powerlessness
Powerlessness, Risk for
Role performance, Ineffective
Self-care deficit (specify)
Self-esteem, Disturbed
Self-esteem, Risk for situational low
Self-esteem, Situational low
Sensory perception, Disturbed (specify)
*Sexual dysfunction
*Sexuality patterns, Ineffective
Social interaction, Impaired
Spiritual distress

*Primary nursing diagnosis for variations in sexual response.
*From North American Nursing Diagnosis Association:* NANDA nursing diagnoses: definitions and classification 2000-2001, *Philadelphia, 2001, The Association.*

**Planning**

Education is the usual method of primary prevention for sexual problems and issues. A Patient Education Plan for teaching about sexual response after an organic illness is presented on page 396.

## DSM-IV-TR Medical Diagnoses Related to Variations in Sexual Response

| DSM-IV-TR Diagnosis | Essential Features |
| --- | --- |
| Hypoactive sexual disorder | Persistent or recurrent deficit or absence of sexual fantasies and desire for sexual activity. |
| Sexual aversion disorder | Persistent or recurrent extreme aversion to and avoidance of all or almost all genital sexual contact with a sexual partner. |
| Sexual arousal disorder | Persistent or recurrent partial or complete failure to attain or maintain the physiological response of sexual activity, or persistent or recurrent lack of a subjective sense of sexual excitement and pleasure during sexual activity. |
| Orgasmic disorder | Persistent or recurrent delay in or absence of orgasm after a normal sexual excitement phase during sexual activity that the clinician judges to be adequate in focus, intensity, and duration, taking into account the individual's age. |
| Premature ejaculation | Persistent or recurrent ejaculation with minimal sexual stimulation, before, during, or shortly after penetration, before the individual desires it. |
| Dyspareunia | Recurrent or persistent genital pain before, during, or after sexual intercourse. |
| Vaginismus | Recurrent or persistent involuntary spasm of the musculature of the outer third of the vagina that interferes with coitus. |
| Sexual dysfunction caused by a general medical condition | Clinically significant sexual dysfunction etiologically related to a general medical condition. |
| Substance-induced sexual dysfunction | Clinically significant sexual dysfunction that developed during significant substance intoxication or withdrawal. |

| Exhibitionism | Persistent association, lasting at least 6 months, between intense sexual arousal, desire, acts, or fantasies and exposing one's genitals to an unsuspecting stranger. |
| Fetishism | Persistent association, lasting at least 6 months, between intense sexual arousal, desire, acts, or fantasies and nonliving objects (e.g., female undergarments). |
| Frotteurism | Persistent association, lasting at least 6 months, between intense sexual arousal, desire, acts, or fantasies and rubbing against a nonconsenting person. |
| Pedophilia | Persistent association, lasting at least 6 months, between intense sexual arousal, desire, acts, or fantasies and one or more children age 13 years or younger. |
| Sexual masochism | Persistent association, lasting at least 6 months, between intense sexual arousal, desire, acts, or fantasies and being humiliated, beaten, bound, or otherwise being made to suffer (real or imagined). |
| Sexual sadism | Persistent association, lasting at least 6 months, between intense sexual arousal, desire, acts, or fantasies and the affliction of real or simulated psychological or physical suffering (including humiliation). |
| Voyeurism | Persistent association, lasting at least 6 months, between intense sexual arousal, desire, acts, or fantasies and observing unsuspecting people who are naked, in the act of disrobing, or engaging in sexual activity. |
| Transvestic fetishism | Persistent association, lasting at least 6 months, between intense sexual arousal, desire, acts, or fantasies and cross-dressing. |
| Gender identity disorder of childhood, adolescence, or adulthood | Persistent and intense distress about being a male or a female, with an intense desire to be the opposite sex, a preoccupation of adulthood with the activities of the opposite sex, and a repudiation of one's own anatomical structures. |

*Modified from American Psychiatric Association: Diagnostic and statistical manual of mental disorders, ed 4, text revision (DSM-IV-TR), Washington, DC, 2000, The Association.*

## Patient Education Plan:  Sexual Response after an Organic Illness

| Content | Instructional Activities | Evaluation |
|---|---|---|
| Describe the variety of human sexual response patterns. | Discuss range of sexual desires, modes of expression, and techniques. | Patient identifies preferences and typical level of sexual functioning. |
| Define patient's primary organic problem. | Provide accurate information on disruption caused by the organic impairment. | Patient understands nature of the organic illness. |
| Clarify relationship between patient's organic problem and level of sexual functioning. | Reframe distorted or confused perceptions about impact of illness on sexual functioning. | Patient accurately describes the impact of illness on sexual functioning. |
| Identify ways to enhance patient's sexual functioning and improve interpersonal communication. | Describe additional experiences that would enhance sexual satisfaction and the relationship between patient and partner. | Patient and partner report reduced anxiety and greater satisfaction with sexual responses. |

## Intervening in Health Education

Before engaging in either health education or counseling, nurses must examine their own values and beliefs about patients who practice sexual behavior that may be different. This can be facilitated by exploring typical myths about human sexuality held by society as listed in Table 19-1.

## Intervening in Sexual Responses in the Nurse-Patient Relationship

Feelings of sexual attraction and sexual fantasies are part of the human experience, and the nurse should address them. Two aspects of this include a nurse's sexual attraction to a patient and the patient's sexual acting out or display of seductive behaviors toward the nurse. Table 19-2 summarizes considerations in sexual responses of patients to nurses.

Patients may also experience maladaptive sexual responses resulting from physical and emotional illness, sexual preference, gender identity, or dysfunctions of the sexual response cycle. A Nursing Treatment Plan Summary for maladaptive sexual responses is presented on pages 403 and 404.

1. Were the nurse's own feelings and values about sexuality explored and handled appropriately in giving patient care?
2. Was the nursing assessment of the patient's sexuality complete, accurate, and done professionally?
3. Have the patient's feelings about self improved during treatment?
4. If the patient was dysfunctional, was functional ability improved or restored?
5. Was health teaching on variations in sexual expression appropriately carried out?
6. Have the patient's interpersonal relationships improved?
7. Did the patient think that the care was helpful in meeting health care goals?
8. Is referral to another health care professional or agency indicated for the patient?

*Text continued on p. 405*

Table 19-1    Ten common myths and facts about human sexuality

| Myth | Result of Myth | Fact |
|---|---|---|
| Patients become embarrassed when nurses bring up the subject of sexuality and would prefer that nurses not ask questions about sex. | If nurses believe this, they deny patients the opportunity to ask questions and clarify concerns related to sexual issues. | Patients would prefer that nurses initiate discussions of sexuality with them. |
| Excessive masturbation is harmful. | Individuals often feel guilty or ashamed about masturbating; some deny themselves this experience because of uncomfortable feelings perpetuated by society. | No evidence indicates that masturbation causes physical problems. If masturbation leads to satisfaction and pleasure, it is unlikely to be a problem. |
| Sexual fantasies about having sex with a partner other than lover or spouse indicate relationship difficulties. | Individuals may become uncomfortable about having a fantasy with a different partner. They may experience guilt feelings and view the fantasy as a sign of infidelity. | Imagining sex with a different partner is a common sexual fantasy and does not necessarily indicate desire to act out the fantasized behavior. |
| Sex during menstruation is unclean and harmful. | Women often view their bodies as unclean and even unfit or inferior during menstruation. Women use menstruation as an excuse to avoid intercourse rather than simply saying no without a "good reason." | Medically, menstrual flow is not harmful or dirty. If women desire, no reason exists to abstain from intercourse during menstrual flow. |

| Oral and anal intercourse are perverted and dangerous. | Many individuals refrain from these behaviors or indulge in them only to feel ashamed and guilty afterward. | Oral and anal intercourse are not harmful if certain precautions are taken when performing anal intercourse, such as avoiding vaginal contamination and wearing a condom to prevent disease transmission. |
| Most homosexuals molest children. | Known homosexuals are often fired from teaching jobs, and many parents will not allow their children to spend time with any homosexual. | Research shows that the adult heterosexual male poses a much greater risk to the underage child than the adult homosexual male. |
| Homosexuals are sick and cannot control their sexual behavior. | Homosexuals are denied jobs and are sometimes jailed for their homosexuality. Homosexual partners may have their children taken away by courts. | Most homosexuals' social and psychological adjustment is the same as that of the heterosexual majority, and objectionable sexual advances are much more likely to be made by a heterosexual (usually male to female) than a homosexual. |

*Continued*

Table 19-1　Ten common myths and facts about human sexuality—cont'd

| Myth | Result of Myth | Fact |
|---|---|---|
| Because of sex education programs, most adolescents and young adults are aware of the risks of acquiring sexually transmitted diseases (STDs) and practice safe sex. | When health educators believe that young adults have adequate knowledge about STDs, they may not take the time to assess further, add to this knowledge, and correct any misconceptions. | A study of more than 500 freshmen at a large university reported that of those who had multiple partners, fewer than 50% used condoms to lower the risk of disease. |
| Advancing age means the end of sex. | Many older adults become victims of this myth not because their bodies have lost the ability to perform, but because they believe they have lost the ability to perform. | Sexually, men and women in good health can function effectively throughout their lives. |
| Alcohol ingestion reduces inhibitions and therefore enhances sexual enjoyment. | Many individuals use alcohol in the hope that it will increase their sexual pleasure and performance. Alcohol ingestion can also provide an excuse for engaging in sexual behaviors, e.g. "I would never have gone to bed with him if I hadn't had all that wine." | Data do not support the belief that alcohol ingestion reduces inhibitions and enhances sexual enjoyment. |

Table 19-2   Nursing interventions in sexual responses of patients to nurses

**Goal: Maintain a professional nurse-patient relationship that will enable nurse to provide therapeutic nursing care.**

| Principle | Rationale | Nursing Interventions |
|---|---|---|
| Establish a trusting relationship. | Atmosphere of trust allows for open, honest communication between patient and nurse; when this occurs, nurse can aid patient in discovering underlying issues related to patient's sexual feelings and behavior. | Express nonsexual caring and concern for patient. Be a responsible listener, especially to feelings and needs that patient may not be able to express directly. Reinforce purpose of professional, therapeutic nurse-patient relationship. |
| Be aware of own feelings and thoughts. | When aware of his or her own feelings and thoughts, the nurse will begin to understand how they influence behavior. With increased self-awareness, nurse increases effectiveness of interactions with patients. | Recognize own feelings and thoughts. Identify any specific patient interaction or behavior that influences feelings and thoughts. Identify influence of feelings and thoughts on behavior to increase effectiveness of interventions. |

*Continued*

Table 19-2  Nursing interventions in sexual responses of patients to nurses —cont'd

| Principle | Rationale | Nursing Interventions |
|---|---|---|
| Decrease patient's inappropriate expressions of sexual feelings and behavior. | If nurse can help patient see that the sexual interactions and behavior are being expressed to an inappropriate partner (nurse), sexual acting out will usually decrease. Nurse can help patient begin to identify reasons for behavior. | Set limits on patient's sexual behavior. Use a calm, matter-of-fact approach without implying judgment. Reaffirm nonsexual caring for patient. Explore meaning of patient's feelings and behavior. |
| Expand patient's insight into sexual feelings and behavior. | Once patient begins to identify reasons for sexual feelings and behaviors, patient can see that nurse is not an appropriate outlet for these feelings and behaviors. Patient then can move toward a more appropriate and therapeutic relationship with nurse. | Clarify misconceptions about any feeling patient may have about nurse as possible sexual partner. Point out futile nature of patient's romantic or sexual interest. Redirect patient's energies toward appropriate health care issues. |

## Nursing Treatment Plan Summary:  Maladaptive Sexual Responses

**Nursing Diagnosis:** Altered sexuality pattern

**Expected Outcome: Patient will obtain the maximal level of adaptive sexual responses to enhance or maintain health.**

| Short-term Goals | Interventions | Rationale |
|---|---|---|
| Patient will describe values, beliefs, questions, and problems regarding sexuality. | Listen to sexual concerns implied and expressed. Help patient explore sexual beliefs, values, and questions. Encourage open communication between patient and partner. | An accepting therapeutic relationship will allow patients to be free to question, grow, and seek help with sexual concerns. Communicate respect, acceptance, and openness to sexual concerns. |
| Patient will relate accurate information about sexual concerns. | Clarify sexual misinformation. Dispel myths. Provide specific education about sexual health practices, behaviors, and problems. Give professional "permission" to continue sexual behavior that is not physically or emotionally harmful. Reinforce positive attitudes of patient. | Accurate information is helpful in changing negative thoughts and attitudes about particular aspects of sexuality. It can also prevent or limit dysfunctional behavior. Giving permission allows patient to continue the behavior and alleviate anxiety about normalcy. Patient can incorporate sexual behavior in a positive and accepting self-concept. |

*Continued*

### Nursing Treatment Plan Summary: Maladaptive Sexual Responses—cont'd

Nursing Diagnosis: Altered sexuality pattern

**Expected Outcome: Patient will obtain the maximal level of adaptive sexual responses to enhance or maintain health.**

| Short-term Goals | Interventions | Rationale |
|---|---|---|
| Patient will implement one new behavior to enhance sexual response. | Set clear goals with patient. Identify specific behaviors that can be carried out, focusing on enhancing self-concept, role functioning, and sexuality. Encourage relaxation techniques, redirection of attention, positional changes, and alternative ways of sexual expression as appropriate. Become familiar with sexuality therapy resources available in the community. Refer patient to a qualified sexuality therapist as needed. | Giving patient direct behavioral suggestions can help relieve a sexual problem or difficulty and is a useful intervention when the problem is of recent onset and short duration. All nurses must screen for maladaptive sexual responses and provide basic nursing care, but should refer complex problems to qualified sexuality therapists for further treatment. |

*your*INTERNET
connection

American Association of Sexuality Educators,
Counselors and Therapists (AASECT):
www.aasect.org

The Kinsey Institute:
www.indiana.edu/~kinsey/index.html

Sexual Health Network:
www.sexualhealth.com

Society for the Scientific Study of Sexuality (SSSS):
www.ssc.wisc.edu/ssss/

## Suggested readings

Committee on Human Sexuality, Group for the Advancement of Psychiatry: *Homosexuality and the mental health professions: the impact of bias,* Report No 144, Hillsdale, NJ, 2000, Analytic Press.

Duffy L: Lovers, loners and lifers: sexuality and the older adult, *Geriatrics* 53:S68, 1998.

Hajagos K et al: Safer-sex education for persons with mental illness, *J Psychosoc Nurs* 36(8):33, 1998.

Hellman R: Issues in the treatment of lesbian women and gay men with chronic mental illness, *Psychiatric Serv* 47:1093, 1996.

Laumann E et al: Sexual dysfunction in the United States: prevalence and predictors, *JAMA* 281:542, 1999.

Moore B, Rothschild A: Treatment of antidepressant induced sexual dysfunction, *Hosp Pract* 34:89, 1999.

Richmond J, McKenna H: Homophobia: an evolutionary analysis of the concept as applied to nursing, *J Adv Nurs* 28:362, 1998.

Stuart G, Laraia M: *Principles and practice of psychiatric nursing,* ed 7, St Louis, 2001, Mosby.

Taylor B: 'Coming out' as a life transition: homosexual identity formation and its implications for health care practice, *J Adv Nurs* 30:523, 1999.

Torkelson D, Dobal M: Sexual rights of people with serious and persistent mental illness: gathering evidence for decision making, *J Am Psychiatr Nurses Assoc* 5:150, 1999.

Warner P et al: Shedding light on the sexual history, *Am J Nurs* 99:34, 1999.

Weingourt R: A comparison of heterosexual and homosexual long-term sexual relationships, *Arch Psychiatr Nurs* 12(2):114, 1998.

# Psycho-pharmacology 20

## Role of the Nurse

The nurse should be knowledgeable about the psychopharmacological strategies available, but this information must be used as one part of a holistic approach to patient care. The nurse's role includes the following:

1. *Patient assessment.* This provides a baseline view of each patient.
2. *Coordination of treatment modalities.* This integrates the varied and often confusing drug treatments for patients.
3. *Administration of psychopharmacological agents.* This provides a professionally designed and individualized drug administration regimen.
4. *Monitoring drug effects.* This includes both desired effects and side effects that patients may experience.
5. *Patient education.* This enables patients to take their medicines safely and effectively.
6. *Drug maintenance program.* This is designed to support the patient in aftercare settings for extended periods.
7. *Participation in interdisciplinary clinical research drug trials.* The nurse is an essential member of the team that researches the drugs used to treat patients with psychiatric disorders.
8. *Prescriptive authority.* Some psychiatric nurses who are qualified by education and experience in accordance with their state practice act are able to prescribe pharmacological agents to treat the symptoms and improve the functional status of patients with psychiatric illness.

# Assessment

Before initiation of psychopharmacological treatment, a thorough psychiatric evaluation must be completed, including the following:
1. Physical examination
2. Laboratory studies
3. Mental status evaluation
4. Medical and psychiatric history
5. Medication history
6. Family history

The Medication Assessment Tool presented in Box 20-1 can be used to take a drug history.

**NURSE ALERT.**  Concurrent use of drugs, or polypharmacy, can enhance a specific therapeutic action, can be necessary to treat concurrent illnesses, and can counteract unwanted effects of the first drug. Unfortunately, several problems are associated with concurrent drug use, including confusion over therapeutic efficacy and side effects and development of drug interactions. Table 20-1 lists some of the more common interactions of psychotropic drugs and other substances.

# Antianxiety and Sedative-Hypnotic Drugs

Antianxiety and sedative-hypnotic drugs are divided into two categories: the benzodiazepines and the nonbenzodiazepines, which include several classes of drugs. The benzodiazepines are the most widely prescribed drugs in the world, and in the last 20 years they have almost entirely replaced the barbiturates in the treatment of anxiety and sleep disorders. Their popularity is related to their effectiveness and wide margin of safety.

## Benzodiazepines

### Mechanism of action

The benzodiazepines are thought to exert their antianxiety effects through their powerful potentiation of the inhibitory neurotransmitter γ-aminobutyric acid (GABA).

*Text continued on p. 413*

**Box 20-1    Medication Assessment Tool**

For each of the following categories of drugs taken by the patient:

- Prescribed psychiatric medications ever taken
- Prescribed nonpsychiatric medication taken in the past 6 months or taken for major medical illnesses if more than 6 months ago
- Over-the-counter medication taken in the past 6 months

- Obtain the following information from the patient and other sources:
  - Name of the drug
  - Reason taken
  - Dates started and stopped
  - Highest daily dose
  - Who prescribed it?
  - Was it effective?
  - Side effects or adverse reactions
  - Was it taken as directed?
  - If not, how was it taken?
  - History of drugs taken by first-degree relative
  - Drugs taken prescribed to others

For each of the following categories of drugs taken by the patient:

- Alcohol
- Tobacco
- Caffeine
- Street drugs

- Obtain the following information from the patient and other sources:
  - Name of substance
  - Dates and schedule of use
  - Summary of effects
  - Adverse reactions/withdrawal symptoms
  - Attempts to stop/treatments to stop
  - Impact of substance on:
    - Quality of life
    - Relationships/spouse/children
    - Occupation/education
    - Health/productivity
    - Self-image
    - Expense

Table 20-1   Interactions of psychotropic drugs and other substances

| Psychotropic Category | Possible Interactions |
|---|---|
| Antianxiety Agents | |
| *Benzodiazepines with:* | |
| Central nervous system (CNS) depressants (alcohol, barbiturates, antipsychotics, antihistamines, cimetidine) | Potential additive CNS effects, especially sedation and decreased daytime performance |
| Selective serotonin reuptake inhibitors (SSRIs), disulfiram, estrogens | Increased benzodiazepine effects |
| Antacids, tobacco | Decreased benzodiazepine effects |
| *Sedative-hypnotics with:* | |
| CNS depressants (alcohol, antihistamines, antidepressants, narcotics, antipsychotics) | Enhancement of sedative effects; impairment of mental and physical performance; may result in lethargy, respiratory depression, coma, death |
| Anticoagulants (oral)* | Decreased coumarin plasma levels and effect; monitor and adjust dose of coumarin |

*Potentially clinically significant.

*Continued*

Table 20-1 Interactions of psychotropic drugs and other substances—cont'd

| Psychotropic Category | Possible Interactions |
|---|---|
| Antidepressants | |
| *Tricyclics (TCAs) with:* | |
| MAOIs* | May cause hypertensive crisis |
| Monoamine oxidase inhibitors | Additive CNS depression; decreased TCA effect |
| Alcohol and other CNS depressants | |
| Antihypertensives* (guanethidine, methyldopa, clonidine) | Antagonism of antihypertensive effect |
| Antipsychotics and antiparkinsonians | Increased TCA effect; confusion, delirium, ileus |
| Anticholinergics | Additive anticholinergic effects |
| Antiarrhythmics (quinidine, procainamide, propranolol) | Additive antiarrhythmic effects; myocardial depression |
| SSRIs* | Increased TCA serum level/toxicity through inhibition of cytochrome P-450 system |
| Anticonvulsants | |
| Tobacco | Decreased TCA effect; seizures |
| *SSRIs with:* | Decreased TCA plasma levels |
| Clomipramine, maprotiline, bupropion, clozapine | Increased risk of seizures |
| MAOIs* | Serotonin syndrome |
| Barbiturates, benzodiazepines, narcotics | Increased CNS depression |
| Carbamazepine | Neurotoxicity: nausea, vomiting, vertigo, tinnitus, ataxia, lethargy, blurred vision |

*MAOIs with:*
Many drugs and foods — Hypertensive crisis

Mood Stabilizers
*Lithium with:*
Diuretics,* marijuana — Increased lithium levels/toxicity
SSRIs — Lithium toxicity; enhanced therapeutic effect
Nonsteroidal antiinflammatory agents* — Increased lithium blood levels/toxicity
Antipsychotics — Increased CNS toxicity
Tetracyclines — Lithium intoxication
Acetylcholinesterase (ACE) inhibitors — Confusion, ataxia, dysarthria, tremor, electrocardiogram (ECG) changes

*Carbamazepine with:*
Lithium — Lithium intoxication; increased effect; inhibits lithium-induced polyuria
Haloperidol — Decreased effect of either drug
Calcium channel blockers — Neurotoxicity; dizziness, nausea, diplopia, headache
Valproate — Decreased valproate serum concentration
Cimetidine, erythromycin, isoniazid — Somnolence, lethargy, dizziness, blurred vision, ataxia, nausea

*Potentially clinically significant.

*Continued*

Table 20-1    Interactions of psychotropic drugs and other substances—cont'd

| Psychotropic Category | Possible Interactions |
| --- | --- |
| *Valproate with:* | |
| SSRIs, erythromycin, cimetidine | Increased valproate serum concentrations |
| Antipsychotics with: | |
| Antacids, tea, coffee, milk, fruit juice | Decreased phenothiazine effects |
| CNS depressants (narcotics, antianxiety drugs, alcohol, antihistamines, barbiturates) | Additive CNS depression |
| Anticholinergic agents (levodopa)* | Additive atropinelike side effects and increased antiparkinsonian effects |
| SSRIs | Increased neuroleptic serum level and extrapyramidal side effects (EPS) |
| Antipsychotics | |
| *Clozapine with:* | |
| Carbamazepine* | Additive bone marrow suppression |
| Benzodiazepines* | Circulatory collapse, respiratory arrest |
| SSRIs* | Increased risk of seizures |

*Potentially clinically significant.

## Clinical use

The benzodiazepines are frequently the drug of choice in the management of anxiety, insomnia, and stress-related conditions. Most experts believe that treatment with benzodiazepines should be brief, during periods of specific stress. With supervision, however, they are often given for extended periods (Table 20-2).

The major indications for benzodiazepine use follow:

1. Generalized anxiety disorder
2. Anxiety associated with depression
3. Sleep disorders
4. Anxiety associated with phobic disorders
5. Posttraumatic stress disorder
6. Alcohol and drug withdrawal
7. Anxiety associated with medical disease
8. Musculoskeletal relaxation
9. Seizure disorders
10. Preoperative anxiety

### Adverse reactions and nursing considerations

The benzodiazepines have a very high therapeutic index; thus overdoses of these drugs alone almost never cause fatalities. Side effects are common, dose related, and almost always harmless. Table 20-3 summarizes these reactions and identifies nursing considerations.

**NURSE ALERT.**   The benzodiazepines generally are not as strongly addictive as thought if their discontinuation is accomplished by gradual tapering, if they have been used for appropriate purposes, and if their use has not been complicated by the use of other substances, such as chronic use of barbiturates or alcohol. Watch particularly for the following:

1. Sedation
2. Ataxia
3. Irritability
4. Memory problems

## Nonbenzodiazepines

The nonbenzodiazepines have been largely replaced by the benzodiazepines although they are used occasionally. Table 20-4 lists

Table 20-2    Antianxiety and sedative-hypnotic drugs: benzodiazepines

| Generic Name (trade name) | Active Metabolites | Half-life (hr) | Equivalents (mg) | Usual Adult Dosage Range (mg/day) | Preparations |
|---|---|---|---|---|---|
| **Antianxiety Drugs** | | | | | |
| Alprazolam (Xanax) | Yes (not significant) | 6-20 | 0.25 | 0.5-10 bid to quid | PO |
| Chlordiazepoxide (Librium) | Yes | 6-100 | 10 | 10-150 bid to quid | PO, IM, IV |
| Clonazepam (Klonopin) | No | >20 | 0.5 | 0.5-10 bid | PO |
| Clorazepate (Tranxene) | Yes | >20 | 7.5 | 7.5-60 bid or quid | PO |
| Diazepam (Valium) | Yes | >20 | 5 | 2-40 bid | PO, SR, IM, IV |
| Halazepam (Paxipam) | Yes | >20 | 20 | 60-160 tid or quid | PO |
| Lorazepam (Ativan) | No | 6-20 | 1 | 1-6 tid | PO, IM, IV |
| Oxazepam (Serax) | No | 6-20 | 15 | 15-120 tid or quid | PO |
| Prazepam (Centrax) | Yes | >20 | 10 | 10-60 tid or quid | PO |
| **Sedative-Hypnotic Drugs** | | | | | |
| Estazolam (ProSom) | No | 6-20 | .33 | 1-2 HS | PO |
| Flurazepam (Dalmane) | Yes | <6 | 5 | 15-60 HS | PO |
| Temazepam (Restoril) | No | 6-20 | 5 | 15-30 HS | PO |
| Triazolam (Halcion) | No | >6 | 0.25 | 0.25-0.5 HS | PO |
| Quazepam (Doral) | Yes | >20 | 5 | 7.5-50 HS | PO |

*IM,* Intramuscular; *IV,* intravenous; *PO,* oral tablet or capsule; *SR,* oral slow-release tablet.

Table 20-3   Side effects and nursing considerations: benzodiazepines

| Side Effects | Nursing Considerations* |
|---|---|
| **Common** | |
| Drowsiness, sedation | Activity helpful; caution patient when using machinery. |
| Ataxia, dizziness | Caution with activity; prevent falls. |
| Feelings of detachment | Discourage social isolation. |
| Increased irritability or hostility | Observe; support; be alert for disinhibition. |
| Anterograde amnesia | Patient unable to recall events that occur while taking drug. |
| Cognitive effects with long-term use | Interference with concentration and memory of new material. |
| Tolerance, dependency, rebound insomnia/anxiety | Short-term use; discontinue, using a slow taper. |
| **Rare** | |
| Nausea | Administer dose with meals; decrease dose. |
| Headache | Patient usually responds to mild analgesic. |
| Confusion | Decrease dose. |
| Gross psychomotor impairment | Dose related; decrease dose. |
| Depression | Decrease dose; antidepressant treatment. |
| Paradoxical rage reaction | Discontinue drug. |

*Benzodiazepines contraindicated in patients with a history of drug or alcohol abuse.

Table 20-4    Newer, nonbenzodiazepine antianxiety and sedative-hypnotic agents

| Generic Name (Trade Name) | Dose (mg) | Half-Life (hr) |
|---|---|---|
| Antianxiety Agents | | |
| *Azaspirone* | | |
| Buspirone (BuSpar) | 10-40 | 2-5 |
| *Beta-adrenergic blocker* | | |
| Propranolol (Inderal) | 10 qid | 3 |
| *Herbal preparation* | | |
| Kava extract | 120-240 | Unknown |
| | | |
| Sedative-Hypnotic Agents | | |
| *Imidazopyridine* | | |
| Zolpidem (Ambien) | 10 | 2.5 |
| *Pyrazolopyrimidine* | | |
| Zaleplon (Sonata) | 5-10 | 1 |
| *Antihistamines* | | |
| Diphenhydramine (Benadryl) | 50 | Unknown |
| Hydroxyzine (Atarax) | 100 tid | Unknown |
| *Antidepressant* | | |
| Trazodone (Desyrel) | 50-200 | 4 |

the newer nonbenzodiazepine antianxiety and sedative-hypnotic agents.

**NURSE ALERT.**    Use of barbiturates has numerous disadvantages, as follows:
1. Tolerance develops to the antianxiety effects of barbiturates.
2. They are more addictive.
3. They cause serious and even lethal withdrawal reactions.
4. They are dangerous in overdose and cause central nervous system (CNS) depression.
5. They have a variety of dangerous drug interactions.

## Antidepressants

The types of antidepressant drugs are tricyclics (TCAs), monoamine oxidase inhibitors (MAOIs), selective serotonin reuptake inhibitors (SSRIs), and a group of other antidepressants not in the first three classes (Table 20-5). The primary clinical indication for the use of antidepressant drugs is major depressive illness. They are also useful in the treatment of panic disorder, other anxiety disorders, and enuresis in children. Preliminary research studies suggest they are useful for attention deficit disorders in children and for bulimia and narcolepsy.

## Tricyclic Antidepressants

### Mechanism of action

The TCAs appear to regulate the brain's use of the neurotransmitters norepinephrine and serotonin.

### Clinical use

With an acceptable cardiac history and an electrocardiogram (ECG) within normal limits, particularly for people more than 40 years old, TCAs are safe and effective in the treatment of acute and long-term depressive illnesses.

### Adverse reactions and nursing considerations

The nurse should know the common side effects of the antidepressants and be aware of toxic effects and their treatment. These drugs cause sedation and anticholinergic side effects, such as dry mouth, blurred vision, constipation, urinary retention, orthostatic hypotension, temporary confusion, tachycardia, and photosensitivity. Most of these are common, short-term side effects and can be minimized with a decrease in dose. Toxic side effects include confusion, poor concentration, hallucinations, delirium, seizures, respiratory depression, tachycardia, bradycardia, and coma.

**NURSE ALERT**
1. Tricyclic antidepressants can be lethal in overdose.
2. They have a 3- to 4-week delay before therapeutic response.
3. They have no known long-term adverse effects.
4. Tolerance to therapeutic effects does not develop.
5. Persistent side effects can often be minimized by a small decrease in dose.

6. TCAs do not cause physical addiction or psychological dependence.
7. They do not cause euphoria; thus they have no abuse potential.
8. They can be conveniently given once a day.

## Monoamine Oxidase Inhibitors (MAOIs)

### Mechanism of action

MAOIs block monoamine oxidase in the brain and the rest of the body. By blocking MAO in the brain, less norepinephrine is metabolized, thus increasing its availability in the synapse.

### Clinical use

MAOIs are very effective antidepressant and antipanic drugs that have been underused and overly feared. Because of the potential for hypertensive crisis when tyramine-containing foods and certain medicines are taken concomitantly with these drugs, careful health teaching of a reliable patient is important. Box 20-2 outlines dietary restrictions with MAOI therapy.

### Adverse reactions and nursing considerations

Side effects of MAOIs include lightheadedness, constipation, sexual dysfunction, muscle twitching, drowsiness, dry mouth, fluid retention, insomnia, urinary hesitancy, and weight gain. Box 20-3 lists signs and treatment of hypertensive crisis during MAOI therapy.

**NURSE ALERT**
1. MAOIs may be lethal in overdose.
2. Dietary restrictions must begin several days before taking the medication, be maintained while taking the medication, and be continued for 2 weeks after discontinuing therapy.
3. These drugs are nonaddicting.
4. Tolerance does not develop for therapeutic effects.
5. MAOIs decrease the body's ability to use vitamin $B_6$; thus supplements may be necessary.

Table 20-5    Antidepressant drugs

| Generic (trade name) | Usual Adult Daily Dose (mg/day) | Preparations |
|---|---|---|
| Selective Serotonin Reuptake Inhibitors | | |
| Citalopram (Celexa) | 20-50 | PO |
| Fluoxetine (Prozac) | 20-80 | PO |
| Fluvoxamine (Luvox) | 50-300 | PO |
| Paroxetine (Paxil) | 20-50 | PO |
| Sertraline (Zoloft) | 25-200 | PO |
| Other Newer Antidepressant Drugs | | |
| Amoxapine (Asendin) | 200-300 | PO |
| Bupropion (Wellbutrin) | 150-450* | PO and SR |
| Maprotiline (Ludiomil) | 50-200* | PO |
| Mirtazapine (Remeron) | 15-45 | PO |
| Trazodone (Desyrel) | 50-600 | PO |
| *Serotonin Antagonist and Reuptake Blocker (SARI)* | | |
| Nefazodone (Serzone) | 200-600 | PO |
| *Serotonin-Norepinephrine Reuptake Inhibitor* | | |
| Venlafaxine (Effexor) | 25-375 | PO and XT |
| *Selective Presynaptic Noradrenergic Reuptake Inhibitor* | | |
| Reboxetine (Vestra) | 4-10 | PO |
| Tricyclic Drugs | | |
| *Tertiary (parent)* | | |
| Amitriptyline (Elavil) | 50-300 | PO, IM |
| Clomipramine (Anafranil) | 50-250 | PO |
| Doxepin (Adapin, Sinequan) | 50-300 | PO, L |
| Imipramine (Tofranil) | 50-300 | PO, IM |
| Trimipramine (Surmontil) | 50-300 | PO |
| *Secondary (metabolite)* | | |
| Desipramine (Norpramin) | 50-300 | PO, L |
| Nortriptyline (Pamelor) | 50-150 | PO |
| Protriptyline (Vivactil) | 30-60 | PO |
| Monoamine Oxidase Inhibitors | | |
| Isocarboxazid (Marplan) | 20-60 | PO |
| Phenelzine (Nardil) | 45-90 | PO |
| Tranylcypromine (Parnate) | 20-60 | PO |

*Antidepressants with a ceiling dose because of dose-related seizures.

*IM,* Intramuscular; *L,* oral liquid; *PO,* oral tablet/capsule; *SR,* sustained release; *XT,* extended release.

## Box 20-2   Dietary Restrictions: 1 Day Before, During, and 2 to 6 Weeks After MAOI Therapy

### Food and Beverages to Avoid

Cheese, especially aged or matured
Fermented or aged protein (meat or fish)
Pickled or smoked fish
Chianti and vermouth wines, tap (draft) beer
Yeast or protein extracts
Fava or broad bean pods
Liver, sausages, pepperoni, salami, canned ham
Spoiled or overripe fruit
Banana peel, sauerkraut

### Food and Beverages to Be Consumed in Moderation

Chocolate
Yogurt, sour cream, cottage and cream cheese
Clear spirits and white wine
Avocado, raspberries
New Zealand spinach
Soy sauce
Aspartame, monosodium glutamate

### Drugs to Avoid

Most other antidepressant drugs
Other MAOIs
Nasal and sinus decongestants
Allergy and hay fever remedies
Narcotics, especially meperidine
Asthma remedies
Local anesthetics with epinephrine
Weight-reducing pills, pep pills, stimulants
Cocaine, amphetamines
Other medications without first checking with clinician

### Medications That May Need Dose Decreased

Insulin and oral hypoglycemics
Oral anticoagulants
Thiazide diuretics
Anticholinergic agents
Muscle relaxants

*Modified from Bernstein JG:* Handbook of drug therapy in psychiatry, *ed 3, St Louis, 1995, Mosby.*

## Box 20-3    Signs and Treatment of Hypertensive Crisis During MAOI Therapy

Warning Signs

Increased blood pressure, palpitations, frequent headaches

Symptoms of Hypertensive Crisis

Sudden elevation of blood pressure
Explosive headache, occipital that may radiate frontally
Head and face flushed and feel "full"
Palpitations, chest pain
Sweating, fever
Nausea, vomiting
Dilated pupils
Photophobia
Intracranial bleeding

Treatment

Hold next MAOI dose.
Do not have patient lie down (elevates blood pressure
   in head).
Administer intramuscular chlorpromazine, 100 mg;
   repeat if necessary (mechanism of action: blocks
   norepinephrine).
Administer intravenous phentolamine slowly in 5-mg
   doses (mechanism of action: binds with norepinephrine
   receptor sites, blocking norepinephrine).
Manage fever with external cooling techniques.
Evaluate diet, adherence to regimen, and education.

## Selective Serotonin Reuptake Inhibitors
### Mechanism of action

The SSRIs inhibit the reuptake of serotonin at the presynaptic membrane. Thus these drugs promote the neurotransmission of serotonin in the brain. One of the newer antidepressants, venlafaxine, raises the levels of serotonin and norepinephrine. Thus it has a broad spectrum of activity and is called a nonselective reuptake inhibitor.

Clinical use

SSRIs not only represent a new approach to the treatment of depression and other disorders (e.g., panic disorder, obsessive-compulsive disorder) but also may provide a safer treatment option than other antidepressants because they are relatively safe in overdose. In addition, the SSRIs have a safer side effect profile than the TCAs and MAOIs.

### Adverse reactions and nursing considerations

The SSRIs have antidepressant effects comparable to the other classes of antidepressant drugs but without significant anticholinergic, cardiovascular, and sedative side effects. The most common side effects include nausea, diarrhea, insomnia, dry mouth, nervousness, headache, sexual dysfunction, drowsiness, dizziness, and sweating. Most of these are short-term side effects and can be minimized by supportive measures, titrating the dose, or changing the medication schedule.

# Mood-Stabilizing Drugs

Table 20-6 lists the major mood-stabilizing drugs.

## Lithium

### Mechanism of action

Lithium is a naturally occurring salt, and the exact mechanism of action is not fully understood. Many neurotransmitter functions are altered.

### Clinical use

Acute episodes of mania and hypomania and recurrent bipolar illness are the most common indications for lithium treatment. Other disorders with an affective component, such as recurrent unipolar depression, schizoaffective disorder, catatonia, rage reactions, and alcoholism, are sometimes effectively treated with lithium, especially when they are periodic or cyclical.

### Adverse reactions and nursing considerations

Patients can take lithium for many years. They must be taught the common causes for an increase in lithium level and ways to stabilize a therapeutic level (Box 20-4). Lithium side effects include fine hand tremor, fatigue, headache, mental dullness, lethargy,

Table 20-6   Mood-stabilizing drugs

| Generic (Trade Name) | Peak Plasma Levels (h) | Half-Life | Usual Adult Daily Dose (mg/day) | Preparations |
|---|---|---|---|---|
| Lithium carbonate (Eskalith, Lithobid, Lithium Citrate, etc.) | 1-4 | 18-36 | 600-2400 | PO, SR, L |
| Carbamazepine (Tegretol) | 1.5-6 | 25-65, 8-29 | 200-1600 | PO, Ch |
| Valproic acid (Valproate, Depakote, Divalproex, etc.) | 2-4 | 9-16 | 750+ | PO, L |
| Lamotrigine (Lamictal) | 1-5 | 26 | 12.5-150+ | PO |
| Gabapentin (Neurontin) | 3 | 5-7 | 300-1800+ | PO |
| Topiramate (Topamax) | 2 | 21 | 25-200+ | PO |
| Olanzapine (Zyprexa) | | 27 | 15-20 | PO |

*Ch*, Chewable tablets; *L*, liquid; *PO*, oral tablet/capsule; *SR*, oral slow-release tablets.

---

### Box 20-4    Lithium Levels

---

Common Causes for Increased Lithium Levels

1. Decreased sodium intake
2. Diuretic therapy
3. Decreased renal functioning
4. Fluid and electrolyte loss: sweating, diarrhea, dehydration
5. Medical illness
6. Overdose
7. Nonsteroidal antiinflammatory drug therapy

Ways to Maintain Stable Lithium Levels

1. Stabilize dosing schedule by dividing doses or using sustained-release capsules.
2. Maintain adequate dietary sodium and fluid intake (2-3 quarts/day).
3. Replace fluid and electrolytes during exercise or gastrointestinal illness.
4. Monitor signs and symptoms of lithium side effects and toxicity.
5. If patients forget a dose, they may take it if they missed dosing time by 2 hours; if longer than 2 hours, skip that dose and take the next dose; never double-up doses.

---

polyuria, polydipsia, gastric irritation, mild nausea, vomiting, diarrhea, acne, ECG changes, and weight gain.

Signs of lithium toxicity are related to lithium levels and include anorexia, nausea, vomiting, diarrhea, coarse hand tremor, twitching, lethargy, dysarthria, ataxia, fever, irregular vital signs, seizures, and coma.

### Anticonvulsants

In the last two decades, several anticonvulsant drugs have been used successfully to treat bipolar illness. Carbamazepine (Tegretol) has a variety of effects in the brain that help to stabilize mood. Side effects include drowsiness, dizziness, ataxia, blurred vision, nausea, vomiting, and skin rash. A rare but serious problem is agranulocytosis; thus blood levels and complete blood counts are monitored frequently. Valproate (Depakote) is another anticonvulsant used in the treatment of bipolar illness. It is well tolerated in general, and side effects include anorexia, nausea, vomiting, diarrhea, tremor, sedation, ataxia, weight gain, and, very rarely, pancreatitis and hepatic dysfunction, which necessitate regular laboratory studies.

---

**NURSE ALERT**
1. Lithium toxicity is a life-threatening emergency.
2. Blood levels must be monitored frequently.
3. Treatment failures may occur.
4. Lithium can also be combined with other antidepressants.
5. Patients need careful education about maintenance of lithium levels.
6. Lithium is sometimes used to augment the efficacy of other antidepressants.

---

## Antipsychotic Drugs

### Mechanism of action

Antipsychotic drugs are dopamine antagonists and block dopamine receptors in various pathways in the brain. Atypical antipsychotics also enhance the effectiveness of serotonin.

### Clinical use

Table 20-7 lists the most frequently prescribed antipsychotic drugs. The chemical classes of the conventional, "typical" antipsychotic drugs are distinguished by the extent, type, and severity of side effects produced. Their overall clinical efficacy at equivalent doses is similar.

The newer, atypical antipsychotic drugs, such as clozapine, risperidone, olanzapine, and ziprasidone, have clinical effects superior to other classes of antipsychotics with minimal acute extrapyramidal side effects.

The major uses of antipsychotic drugs are to manage schizophrenia, organic brain syndrome with psychosis, the manic phase of manic-depressive illness, and severe depression with psychosis. They are also useful for patients with severe anxiety who abuse

Table 20-7 Antipsychotic drugs

| Generic Name (Trade Name) | Drug Dosage: Equivalence (mg) | Usual Adult Dosage Range (mg/day) | Preparations |
|---|---|---|---|
| *Atypical Antipsychotics* | | | |
| Clozapine (Clozaril) | 50 | 25-600+ | PO |
| Risperidone (Risperdal) | 1-2 | 2-8 | PO, L |
| Olanzapine (Zyprexa) | 2-3 | 5-20 | PO |
| Quetiapine (Seroquel) | 50-100 | 150-750 | PO |
| Ziprasidone (Geodon) | | 80-160 | PO |
| *Typical Antipsychotics* | | | |
| *Phenothiazines* | | | |
| Chlorpromazine (Thorazine) | 100 | 200-1000 | PO, IM, L |
| Thioridazine (Mellaril) | 100 | 200-600* | PO, IM, L |
| Mesoridazine (Serentil) | 50 | 100-400 | PO, IM, L |
| Perphenazine (Trilafon) | 10 | 8-64 | PO, IM, L |
| Trifluoperazine (Stelazine) | 5 | 5-30 | PO, IM, L |
| Fluphenazine (Prolixin) | 2 | 2-20 | PO, IM, L |
| Fluphenazine decanoate (Prolixin Decanoate) | 12.5-50 | 2.5-50 q2-4 weeks | L-A |

| | | | |
|---|---|---|---|
| *Thioxanthene* | | | |
| Thiothixene (Navane) | 5 | 5-30 | PO, L |
| *Butyrophenone* | | | |
| Haloperidol (Haldol) | 2 | 2-20 + | PO, IM, L |
| Haloperidol decanoate (Haldol Decanoate) | 50-300 | 50-300 q3-4 weeks | L-A |
| *Dibenzoxazepine* | | | |
| Loxapine (Loxitane) | 15 | 20-100+ | PO, IM, L |
| *Dihydroindolone* | | | |
| Molindone (Moban) | 10 | 20-100+ | PO, L |
| Diphenybutylpiperidine | | | |
| Pimozide (Orap) | 2 | 2-16 | PO |

*Upper limit to avoid retinopathy.

*IM*, Intramuscular; *L*, oral liquid, concentrate, suspension, or elixir; *L-A*, long-acting injectable preparations; *PO*, oral tablet or capsule.

drugs or alcohol because the benzodiazepines are contraindicated for them.

## Adverse reactions and nursing considerations

The side effects of antipsychotic drugs are many and varied and demand much clinical attention from the nurse for optimal care. Some side effects are merely uncomfortable for the patient, and most are easily treated, but some are life threatening. The nurse should pay particular attention to the extrapyramidal symptoms or syndromes (EPS), both short term and long term. The most common drugs to treat short-term EPS follow:

1. Benztropine, 1 to 6 mg/day
2. Trihexyphenidyl, 1 to 10 mg/day
3. Diphenhydramine, 25 to 150 mg/day

The most serious adverse effect of clozapine is agranulocytosis, which occurs in approximately 1% to 2% of patients. Table 20-8 lists some of the more common side effects and nursing considerations.

**NURSE ALERT**
Guidelines for antipsychotic drug administration:

1. Individualized dosage requirements for antipsychotic drugs vary greatly.
2. After initial divided doses, patients can receive doses once a day.
3. Symptom improvement usually occurs in 2 or 3 days to 2 weeks. Optimal effects may take several months.
4. Some patients require a lifetime of continuous antipsychotic medication treatment.
5. Observation for tardive dyskinesia (long-term EPS) should be done about monthly during long-term treatment with conventional antipsychotics.
6. Good clinical care for patients taking clozapine includes weekly complete blood counts to monitor for decreased white cell count and clozapine prescriptions given for 1 week at a time.

Table 20-8  Side effects and nursing considerations: antipsychotic drugs

| Side Effects | Nursing Care and Teaching Considerations |
|---|---|
| **Extrapyramidal symptoms (EPS)** | General treatment principles:<br>1. Tolerance usually develops by third month.<br>2. Decrease dose of drug.<br>3. Add a drug to treat EPS, then taper before 3 months of antipsychotic administration.<br>4. Use a drug with a lower EPS profile.<br>5. Provide patient education and support. |
| 1. Acute dystonic reactions: oculogyric crisis, torticollis (wryneck) | Frightening, painful spasms of major muscle groups of neck, back, and eyes; more common in children and young males and with high-potency drugs.<br>Medicate with drugs to treat EPS; have respiratory support available.<br>Taper dose gradually when discontinuing antipsychotics to avoid withdrawal dyskinesia. |
| 2. Akathisia | Patient cannot remain still; pacing, inner restlessness, and leg aches are relieved by movement.<br>Rule out anxiety or agitation; medicate. |
| 3. Parkinson's syndrome: akinesia, cogwheel rigidity, fine tremor | More common in males and elderly patients; tolerance may not develop.<br>Medicate with amantadine, a dopamine (DA) agonist; patient must have good renal function. |

*Continued*

Table 20-8 Side effects and nursing considerations: antipsychotic drugs—cont'd

| Side Effects | Nursing Care and Teaching Considerations |
|---|---|
| 4. Tardive dyskinesia (TD) | Can occur after use (usually long use) of conventional antipsychotics; stereotyped involuntary movements: tongue protrusion, lip smacking, chewing, blinking, grimacing, choreiform movements of limbs and trunk, foot tapping. Assess patient often; consider changing to atypical antipsychotic drug. |
| **Neuroleptic malignant syndrome (NMS)** | Potentially fatal, with fever, tachycardia, sweating, muscle rigidity, tremor, incontinence, stupor, leukocytosis, elevated creatinine phosphokinase, renal failure; more common with high-potency drugs and in dehydrated persons. Discontinue all drugs; provide supportive symptomatic care: hydration, renal dialysis, ventilation, and fever reduction as appropriate; can treat with dantrolene or bromocriptine; antipsychotic drugs can be cautiously reintroduced eventually. |
| **Seizures** | Occur in approximately 1% of patients taking antipsychotics; clozapine has a 5% seizure rate in patients taking 600-900 mg/day; may have to discontinue clozapine. |

**Other side effects**

| | |
|---|---|
| 1. Agranulocytosis | This is an emergency; it develops abruptly, with fever, malaise, ulcerative sore throat, and leukopenia. High incidence (1%-2%) is associated with clozapine; must do weekly complete blood counts and prescribe only 1 week of drug at a time; discontinue drug immediately; patient may need reverse isolation and antibiotics. |
| 2. Photosensitivity | Use sunscreen and sunglasses; cover body with clothing. |
| 3. Anticholinergic effects | Symptoms include constipation, dry mouth, blurred vision, orthostatic hypotension, tachycardia, urinary retention, nasal congestion. Decrease dose; use alternate drug. |
| 4. Sedation, weight gain | Decrease dose; change drug; keep patient active; reduce calories. |

*your* **INTERNET**
c o n n e c t i o n

**Nurse PDR:**
www.NursesPDR.com/members/database/index.html

**Psychopharmacology Tips:**
www.dr-bob.org/tips

**RX List:**
www.rxlist.com

**US Food and Drug Administration:**
www.fda.gov/cder/drug/infopage/lotronex/
lotronex.htm

**Virtual Drug Store:**
www.virtualdrugstore.com

## Suggested readings

Benkert O et al: Public opinion on psychotropic drugs: an analysis of the factors influencing acceptance or rejection, *J Nerv Ment Dis* 3:151, 1997.

Chou J et al: Clinical research on antipsychotics in bipolar disorder, *J Psychiatr Pract* 6:310, 2000.

Cornwell C, Chiverton P: The psychiatric advanced practice nurse with prescriptive authority: role development, practice issues, and outcomes measurement, *Arch Psychiatr Nurs* 2:57, 1997.

Keltner N: Catastrophic consequences secondary to psychotropic drugs, *J Psychosoc Nurs* 35:41, Part I and Part II, 1997.

Keltner N: Neuroreceptor function and psychopharmacologic response, *Issues Ment Health Nurs* 21:31, 2000.

Keltner N et al: Atypical antipsychotic drugs, parts 1 and 2, *Perspect Psychiatr Care* 36(3):101, 2000, 36(4):139, 2000.

Keltner N, Folks D: *Psychotropic drugs,* ed 3, St Louis, 2001, Mosby.

Lieberman J, Tasman A (eds): *Psychiatric drugs,* Philadelphia, 2000, WB Saunders.

Lin KM, Poland RE, Nakasaki G: *Psychopharmacology and psychobiology of ethnicity,* Washington, DC, 1993, American Psychiatric Press.

Preston J, Johnson J: *Clinical psychopharmacology made ridiculously simple,* ed 4, Miami, 2000, MedMaster, Inc.

Stuart G, Laraia M: *Principles and practice of psychiatric nursing,* ed 7, St Louis, 2001, Mosby.

Van Dongen CJ: Is the treatment worse than the cure? Attitudes toward medications among persons with severe mental illness, *J Psychosoc Nurs* 35:21, 1997.

Weiden PJ: How to evaluate for acute medication-induced movement disorders, *J Pract Psychiatry Behav Health* 2:176, 1996.

Weiden PJ: Prevention for acute extrapyramidal side effects, *J Pract Psychiatry Behav Health* 2:240, 1996.

Weiden P, Miller A: Which side effects really matter? Screening for common and distressing side effects of antipsychotic medications, *J Psychiatr Pract* 7(1):41, 2001.

# Somatic and Alternative Therapies

Many somatic treatments have been used in psychiatric settings. As research into the pathophysiology of mental illness continues, more and increasingly sophisticated somatic treatment modalities are being developed. At the same time, treatment modalities such as restraint, which was among the earliest means of providing nursing care for psychiatric patients, are still used judiciously. This chapter discusses the somatic therapies of mechanical restraints, seclusion, electroconvulsive therapy, and phototherapy. It also reviews current knowledge about alternative and complementary therapies.

## Physical Restraints

Physical restraint includes the use of mechanical restraints, such as wrist or ankle cuffs and restraining sheets, and seclusion, which is confinement to a room from which the patient is unable to exit at will. In this era of sensitivity to civil liberties and individual rights, restraint should be used with great discretion.

### Mechanical Restraints

Types of mechanical restraints are (1) camisoles (straitjackets), (2) wrist cuff restraints, (3) ankle cuff restraints, and (4) sheet restraints.

> **NURSE ALERT.** *Prevention* of behavior necessitating restraints is the most important nursing action. Restraint is always an intervention of last resort.

## Indications for Restraint

Indications for restraint are as follows:

1. Violent behavior that is dangerous to the patient or others
2. Agitated behavior that cannot be controlled by medication
3. Threat to physical integrity related to the patient's refusal to rest or eat and drink
4. Patient's request for external behavioral controls, provided this is assessed to be therapeutically indicated

Table 21-1 presents nursing interventions for restrained patients.

> **NURSE ALERT.**   Patients in any type of physical restraint are highly vulnerable and must be protected.

## Seclusion

Seclusion is confinement in a room that the patient is unable to leave at will. Degrees of seclusion may range from confinement in a room with a closed but unlocked door to a locked room with a mattress without linens on the floor, limited opportunity for communication, and the patient dressed in a hospital gown or a heavy canvas coverall. The latter are minimally acceptable conditions for seclusion and are used only when essential for the protection of the patient or others.

Indications for seclusion follow:

1. Control of violent behavior that is potentially dangerous to the patient or others and cannot be controlled by other, less restrictive interventions such as interpersonal contact or medications
2. Reduction of environmental stimuli, particularly if requested by the patient

Contraindications include the following:

1. Need for observation for a medical problem
2. High suicide risk
3. Potential for intolerance of sensory deprivation
4. Punishment

Table 21-1 presents nursing interventions for secluded patients. Box 21-1 outlines the procedure for managing psychiatric emergencies.

Table 21-1    Nursing interventions for a secluded or mechanically restrained patient

| Principle | Rationale | Nursing Interventions |
|---|---|---|
| Patient has a right to least restrictive treatment. | This is a constitutional right of all patients. | Identify precipitating events. Observe patient for agitated behavior. Attempt alternative interventions. Document patient behavior and nursing interventions. |
| Protect patient from physical injury. | An individual who is not in control of behavior is at risk of injury and needs external limits, safely applied. | Provide adequate staff resources to control patient. Be sure staff is trained to manage violent behavior. Plan the approach to patient. Use safe physical restraint techniques. |
| Provide a safe environment. | An individual who is not in control of behavior may have impaired judgment and may harm self accidentally or purposefully. | Observe patient constantly or very frequently, depending on condition. Remove dangerous objects from area. |
| Maintain biological integrity. | Physically restrained patients are not able to attend to their own biological needs and are at risk for complications related to immobility. | Check vital signs. Bathe patient and provide skin care. Take patient to bathroom or provide bedpan or urinal. Regulate room temperature. Position patient anatomically. Pad restraints. Offer food and fluids. Release restraints at least every 2 hours. |
| Maintain dignity and self-esteem. | Loss of control and imposition of physical restraint may be embarrassing to patient. | Provide privacy. Explain situation to other patients without revealing confidential patient information. Maintain verbal contact with patient at regular intervals while awake. Assign consistent staff member of same sex to provide personal care. Involve patient in plans to terminate physical restraint. Wean patient from protected setting. |

---

**Box 21-1**  **Procedure for Managing Psychiatric Emergencies**

1. Identify crisis leader.
2. Assemble crisis team.
3. Notify security officers if necessary.
4. Remove all other patients from area.
5. Obtain restraints if appropriate.
6. Devise a plan to manage crisis and inform team.
7. Assign securing of patient's limbs to crisis team members.
8. Explain necessity of intervention to patient and attempt to enlist cooperation.
9. Restrain patient when directed by crisis leader.
10. Administer medication if ordered.
11. Maintain calm, consistent approach to patient.
12. Review crisis management interventions with crisis team.
13. Process events with other patients and staff as appropriate.
14. Gradually reintegrate patient into milieu.

---

## Electroconvulsive Therapy

Electroconvulsive therapy (ECT) artificially induces a grand mal seizure by passing an electrical current through electrodes applied to one or both temples. The number of treatments given in a series varies according to the patient's initial problem and therapeutic response as assessed during treatment. The most common range for affective disorders is 6 to 12 treatments, whereas as many more may be given for a patient with schizophrenia. ECT is usually administered two to three times a week on alternate days, although it can be given more or less frequently.

Indications for ECT follow:

1. Patients with major depressive illness who have not responded to antidepressant medication or who are unable to take medication
2. Patients with bipolar disorder who have not responded to medication

3. Acutely suicidal patients who have not received medication long enough to achieve a therapeutic effect

4. When the anticipated side effects of ECT are less than those associated with drug therapy, such as with elderly patients, for patients with heart block, and during pregnancy

The following is a summary of correct ECT procedures:

1. Provide patient and family education about the procedure.
2. Obtain informed consent.
3. Ensure NPO (nothing by mouth) status of the patient after midnight.
4. Ask the patient to remove jewelry, hairpins, eyeglasses, and hearing aids. Full dentures are removed; partial plates remain in place.
5. Dress the patient in loose, comfortable clothing.
6. Have the patient empty bladder.
7. Administer pretreatment medications.
8. Ensure necessary drugs and equipment are available and in working order (Box 21-2).
9. Assist with administration of ECT.
   - Reassure the patient.
   - The physician or anesthesiologist administers oxygen to prepare the patient for the period of apnea that results from the muscle relaxant.
   - Administer medications.
   - Position padded mouth gag to protect the patient's teeth.
   - Position electrodes. The shock is then given.
10. Monitor the patient during the recovery period.
    - Assist as needed with the administration of oxygen and suctioning.
    - Monitor vital signs.
    - After respiration is established, position the patient on side until conscious. Maintain a patent airway.
    - When the patient is responsive, provide orientation.
    - Ambulate with assistance, after checking for postural hypotension.
    - Allow the patient to sleep for a short time if desired.
    - Provide a light meal.
    - Involve in usual daily activities, providing orientation as needed.
    - Offer prescribed analgesia for headache as necessary.

---

**Box 21-2**  Equipment for Electroconvulsive
Therapy (ECT)

---

- Treatment device and supplies, including electrode paste and gel, gauze pads, alcohol preps, saline, electroencephalogram (EEG) electrodes, and chart paper
- Monitoring equipment, including electrocardiogram (ECG) and ECG electrodes
- Blood pressure cuffs (2), peripheral nerve stimulator, and pulse oximeter
- Stethoscope
- Reflex hammer
- Intravenous and venipuncture supplies
- Bite blocks with individual containers
- Stretcher with firm mattress and siderails and capability to elevate head and feet
- Suction device
- Ventilation equipment, including tubing, masks, Ambu bags, oral airways, and intubation equipment with an oxygen delivery system capable of providing positive-pressure oxygen
- Emergency and other medications as recommended by anesthesia staff
- Miscellaneous medications not supplied by the anesthesia staff for medical management during ECT, such as labetalol, esmolol, glycopyrrolate, caffeine, curare, midazolam, diazepam, thiopental sodium (Pentothal Sodium), methohexital sodium (Brevital Sodium), and succinylcholine

---

Table 21-2 summarizes nursing interventions for the patient receiving ECT.

## Phototherapy

Phototherapy, or light therapy, consists of exposing patients to artificial therapeutic lighting about 5 to 20 times brighter than indoor

Table 21-2 Nursing interventions for a patient receiving electroconvulsive therapy (ECT)

| Principle | Rationale | Nursing Interventions |
|---|---|---|
| Obtain informed participation in the procedure. | A patient who understands the treatment plan will be more cooperative and experience less stress than one who does not. An informed family is able to provide patient with emotional support. | Educate about ECT, including procedure and expected effects. Teach family about treatment. Encourage expression of feelings by patient and family. Reinforce teaching after each treatment. |
| Maintain biological integrity. | General anesthesia and an electrically induced seizure are physiological stressors and require supportive nursing care. | Check emergency equipment before procedure. Keep patient NPO several hours before treatment. Remove potentially harmful objects (e.g., jewelry, dentures). Check vital signs. Maintain patent airway. Position on side until reactive. Assist to ambulate. Offer analgesia or antiemetic as needed. |
| Maintain patient's dignity and self-esteem. | Patients are usually fearful before the treatment. Amnesia and confusion may lead to fear of becoming insane. Patient will need assistance to function appropriately in the milieu. | Remain with patient and offer support before and during treatment. Maintain patient's privacy during and after treatment. Reorient patient. Assist family members and other patients to understand behavior related to amnesia and confusion. |

lighting. Patients usually sit with eyes open, about 3 feet away from and at eye level with broad-spectrum fluorescent bulbs designed to produce the intensity and color composition of outdoor light. The timing and dosage of light therapy vary for each patient. The brighter the light, the more effective is the treatment per unit of time.

## Effectiveness

Treatment is rapid and can be effective. Most patients feel relief after 3 to 5 days and relapse when treatment is stopped. Patients do not appear to develop tolerance to phototherapy, but its long-term efficacy has not been fully evaluated.

## Indications

Phototherapy has a 50% to 60% response rate in patients with well-documented nonpsychotic winter depression or seasonal affective disorder (SAD). Light therapy should be administered by a professional with experience and training.

# Sleep Deprivation Therapy

It has been reported that as many as 60% of depressed patients improve immediately after one night of total sleep deprivation. However, few randomized controlled clinical studies have been conducted on sleep deprivation, thus these reports should be considered with caution. Unfortunately, many patients who respond to this therapy become depressed again when they resume sleeping even as little as 2 hours a night.

# Transcranial Magnetic Stimulation

Transcranial magnetic stimulation (TMS) is a noninvasive procedure in which a changing magnetic field is introduced into the brain in order to influence the brain's activity. The field is generated by passing a large electric current through a wire stimulation coil for a brief period of time. The insulated coil is placed on or close to a specific area of the patient's head, allowing the magnetic field to pass through the skull and into target areas of the brain. The most frequently cited indication for TMS is in the treatment of mood disorders.

# Vagus Nerve Stimulation

Vagus nerve stimulation (VNS) is the newest of the somatic therapies currently under investigation. A recent multicenter study showing a 40% to 50% reduction in depressive symptoms using VNS validates its potential as a promising new somatic therapy in psychiatry. VNS involves surgically implanting a small (pocket watch–sized) generator into the patient's chest. An electrode is threaded subcutaneously from the generator to the vagus nerve on the left side of the patient's neck. The end of the electrode is wrapped around the nerve. Once implanted, the generator is programmed via computer for the frequency and intensity of the stimulus. At present VNS is only approved for clinical use in the treatment of epilepsy. The most compelling use of VNS in psychiatry is in the treatment of affective disorders, particularly depression.

# Alternative Therapies

*Complementary and alternative medicine (CAM)* is the term commonly used to describe a broad range of healing philosophies, approaches, and therapies that focus on the whole person, including biopsychosocial and spiritual aspects. CAM therapies are often used alone (often referred to as *alternative*), in combination with other CAM therapies, or in combination with other conventional therapies (sometimes referred to as *complementary*). Some therapies are consistent with principles of Western medicine, whereas others involve healing systems with a different origin. Although some therapies are outside the realm of accepted Western medical practice, others are becoming established in mainstream health care. The National Center of Complementary and Alternative Medicine has developed a classification system of seven major categories for CAM therapies. Table 21-3 lists the seven categories, a description of each, and specific examples of CAM therapies that fall under each classification.

There are only a modest number of well-designed CAM research studies in mental health. In addition, ethical concerns about CAM therapies include issues of safety and effectiveness and the expertise and qualifications of the practitioner. Of equal importance is the communication between the CAM provider and the traditional health care provider. Table 21-4 provides information health consumers should consider in trying to decide on a complementary or alternative therapy.

Table 21-3  NCCAM's classification system for complementary and alternative medicine

**Classification:** Mind-Body Medicine

**Definition:** Mind-body medicine involves behavioral, psychological, social, and spiritual approaches to health. It is divided into four subcategories: mind-body systems, mind-body methods, religion and spirituality, and social and contextual areas.

**CAM Therapy:** Yoga, meditation, relaxation, imagery, hypnosis, biofeedback, spiritual healing

**Classification:** Alternative Medical Systems

**Definition:** This category involves complete systems of theory and practice that have been developed outside the Western biomedical approach. It is divided into four subcategories: acupuncture and Oriental medicine, traditional indigenous systems, unconventional Western systems, and naturopathy.

**CAM Therapy:** Acupuncture, homeopathy

**Classification:** Lifestyle and Disease Prevention

**Definition:** This category involves theories and practices designed to prevent the development of illness, identify and treat risk factors, or support the healing and recovery process. Lifestyle and disease prevention is concerned with integrated approaches for the prevention and management of chronic disease in general or the common determinants of chronic disease. It is divided into three subcategories: clinical preventative practices, lifestyle therapies, and health promotion.

**CAM Therapy:** Exercise, stress management

*Continued*

Table 21-3 NCCAM's classification system for complementary and alternative medicine—cont'd

**Classification:** Biologically Based Therapies

**Definition:** This category includes natural and biologically based practices, interventions, and products. Many overlap with conventional medicine's use of dietary supplements. This category is divided into four subcategories: phytotherapy of herbalism, special diet therapies, orthomolecular medicine, and pharmacological, biological, and instrumental interventions.

**CAM Therapy:** Herbs, diet therapies, megavitamins

**Classification:** Manipulative and Body-Based Systems

**Definition:** This category refers to systems that are based on manipulation or movement of the body and is divided into three subcategories: chiropractic medicine, massage and body work, and unconventional physical therapies.

**CAM Therapy:** Chiropractic, massage and body work, reflexology

**Classification:** Biofield

**Definition:** Biofield medicine involves systems that use subtle energy fields in and around the body for medical purposes.

**CAM Therapy:** Therapeutic touch, SHEN, Reiki

**Classification:** Bioelectromagnetics

**Definition:** Bioelectromagnetics refers to the unconventional use of electromagnetic fields for medical purposes.

**CAM Therapy:** Electromagnets

Table 21-4    Approaching complementary and alternative therapies

- Ask a health care provider about the safety and effectiveness of the desired therapy or treatment. Information can also be found in current publications and on the Web site of the NCCAM at the National Institutes of Health

- Contact a state or local regulatory agency with authority over practitioners who practice the therapy or treatment being sought. CAM usually is not as regulated as the practice of conventional medicine, but licensing, accreditation, and regulatory laws are increasingly being implemented. Check to see if the practitioner is licensed to deliver the identified services.

- Talk with those who have had experience with this practitioner, both health care providers and other patients. Find out about the confidence and competence of the practitioner and whether there have been any complaints from patients.

- Talk with the practitioner in person. Ask about education, additional training, licenses, and certifications, both conventional and unconventional. Find out how open the practitioner is to communicating with patients about technical aspects of methods, possible side effects, and potential problems.

- Visit the practitioner's office, clinic, or hospital. Ask how many patient are typically seen in a day or week and how much time is spent with each patient. Look at the conditions of the office or clinic. The primary issue here is whether the service delivery adheres to regulated standards for medical safety and care.

- Find out what several practitioners charge for the same treatment to get a better idea about the appropriateness of costs. Regulatory agencies and professional associations may also provide cost information.

- Most importantly, discuss all issues concerning therapies and treatments with your usual health care provider, whether a practitioner of conventional or alternative medicine. Competent health care management requires knowledge of both conventional and alternative therapies for the provider to have a complete picture of your treatment plan.

## Depression

Depression is one of the most common conditions for which people use alternative therapies. A review of the most beneficial CAM therapies for depression finds that there is evidence to support the use of exercise, herbal therapy, acupuncture, and massage therapy.

## Anxiety

Anxiety disorders are cited as one of the major reasons people use CAM therapies. Anxiety disorders that have been investigated using CAM therapies include generalized anxiety disorders, social and specific phobias, panic disorder, obsessive-compulsive disorder, and posttraumatic stress disorder. Evidence suggests that relaxation, therapeutic touch, yoga, herbal products, and eye movement desensitization and reprocessing can reduce anxiety.

## Substance Use Disorders

One of the most widely researched CAM therapies for addiction is acupuncture, and many chemical dependency programs in the United States use acupuncture as an additional therapy. One study supports the use of yoga in reducing drug use, and there are some small studies reporting the efficacy of biofeedback for the treatment of addictions.

In summary, CAM therapies can have an important impact on psychiatric nursing practice. They can be beneficial, safe, cost-effective, and easily implemented throughout psychiatric settings. Nurses should continue to follow the research literature to track the emerging evidence about the effectiveness of these therapies. Critically evaluations clinical trial studies will be important to ensure that patients receive treatment with a strong evidence base.

*your* **INTERNET**
c o n n e c t i o n

**Acupuncture.com:**
www.acupuncture.com

**Alternative Medicine Center:**
www.healthy.net/clinic/therapy/index.html

**Dr. Ivan's Depression Central—ECT:**
www.psychom.net/depression.central.ect.html

**Dr. Ivan's Depression Central—TMS:**
www.psychom.net/depression.central.
transcranial.html

**National Center for Complementary and Alternative Medicine:**
nccam.nih.gov

**The Surgeon General's Report on Mental Health:**
www.surgeongeneral.gov/library/mentalhealth/
home.html

## Suggested readings

American Psychiatric Association: *The practice of electroconvulsive therapy: recommendations for treatment, training, and privileging,* ed 2, Washington, DC, 2000, The Association.

Astin J: Why patients use alternative medicine: results of a national study, *JAMA* 279(19):1548, 1998.

Canatsey K, Roper J: Removal from stimuli for crisis intervention: using least restrictive methods to improve the quality of patient care, *Issues Ment Health Nurs* 18:35, 1997.

Chandler D et al: Performance improvement through monitoring seclusion and restraint practices, *Adm Policy Ment Health* 25(5):525, 1998.

Clark C: *Encyclopedia of complementary health practice,* New York, 1999, Springer Publishing.

Cupp M: Herbal remedies: adverse effects and drug interactions, *Am Fam Physician* 59(5):1239-1245, 1999.

Fink M: *Electroshock: restoring the mind,* New York, 1999, Oxford University Press.

Forster P et al: Staff training decreases use of seclusion and restraint in an acute psychiatric hospital, *Arch Psychiatr Nurs* 13(5):269, 1999.

Fox H: Electroconvulsive therapy: an overview, *J Pract Psychiatry Behav Health* 2:223, 1996.

George M et al: Transcranial magnetic stimulation: applications in neuropsychiatry, *Arch Gen Psychiatry* 56:300, 1999.

George M et al: Vagus nerve stimulation: a new tool for brain research and therapy, *Biol Psychiatry* 47(4):287, 2000.

Gillig P et al: A comparison of staff and patient perceptions of the causes and cures of physical aggression on a psychiatric unit, *Psychiatr Q* 69(1):45, 1998.

Harrison B, Kaarsemaker B: Continuous quality improvement to an electroconvulsive therapy delivery system, *J Psychosoc Nurs* 38(3):27, 2000.

Hatcher T: The proverbial herb, *AJN* 101(2):36-43, 2001.

Hermann R et al: Diagnoses of patients treated with ECT: A comparison of evidence-based standards with reported use, *Psychiatr Serv* 50(8):1059, 1999.

Johnson M: Being restrained: a study of power and powerlessness, *Issues Ment Health Nurs* 19:191, 1998.

Joint Commission on Accreditation of Healthcare Organizations: *Revised standards and scoring guidelines for restraint and seclusion*, Oakbrook Terrace, Ill, 1996, The Commission.

Kellner C, Pritchett J, Coffey C: *Handbook of ECT*, Washington, DC, 1997, American Psychiatric Press.

Kessler R et al: The use of complementary and alternative therapies to treat anxiety and depression in the United States, *Am J of Psych* 158(2):289-294, 2001.

Lendemaijer B, Shortridge-Baggett L: The use of seclusion in psychiatry: a literature review, *Schol Inquiry Nurs Pract* 1(4):299, 1997.

Littrell K, Littrell S: Current understanding of violence and aggression: assessment and treatment, *J Pychosoc Nurs* 36(12):18, 1998.

McEnany G: Herbal psychotropics: Focus on St. John's wort and SAMe, *J Am Psych Nurses Assoc* 5(6):192, 1999.

McEnany G: Phototherapy & sleep manipulations: an examination of two nondrug biologic interventions for depression, *J Am Psychiatr Nurs Assoc* 2:86, 1996.

Mohr W, Mohr B: Mechanisms of injury and death proximal to restraint use, *Archives of Psychiatric Nursing* 14(6):285-295, 2000.

Morrison E: The culture of caregiving and aggression in psychiatric settings, *Arch Psychiatr Nurs* 12(1):21, 1998.

Post R et al: Repetitive transcranial magnetic stimulations—a neuropsychiatric tool: present status and future potential, *J ECT* 15(1):39-59, 1999.

Rosenthal N: *Winter blues: SAD—what it is and how to overcome it*, New York, 1993, Guilford.

Rush A et al: Vagus nerve stimulation (VNS) for treatment-resistant depressions: a multicenter study, *Biol Psychiatry* 47(4):276, 2000.

Shelton R, Keller M, Gelenberg A et al: Effectiveness of St John's Wort in major depression, *JAMA* 285:1978-1986, 2001.

Skiba-King W: Vitamins, herbs, and supplements: tools of empowerment, *J Psychosocial Nursing* 39:35, 2001.

Spencer J, Jacobs J: *Complementary/alternative medicine: an evidence-based approach,* St Louis, 1999, Mosby.

Stuart G, Laraia M: *Principles and practice of psychiatric nursing,* ed 7, St Louis, 2001, Mosby.

Terman M et al: Seasonal affective disorder and its treatments, *J Pract Psychiatry Behav Health* 5:287, 1998.

The mainstreaming of alternative medicine, *Consumer Reports,* May 17-25, 2000.

Unutzer J et al: Mental disorders and the use of alternative medicine: results from a national survey, *American Journal of Psychiatry* 157(11): 1851-1857, 2000.

Visalli H, et al: Reducing high-risk interventions for managing aggression in psychiatric settings, *J Nurs Care Quality* 11(3):54,1997.

Wong, A et al: Herbal remedies in psychiatric practice, *Arch Gen Psychiatry* 55:1033, 1998.

Yager J et al: Use of alternative remedies by psychiatric patients: illustrative vignettes and a discussion of the issues, *Am J Psychiatry* 156(9):1432, 1999.

# Index

Page numbers followed by f indicate
figures; t, tables; b, boxes.

# NANDA Diagnoses

Activity intolerance
Activity intolerance, Risk for
Adjustment, Impaired
Airway clearance, Ineffective
Allergy response, Latex
Allergy response, Risk for latex
Anxiety
Anxiety, Death
Aspiration, Risk for
Attachment, Risk for impaired
  parent/infant/child
Autonomic dysreflexia
Autonomic dysreflexia, Risk for
Body image, Disturbed
Body temperature, Risk for imbalanced
Bowel incontinence
Breastfeeding, Effective
Breastfeeding, Ineffective
Breastfeeding, Interrupted
Breathing pattern, Ineffective
Cardiac output, Decreased
Caregiver role strain
Caregiver role strain, Risk for
Comfort, Impaired
Communication, Impaired verbal
Conflict, Decisional
Conflict, Parental role
Confusion, Acute
Confusion, Chronic
Constipation
Constipation, Perceived
Constipation, Risk for
Coping, Ineffective
Coping, Ineffective community
Coping, Readiness for enhanced community
Coping, Defensive
Coping, Compromised family
Coping, Disabled family
Coping, Readiness for enhanced family
Denial, Ineffective
Dentition, Impaired
Development, Risk for delayed
Diarrhea

Disuse syndrome, Risk for
Diversional activity, Deficient
Energy field, Disturbed
Environmental interpretation syndrome,
  Impaired
Failure to thrive, Adult
Falls, Risk for
Family processes: alcoholism, Dysfunctional
Family processes, Interrupted
Fatigue
Fear
Fluid volume, Deficient
Fluid volume, Excess
Fluid volume, Risk for deficient
Fluid volume, Risk for imbalanced
Gas exchange, Impaired
Grieving
Grieving, Anticipatory
Grieving, Dysfunctional
Growth and development, Delayed
Growth, Risk for disproportionate
Health maintenance, Ineffective
Health-seeking behaviors
Home maintenance, Impaired
Hopelessness
Hyperthermia
Hypothermia
Identity, Disturbed personal
Incontinence, Functional urinary
Incontinence, Reflex urinary
Incontinence, Stress urinary
Incontinence, Total urinary
Incontinence, Urge urinary
Incontinence, Risk for urge urinary
Infant behavior, Disorganized
Infant behavior, Risk for disorganized
Infant behavior, Readiness for enhanced
  organized
Infant feeding pattern, Ineffective
Infection, Risk for
Injury, Risk for
Injury, Risk for perioperative-positioning
Intracranial adaptive capacity, Decreased